Inflammatory Bowel Disease

Editor

KERRY L. HAMMOND

SURGICAL CLINICS OF NORTH AMERICA

www.surgical.theclinics.com

Consulting Editor
RONALD F. MARTIN

December 2015 • Volume 95 • Number 6

ELSEVIER

1600 John F. Kennedy Boulevard • Suite 1800 • Philadelphia, Pennsylvania, 19103-2899

http://www.surgical.theclinics.com

SURGICAL CLINICS OF NORTH AMERICA Volume 95, Number 6
December 2015 ISSN 0039–6109, ISBN-13: 978-0-323-40272-9

Editor: John Vassallo, j.vassallo@elsevier.com
Developmental Editor: Colleen Viola

Surgical Clinics of North America (ISSN 0039–6109) is published bimonthly by Elsevier Inc., 360 Park Avenue South, New York, NY 10010-1710. Months of publication are February, April, June, August, October, and December. Business and Editorial Offices: 1600 John F. Kennedy Blvd., Suite 1800, Philadelphia, PA 19103-2899. Periodicals postage paid at New York, NY and additional mailing offices. Subscription prices are $370.00 per year for US individuals, $627.00 per year for US institutions, $180.00 per year for US students and residents, $455.00 per year for Canadian individuals, $793.00 per year for Canadian institutions, $510.00 for international individuals, $793.00 per year for international institutions and $250.00 per year for Canadian and foreign students/residents. To receive student/resident rate, orders must be accompanied by name of affiliated institution, date of term, and the *signature* of program/ residency coordinator on institution letterhead. Orders will be billed at individual rate until proof of status is received. Foreign air speed delivery is included in all *Clinics* subscription prices. All prices are subject to change without notice. POSTMASTER: Send address changes to *Surgical Clinics*, Elsevier Health Sciences Division, Subscription Customer Service, 3251 Riverport Lane, Maryland Heights, MO 63043. **Customer Service (orders, claims, online, change of address): Telephone: 1-800-654-2452 (U.S. and Canada); 314-447-8871 (outside U.S. and Canada). Fax: 314-447-8029. E-mail: journalscustomerservice-usa@elsevier.com (for print support); journalsonline support-usa@elsevier.com (for online support)**.

Reprints. For copies of 100 or more, of articles in this publication, please contact the Commercial Reprints Department, Elsevier Inc., 360 Park Avenue South, New York, New York 10010-1710. Tel. 212-633-3874, Fax: 212-633-3820, E-mail: reprints@elsevier.com.

The Surgical Clinics of North America is also published in Spanish by McGraw-Hill Interamericana Editores S.A., P.O. Box 5-237 06500 Mexico D.F. Mexico; and in Portuguese by Interlivros Edicoes Ltda., Rua Comandante Coelho 1085, CEP 21250, Rio de Janeiro, Brazil; and in Greek by Paschalidis Medical Publications, Athens Greece.

The Surgical Clinics of North America is covered in *MEDLINE/PubMed (Index Medicus), EMBASE/Excerpta Medica, Current Contents/Clinical Medicine, Current Contents/Life Sciences, Science Citation Index,* and *ISI/BIOMED.*

Contributors

CONSULTING EDITOR

RONALD F. MARTIN, MD, FACS
Director of Surgical Education, Marshfield Clinic and Saint Joseph's Hospital, Marshfield, Wisconsin; Clinical Adjunct Professor of Surgery, University of Wisconsin School of Medicine and Public Health, Madison, Wisconsin; Colonel (ret.), United States Army Reserve, Medical Corps

EDITOR

KERRY L. HAMMOND, MD, FACS, FASCRS
Associate Professor, Colon and Rectal Surgery, Medical University of South Carolina, Charleston, South Carolina

AUTHORS

EBELE ACHEBE, MS
University of Texas Health Science Center in San Antonio, San Antonio, Texas

ABDUL ALARHAYEM, MD
General Surgery Resident, University of Texas Health Science Center in San Antonio, San Antonio, Texas

ELLEN H. BAILEY, MD
Assistant Professor of Surgery, Mount Carmel Health System, Columbus, Ohio; Section of Colon and Rectal Surgery, Department of Surgery, Washington University School of Medicine, St Louis, Missouri

JAIME L. BOHL, MD
Assistant Professor of Surgery, Department of Surgery, Wake Forest School of Medicine, Winston Salem, North Carolina

SHAUN R. BROWN, DO
Colorectal Surgery Fellow, Oschner Clinic Foundation, New Orleans, Los Angeles; Assistant Professor of Surgery, Department of Surgery, Uniformed Services University of Health Sciences, Bethesda, Maryland

JAMIE CANNON, MD, FACS
Associate Professor of Surgery, University of Alabama at Birmingham, Birmingham, Alabama

DANIEL I. CHU, MD, FACS
Assistant Professor of Surgery, Department of Surgery, University of Alabama, Birmingham, Alabama

CLARENCE CLARK, MD, FACS, FASCRS
Department of Surgery, Division of Colon and Rectal Surgery, Morehouse School of Medicine, Atlanta, Georgia

LISA C. COVIELLO, DO
Colorectal Surgery Service, Department of Surgery, National Capital Region Medical Directorate, Ft. Belvoir, Virginia; Assistant Professor of Surgery, Department of Surgery of the Uniformed Services University of Health Sciences and the Walter Reed National Military Medical Center, Bethesda, Maryland

KURT G. DAVIS, MD
Chief, Colon and Rectal Surgery, Department of Surgery, William Beaumont Army Medical Center, El Paso, Texas

SEAN C. GLASGOW, MD
Assistant Professor of Surgery, Section of Colon and Rectal Surgery, Department of Surgery, Washington University School of Medicine, St Louis, Missouri

PANAYIOTIS GREVENITIS, MD
Division of Gastroenterology and Hepatology, Medical University of South Carolina, Charleston, South Carolina

WILLIAM J. HARB, MD, FACS, FASCRS
The Colorectal Center, Nashville, Tennessee

NILESH LODHIA, MD
Division of Gastroenterology and Hepatology, Medical University of South Carolina, Charleston, South Carolina

ALICIA J. LOGUE, MD, FACS
Assistant Professor, Associate Program Director, Department of Surgery, University of Texas Health Science Center in San Antonio, San Antonio, Texas

TALHA A. MALIK, MD, MSPH
Departments of Medicine-Gastroenterology and Epidemiology, University of Alabama at Birmingham, Birmingham, Alabama

PINKNEY J. MAXWELL IV, MD, FACS, FASCRS
Department of Surgery, Medical University of South Carolina, Charleston, South Carolina

STEPHANIE C. MONTGOMERY, MD, FACS
Department of Surgery, Saint Francis Hospital and Medical Center, Hartford, Connecticut

MELANIE S. MORRIS, MD, FACS, FASCRS
Assistant Professor of Surgery, Department of Surgery, University of Alabama, Birmingham, Alabama

KATHRYN SOBBA, MD
General Surgery Resident, Department of Surgery, Wake Forest School of Medicine, Winston Salem, North Carolina

ARUL THOMAS, MD
Division of Gastroenterology and Hepatology, Medical University of South Carolina, Charleston, South Carolina

JACQUELYN TURNER, MD
Department of Surgery, Division of Colon and Rectal Surgery, Morehouse School of Medicine, Atlanta, Georgia

CAYLA M. WILLIAMS, MD
Western Michigan University, Kalamazoo, Michigan

Contents

Inflammatory bowel disease (IBD) describes a group of closely related yet heterogeneous predominantly intestinal disease processes that are a result of an uncontrolled immune mediated inflammatory response. It is estimated that approximately one and a half million persons in North America have IBD. Pathogenesis of IBD involves an uncontrolled immune mediated inflammatory response in genetically predisposed individuals to a still unknown environmental trigger that interacts with the intestinal flora. There continues to be an enormous amount of information emanating from epidemiological studies providing expanded insight into the occurrence, distribution, determinants, and mechanisms of inflammatory bowel disease.

The evaluation, diagnosis, and monitoring of inflammatory bowel disease (IBD) has improved significantly over the past few decades. However, differentiation and management of the subtypes of IBD (Crohn's disease, ulcerative colitis, and indeterminate colitis) can still be challenging. The evolution of serologic markers has improved our understanding of the pathogenesis and natural history of IBD. In addition, advancements in endoscopy and endoscopic scoring systems have improved the accuracy of diagnosis and the efficacy of surveillance of IBD patients. This article reviews the recent literature on serologic markers, endoscopy, and endoscopy scoring systems.

Multiple imaging modalities exist for inflammatory bowel disease. This article explores the use of plain radiographs, contrast radiologic imaging, computed tomography, MRI, ultrasound, and capsule endoscopy. History, technique, indications for use, limitations, and future directions are discussed for each modality.

Inflammatory bowel disease patients will likely come to the surgeon's attention at some point in their course of disease, and they present several unique anatomic, metabolic, and physiologic challenges. Specific and well-recognized complications of chronic Crohn's disease and ulcerative colitis are presented as well as an organized and evidence-based approach to the medical and surgical management of such disease sequelae. Topics addressed in this article include intestinal fistula and short bowel syndrome, pouch complications, and deep venous thrombosis with emphasis placed on optimization of the patient's physiologic state for best outcomes.

Inflammatory bowel disease (IBD) affects multiple organ systems outside of the gastrointestinal tract. The clinician treating patients with IBD should be acutely aware of the diagnosis and treatment of extraintestinal manifestations in order to decrease morbidity. The management can be difficult and often times requires a multidisciplinary approach. Future research investigating the pathophysiology, diagnosis, and treatment is needed to further the care of these patients.

Inflammatory bowel disease is associated with an increased risk of gastrointestinal neoplasia. Ulcerative colitis increases the risk of colorectal cancer, and patients with this condition should undergo routine colonoscopic surveillance to detect neoplasia. Crohn's disease increases the risk of malignancy in inflamed segments of bowel, which may include small bowel, colon, rectum, and anus.

Ideally, surgical patients should be nutritionally optimized, as better nutritional status correlates with favorable outcomes during the perioperative period. As inflammatory bowel disease often leads to overall malnutrition, special consideration should be given to this patient population by surgeons. In this article, we review methods for nutritional assessment and provide nutritional recommendations for this special surgical population.

Inflammatory bowel disease (IBD) is a chronic, debilitating disease whose effects spread far beyond the gut. IBD does not generally result in excess mortality; health care providers should thus focus their efforts on improving health-related quality of life and minimizing associated morbidity. A bidirectional relationship exists between IBD and psychiatric conditions; chronic inflammation can produce neuromodulatory effects with resultant mood disorders, and the course of IBD is worse in patients with anxiety and depression. Screening for the early signs of depression or anxiety and initiating appropriate treatment can lead to improved functioning and positively impact disease course.

SURGICAL CLINICS
OF NORTH AMERICA

THE CLINICS ARE AVAILABLE ONLINE!
Access your subscription at:
www.theclinics.com

Foreword

Inflammatory Bowel Disease

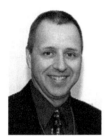

Ronald F. Martin, MD, FACS
Consulting Editor

When I began as the Consulting Editor for the *Surgical Clinics of North America*, one of the main issues I wanted to explore was what it means to be a general surgeon. It has been a very long time since then, and I regret to say that I am not much further along in answering that question to myself or to anybody else than I was when I began. We have covered issues of the *Surgical Clinics of North America* that deal with clinical conditions, organ systems, large system issues such as disaster response and war, and even the business of surgery. Still, what truly defines a general surgeon eludes me. Of all the concepts we address, there is one topic that gives me the greatest pause—the concept of the autonomous surgeon.

Autonomy, or the perceived loss of it more correctly stated, has become a battle cry of our training institutions since the work hours changes started becoming enforced (and yes, I use the word enforced since that well lagged the rules instituting them). There has been a collective wail about how we no longer "let our residents have autonomy" and "they don't get the opportunity to function autonomously" and that is why they are not as prepared at the completion of either residency or fellowship training as some believe they were, usually followed by "back in my day." The corollary to this seems to be if we could only let residents be "autonomous" again, then they would be as good as we were—back in my day.

I, for one, don't buy it.

I realize I am in the minority on this point but not without reason. I don't believe we were ever autonomous. We certainly were less supervised but not autonomous. We were allowed to make and effect decisions, and afterward, our thought process and actions would be criticized either positively or negatively, more often the latter. But we rarely, if ever, acted autonomously. We had teams of people that we played our hierarchical positions on and to whom we answered or for whom we were responsible. We had access to operating rooms and the staff personnel who worked in them. We had the capacity to do many things, which are now reserved for staff surgeons. But we weren't autonomous. We were learning by trial and error, again with much of the

Surg Clin N Am 95 (2015) xi–xii
http://dx.doi.org/10.1016/j.suc.2015.10.001
0039-6109/15/$ – see front matter © 2015 Published by Elsevier Inc.

latter, to become leaders. We weren't learning to be autonomous; we were learning to be surgeons.

To my observation, much of the criticism that was levied before the work-hours cultural shift was after the fact, and precious little occurred in real time. While that was not as helpful in preventing suboptimal decisions, it did have the benefit of the retrospective clarity that illuminates the better and worse choices that were made. The other feature of that kind of feedback was that since it was outside of the "fog of war" and outside of the time constraints of actually getting something done, it provided the opportunity for a much more thorough exploration of our thought processes. In other words, it gave people a chance to really find out if you knew what you were talking about and whether you really knew what you doing. That kind of training works best when one lives in a world of immersion and a world of continuity—both of which are now gone in the training environment.

Not lost, however, is that capacity to know what one is talking about. Continuity is not likely to return soon, if ever. Total immersion in the discipline is also unlikely to make a comeback anytime soon, if ever. That would suggest that, if we wish to learn things well, we have to replace continuity and immersion with structured learning, better quality information, and heavier reliance on team knowledge over individual knowledge; in other words, diminish our concept of the importance of autonomy.

Some forms of structure and team performance will lie predominantly within the surgical world, while others will require cross-disciplinary or multi-disciplinary efforts. I can think of few better clinical examples that illustrate the necessity of working in teams with members of varying expertise than inflammatory bowel disease. A sound working knowledge of basic science, applied science, medical knowledge, and procedural and operative capabilities is required and must be applied systematically to assure the best and most timely outcomes for our patients. Dr Hammond and her colleagues have compiled an excellent collection of reviews that should give a superb foundation to anyone, whether a surgeon or not, who needs to know what matters when we care for patients with these frequently devastating disorders. In every issue, we try to find the correct balance between depth and breadth of exploration of topics to address the concern of the training and practicing surgeons. This issue does an excellent job of walking that tightrope. We are deeply grateful for the team of Dr Hammond and her efforts to put this issue together.

Ronald F. Martin, MD, FACS
Department of Surgery
Marshfield Clinic
1000 North Oak Avenue
Marshfield, WI 54449, USA

E-mail address:
martin.ronald@marshfieldclinic.org

Preface

Inflammatory Bowel Disease

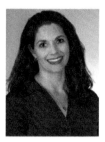

Kerry L. Hammond, MD, FACS, FASCRS
Editor

Current data estimate that over 1.4 million Americans, 2.2 million Europeans, and several hundred thousand additional patients worldwide are presently affected by Crohn's disease or ulcerative colitis.[1] These chronic inflammatory conditions of the gastrointestinal tract are collectively referred to as inflammatory bowel disease (IBD). In addition to gastrointestinal symptoms, the debilitating effects of IBD include nutritional deficiencies, painful extraintestinal manifestations, and negative psychological consequences.

While the exact cause of IBD has not been determined, significant advances in basic science and clinical research in recent years have elucidated genetic and environmental factors involved in disease pathogenesis. Proposed pathways to chronic inflammation of the intestinal mucosa in genetically susceptible individuals include deregulation of the innate immune response to enteric microorganisms and pathogens, increased permeability of the epithelial barrier, and overexpression of pro-inflammatory molecules, including IL-1β, IL-6, IL-12, and TNF-α.[2,3] Based on these mechanisms, options for pharmacologic management of IBD have expanded, and successful long-term disease management with individualized medical therapies has become a reality for many patients.

Multidisciplinary therapy is essential in the successful management of IBD. In this issue of *Surgical Clinics of North America* dedicated to Inflammatory Bowel Disease, talented authors from the fields of Gastroenterology and Colon and Rectal Surgery have contributed their expertise in the various facets of these often vexing clinical disorders. It has been a privilege and a pleasure to work with this group of physicians and

Surg Clin N Am 95 (2015) xiii–xiv
http://dx.doi.org/10.1016/j.suc.2015.09.012
0039-6109/15/$ – see front matter © 2015 Published by Elsevier Inc.

surgical.theclinics.com

the supportive editorial staff at Elsevier to compile this comprehensive review. I hope that the reader will find these articles as educational as I have.

Kerry L. Hammond, MD, FACS, FASCRS
Colon and Rectal Surgery
Medical University of South Carolina
25 Courtenay Drive
MSC 290, Suite 7100A
Charleston, SC 29425, USA

E-mail address:
hammonkl@musc.edu

REFERENCES

1. Cosnes J, Gower-Rousseau C, Seksik P, et al. Epidemiology and natural history of inflammatory bowel diseases. Gastroenterology 2011;140(6):1785–94.
2. Sobczak M, Fabisiak A, Murawska N, et al. Current overview of extrinsic and intrinsic factors in etiology and progression of inflammatory bowel diseases. Pharmacol Rep 2014;66(5):766–75.
3. Goyette P, Labbé C, Trinh TT, et al. Molecular pathogenesis of inflammatory bowel disease: genotypes, phenotypes and personalized medicine. Ann Med 2007; 39(3):177–99.

Inflammatory Bowel Disease
Historical Perspective, Epidemiology, and Risk Factors

Talha A. Malik, MD, MSPH[a,b,]*

KEYWORDS

- Inflammatory bowel disease • Crohn's disease • Ulcerative colitis
- Historical perspective • Epidemiology • Risk factors

KEY POINTS

- Inflammatory bowel disease describes 2 well-established but not entirely discrete disease entities, Crohn's disease (CD) and ulcerative colitis (UC), which are represented by an uncontrolled immune-mediated inflammatory response in genetically predisposed individuals to an unknown environmental trigger that interacts with the intestinal flora and primarily affects the alimentary tract.
- Approximately 1.5 million persons in North America have inflammatory bowel disease.
- Several potential risk factors of inflammatory bowel disease have been studied and include particular environmental triggers, intestinal immune mechanisms, heritable factors, gut flora, diet, mesenteric fat, medications, nicotine, infectious agents, immunization, hygiene, pregnancy, breastfeeding, stress, and lifestyle.
- There are data to suggest a higher mortality in CD compared with the general population; however, there is no definitive evidence to suggest higher mortality among patients with UC compared with the general population.
- Epidemiologic studies have expanded understanding of the occurrence, distribution, determinants, and mechanisms of inflammatory bowel disease and this allows clinicians to identify safer and more effective approaches to management and therapeutics.

INTRODUCTION

Inflammatory bowel disease (IBD) consists of 2 well-established but not entirely discrete disease entities, Crohn's disease (CD) and ulcerative colitis (UC). They together are a group of closely related but heterogeneous disease processes. The

Conflicts of interest: None.
[a] Department of Medicine-Gastroenterology, University of Alabama at Birmingham, 1808 7th Avenue South, BDB 391, Birmingham, AL 35294, USA; [b] Department of Epidemiology, University of Alabama at Birmingham, 1808 7th Avenue South, BDB 391, Birmingham, AL 35294, USA
* Department of Medicine-Gastroenterology, University of Alabama at Birmingham, 1808 7th Avenue South, BDB 391, Birmingham, AL 35294.
E-mail address: tmalik@uabmc.edu

Surg Clin N Am 95 (2015) 1105–1122
http://dx.doi.org/10.1016/j.suc.2015.07.006
0039-6109/15/$ – see front matter © 2015 Elsevier Inc. All rights reserved.

surgical.theclinics.com

mechanism of IBD involves an uncontrolled immune-mediated inflammatory response in genetically predisposed individuals to an unknown environmental trigger that interacts with the gut microbiome (intestinal flora) and primarily affects the alimentary tract **(Fig. 1)**.[1–6] It is estimated that more than 1.5 million Americans have IBD, approximately half represented in each of these 2 discrete IBD subgroups.[2]

HISTORICAL PERSPECTIVE
Background

It is thought that Alfred the Great, who is commonly considered to be the first King of England (849–899 CE), may have had CD.[7] However, it was not until 1913 that a discrete disease condition resembling what is now considered to be CD was identified, when Kennedy Dalziel, a British physician, described patients with transmural inflammation of the small and large intestines.[7,8] Subsequently in 1932, Dr Burrill Crohn, Dr Leon Ginzburg, and Dr Gordon Oppenheimer published articles describing a condition that caused inflammation of the terminal ileum and which they called regional or terminal ileitis. This disease entity later began to be referred as CD.[7–10]

UC was first described in ancient Greece by Hippocrates as a condition characterized by chronic diarrhea and bloody stools.[7,8] This condition was thought to be related to ulceration and inflammation of the large intestine. In the 1600s, Thomas Sydenham, a British physician, named this disease bloody flux. In 1859, Samuel Wilks, another British physician, identified UC as a discrete disease entity.[7,8]

The first breakthrough that established IBD as the prime intestinal autoimmune disease occurred in the 1950s when it was noted that symptoms in patients with both CD and UC responded to corticosteroids.[3] In the 1970s, traditional immune modulators, predominantly thiopurine analogues, began to be used and eventually became first-line steroid-sparing agents.[3] In 1997, Targan and colleagues[11] published findings of the so-called Crohn's Disease cA2 Study, which assessed the effectiveness of the biologic antibody against tumor necrosis factor (TNF) cA2 (infliximab) in induction of remission in luminal CD. This study began the era of biologics. During the first decade of the twenty-first century, biologics began to gradually emerge as the most effective

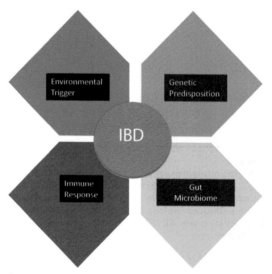

Fig. 1. IBD mechanism.

and central therapeutic agents used to induce and maintain remission in moderate to severe CD and UC.[12–16]

Trends in Occurrence and Distribution

In the past, IBD had been considered a condition that mainly occurred in white populations of Europe, North America, and Australia.[1] For this reason earlier data on CD and UC emanated from these regions.[1] The incidence of CD and UC has stabilized in these regions but still remains higher than it is in the rest of the world.[1] There has been an increasing incidence predominantly of CD in parts of the developing world that include the Middle East, south and southeast Asia, and the Asia-Pacific region.[17,18] However, South America and Africa still have very low incidence rates despite a few case reports that have suggested increasing incidence (**Fig. 2**).[19,20]

Trends in Classification

In 2000, the Working Party for the World Congresses of Gastroenterology proposed the Vienna classification, which attempted to classify CD based on objective variables that included age of onset, disease location, and disease behavior (**Table 1**).[21] In 2005, Silverberg and colleagues[22] presented the report of the Working Party of the Montreal World Congress of Gastroenterology, in which they put forth the Montreal classification of IBD (see **Table 1**; **Table 2**). The Montreal group added classification of UC based on the extent and severity of the disease (see **Table 2**).[3]

Trends in the Course of Disease

With regard to phenotype by location, of all patients diagnosed with CD at the time of their diagnosis, one-third have ileal involvement, one-third have colonic involvement, and one-third have ileocolonic disease.[2] At diagnosis, about 10% to 20% have perianal disease, whereas in 5% to 10% inflammation occurs in the region proximal to the terminal ileum.[2] With regard to phenotype by behavior of disease, of all patients diagnosed with CD, at the time of their diagnosis, 80% have nonpenetrating/nonstricturing disease and the remaining 20% have stricturing or penetrating disease.[23] Although location of CD has been noted to largely remain stable through the disease course, up to one-third of those who are diagnosed with nonpenetrating/nonstricturing disease go on to

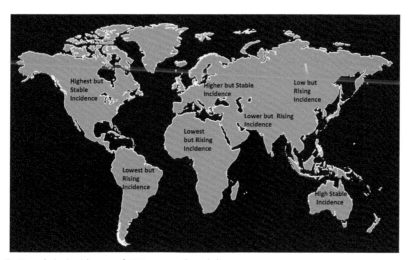

Fig. 2. Trends in incidence of IBD across the globe.

Table 1		
Vienna and Montreal classification of CD		
	Vienna Classification	**Montreal Classification**
Age at Diagnosis (y)	A1: <40 A2: >40	A1: <16 A2: b17–40 A3: >40
Location	L1: ileal L2: colonic L3: ileocolonic L4: upper	L1: ileal L2: colonic L3: ileocolonic L4: upper disease modifier or isolated upper disease
Behavior	B1: nonstricturing, nonpenetrating B2: stricturing B3: penetrating	B1: nonstricturing, nonpenetrating B2: stricturing B3: penetrating P: perianal disease modifier

Adapted from Gasche C, Scholmerich J, Brynskov J, et al. A simple classification of Crohn's disease: report of the Working Party for the World Congresses of Gastroenterology, Vienna 1998. Inflamm Bowel Dis 2000;6(1):8–15; and Silverberg MS, Satsangi J, Ahmad T, et al. Toward an integrated clinical, molecular and serological classification of inflammatory bowel disease: report of a Working Party of the 2005 Montreal World Congress of Gastroenterology. Can J Gastroenterol 2005;19(Suppl A):5A–36A.

develop penetrating or stricturing complications by 5 years, with half of all patients with CD having complicated disease at 20 years of follow-up.[24] With regard to disease activity, based on data from the prebiologic era, of all patients diagnosed with CD, approximately two-thirds have a remitting and relapsing coarse, one-fifth remain active most of the time, and about 13% go into long-term remission.[25]

With regard to patients with UC, at the time of diagnosis, one-third have inflammation that does not extend proximal to the rectosigmoid junction; one-third have disease up to the splenic flexure, and the remaining third has UC pancolitis (contiguous inflammation extending proximal to the splenic flexure).[2] Although data are variable, it has been observed that up to 50% of patients diagnosed with proctitis or proctosigmoiditis progress to more extensive disease by 25 years of follow-up.[26] In the same cohort, up to 75% of patients diagnosed with extensive colitis or pancolitis experienced variable degrees of disease extent regression during the same follow-up period.[27] With regard to disease activity, based on data from the prebiologic era, of all patients diagnosed with UC, more than one-half (57%) have a remitting and relapsing

Table 2		
Montreal classification of UC		
Class	**Extent**	**Description**
E1	Ulcerative proctitis	Proximal extent of inflammation distal to rectosigmoid junction
E2	Left-sided UC (distal UC)	Involvement limited to proportion of colorectum distal to the splenic
E3	Extensive UC (pancolitis)	Involvement extending proximal to splenic flexure

From Silverberg MS, Satsangi J, Ahmad T, et al. Toward an integrated clinical, molecular and serological classification of inflammatory bowel disease: report of a Working Party of the 2005 Montreal World Congress of Gastroenterology. Can J Gastroenterol 2005;19(Suppl A):5A–36A.

disease course, about one-quarter go into long-term remission, and about one-fifth of patients have disease activity most of the time.[28]

Trends in Goals of Management

The historical goals of IBD treatment were to induce and maintain clinical remission.[29] However, it is now evident that the natural course of disease progression of CD and UC is not affected if clinicians only focus on induction and maintenance of clinical remission. Therefore the goals of treatment have changed during the past years.

Conventional therapy for IBD has not accomplished a reduction in the need for surgical intervention. Goals of medical management of IBD now include inducing and maintaining endoscopic remission; decreasing rates of hospitalization, surgery and infection; avoiding steroids; improving health-related quality of life; and decreasing risk of cancer and mortality.[29]

EPIDEMIOLOGY
Incidence

There is a lot of variation in data with regard to the incidence of CD and UC across the globe based on geographic region, environment, immigration trends, and ethnic group.[1–3] There is variation in data even within the same geographic region. In the past, UC was generally considered to be slightly more common; however, with increasing incidence of CD in the past few decades, this trend has changed. The annual incidence in North America of both CD and UC is now fairly stable and estimated to be between 0 and 20 per 100,000 persons.[30]

Prevalence

There is also a lot of variation in prevalence data with regard to CD and UC across the globe based on geographic region, environment, immigration trends, and ethnic group.[1–3] As is the case with the incidence of CD and UC, there is variation in prevalence data even within the same geographic region. Although in the past UC was considered to be slightly more prevalent, with the increase in incidence that occurred in CD in the past few decades more recent prevalence data show that CD and UC may be equally prevalent in North America. The estimates for prevalence of CD and UC in North America are 25 to 300 per 100,000 and 35 to 250 per 100,000 respectively.[31–33]

Distribution by Age

Although CD and UC can occur at any age, the peak age of onset for CD is generally considered to be between 20 and 30 years of age and for UC, it is between 30 and 40 years.[1,3,5,30]

There is another peak, especially for UC between 60 and 70 years of age based on some European cohorts.[34–36]

Based on earlier North American population cohorts, the median age of diagnosis of CD was estimated at around 30 years whereas the mean age of diagnosis of CD ranged between 33 and 45 years.[37,38] According to North American UC cohorts, median and mean age of diagnosis of UC ranged between 40 and 45 years.[37,38]

Distribution by Gender

A consistent significant difference has not been observed in the incidence and prevalence of CD and UC between North American men and women.[1,39] Note that several cohorts have indicated a female predominance in CD and a male predominance in UC. However, these findings are not consistent, especially in some low-incidence areas, where CD may be more prevalent among men.[32,40]

The overall incidence of UC has stabilized. A study from northern France suggested a higher incidence of UC versus CD among boys between the ages of 14 and 17 years compared with girls, although at a younger age the reverse was noted.[41] Moreover, men are more likely to be diagnosed with IBD, specifically UC, later in life compared with women.[5]

Racial and Ethnic Disparity

IBD was first studied specifically in African Americans (AAs) by Mendeloff and colleagues[42] in 1966. They observed a lower incidence of IBD among AAs compared with white Americans. Whether the incidence of IBD was low or whether its true incidence and prevalence were under-reported is unclear; however, a higher incidence of both CD and UC has since been observed.[42] In 1992, Kurata and colleagues[31] found a higher incidence of CD among AAs than had previously been noted. This finding was later confirmed by Ogunbi and colleagues[43] in 1998. In a 1986 study of 15 AA patients with CD, Goldman and colleagues[44] noted that disease in AAs was more aggressive with earlier age of onset and resulted in more complications over time. In a 2000 case-control study that attempted to adequately match and control for confounders, Straus and colleagues[45] concluded that disparities in disease severity were a result of social and economic inequalities, such as affordability of health care, delayed appointments because of financial concerns, and difficulties with traveling to provider's office, rather than biological or genetic differences. These results were later confirmed by other studies, including a 2008 systematic review by Mahid and colleagues,[46] which pooled more than 2000 patients with IBD from 8 different studies.

A particularly vulnerable ethnic group has been the Ashkenazi Jewish population. IBD is more common among Ashkenazi Jews than among the Sephardim and the general population, with estimates of prevalence being 17 and 80 per 100,000 among the Ashkenazi in Israel versus 19 and 55 per 100,000 among the Sephardim living in Israel.[47] Moreover, North American Jewish populations are more likely to have IBD than their counterparts living in the Middle East.[1]

RISK FACTORS
Cause and Pathogenesis

The most popular theory regarding pathogenesis of IBD considers it to be a result of an uncontrolled immune-mediated inflammatory response in genetically predisposed individuals to an unknown environmental trigger that interacts with the intestinal flora and primarily affects the alimentary tract.[6]

Postulated Environmental Triggers

Different triggers have been implicated, both external antigens and autoantigens. External antigens include infectious agents such as viruses and bacteria as well as dietary components.[1,6,17] Autoantigens on bacterial flora have also been implicated in the pathogenesis of IBD.[1,6]

Intestinal Immune Mechanism

The main mechanism of inflammatory injury in IBD is immune mediated. There are various mechanisms by which immune-mediated injury takes place. An important factor is abnormal or exaggerated immune response.[6,17,29] For example, human leukocyte antigen (HLA) class II molecules that mediate autoimmune injury are found in high numbers within the intestinal epithelial cells of patients with active IBD. The HLA class II molecules are responsible for antigen processing and presentation. Activated macrophages, which are also sites of HLA class II molecules, also secrete increased amounts of proinflammatory cytokines, including interleukin (IL)-1, IL-6, IL-8, and TNF-alpha, within the lamina propria of the intestinal wall. IFN-gamma is also produced and it increases intestinal permeability. There is decreased production of IL-2, IL-10, TNF-beta, and transforming growth factor beta, which are downregulatory cytokines, in patients with IBD, and this may explain chronic inflammation in these patients.[4,6,17]

Genetic Predisposition

Up to 15% persons with IBD (both CD and UC) have a first-degree relative who also has IBD.[1,48] The lifetime risk of developing IBD in first-degree relatives has been estimated at 5% in CD and about 2% in UC among non-Jewish populations and 8% and 5% among Jewish populations respectively.[48] In children and siblings, it is generally estimated to be approximately 8% in both CD and UC.[6]

In CD, the concordance rates among monozygotic and dizygotic twins are 50% and 10% respectively, which is suggestive of significant but not complete genetic predisposition. In UC, the concordance rates among monozygotic and dizygotic twins are 16% and 4% respectively, which is suggestive of weaker, albeit definite, genetic predisposition.[48,49]

Gut Flora

Several reviews on the topic of gut flora have suggested that the unknown environmental trigger in IBD (from the external environment) interacts with the intestinal flora within the internal environment to cause disease.[50–52]

Some clues to the veracity of this association emanate from the observations that bigger family size, early life exposure to pets and farm animals, and greater number of siblings is inversely associated with risk of IBD.[1] It has been shown that patients with IBD have reduced diversity of gut microbiota.[1] Another postulated mechanism of pathogenesis of IBD includes the proinflammatory properties of certain microbiota.[53] For example, a 2004 study revealed that adherent-invasive *Escherichia coli* were found in the ileum of 22% of patients with CD versus 6% of controls.[53] It has also been postulated that Firmicutes may confer protection against IBD.[1,51] The study of gut flora and IBD is in flux and it can safely be assumed that, in addition to gut bacteria, viruses and fungi may also play a role.[1]

Role of Diet

Martini and Brandes[54] published a case-control study in 1976 that suggested higher incidence of IBD in those who took larger amounts of refined carbohydrates in their diets. In addition to increased intake of refined sugars, it was also observed that newly diagnosed patients with IBD consumed less dietary fiber, raw fruit, and vegetables compared with healthy controls.[55] Asakura and colleagues[56] subsequently performed a systematic review of past epidemiologic surveys and case-control studies done to study the effect of diet on pathogenesis of CD in Japanese patients and noted an association between increased consumption of animal meat in addition to carbohydrates as potential risk for development of active CD.

Role of Mesenteric Fat and Obesity

Adipose tissue is an active endocrine organ that is made up of elements of connective tissue as well as cells represented by preadipocytes and adipocytes that can be prominent mediators of inflammation in the human body.[57–60] Blain and colleagues[61] found an association between obesity and rapid progression of disease (measured clinically) in patients with CD. In a subsequent study by Hass and colleagues[62] overweight or obese patients with CD experienced more rapid progression to first surgical intervention compared with underweight patients.

Role of Smoking

The association between smoking and IBD was first noted in 1982.[63] Smoking has been associated with a 2-fold increase in the risk for CD and this association includes early-life exposure as well as passive smoking. In addition to causing exacerbations of CD, smoking has been linked to earlier age of onset, increased need for immunosuppression, overall more aggressive disease, increased requirement for surgery, and higher risk of postresection recurrence of disease.[64–66]

With regard to UC, it has been observed that it is smoking cessation that may cause an exacerbation.[67] Moreover, studies have shown that smokers with UC may have a milder disease course, may require less immune suppression, and have reduced need for surgery.[66,68,69] However, the mechanism underlying these divergent effects on the 2 subtypes of IBD is not well understood.[1] Nicotine replacement in UC has not been reliably found to reduce disease activity, suggesting an effect of smoking on IBD that is independent of nicotine.[70,71]

Medications and Inflammatory Bowel Disease

Medications suggested to be potential risk factors for IBD include oral contraceptives, hormonal replacement therapy, nonsteroidal antiinflammatory drugs (including aspirin), as well as antibiotics.[72–77] There is a single study that implicates the role of excess iron in the water supply in the development of IBD.[78] Zinc has been noted to potentially protect against relapses in IBD based on another unpublished study.[1] Studies of the relationship between vitamin D and development of IBD have been equivocal.[1]

Infections and Inflammatory Bowel Disease

There has been interest in studying the association between *Mycobacterium avium* subspecies *paratuberculosis* and CD but this association has not been consistent.[79,80] Other studies have suggested an association between salmonella and campylobacter infections with an increased risk of IBD.[81] With regard to viruses, measles virus was initially thought to be a risk factor for subsequent development of IBD. However, subsequent studies were not able to detect an association.[82–84] *Clostridium difficile* infection, cytomegalovirus infection, and other causes of sepsis have been noted to cause exacerbation of IBD but no causal link between them has been detected.[85,86]

Role of Immunization

In addition to the measles infection, it was proposed in the 1960s that the attenuated live measles virus vaccine might be associated with IBD because prevalence of IBD had been noted to be much higher in a cohort of patients who received the vaccines compared with those who had not.[82] However, subsequent studies did not confirm this finding and several questions were raised about the methodology used to conduct that study.[87,88] A more recent study noted an inverse relationship between measles vaccination and the risk of IBD.[84]

Hygiene Hypothesis

Some observational studies have shown a protective role of poor hygiene against the development of IBD.[89–92] For example, large number of siblings, large family size, not having access to running water, drinking unpasteurized milk, living on a farm, and early exposure to pets have all been associated with a reduced risk of IBD.[1,39,90–92]

However, these studies have been done in the West. The few studies that have assessed this association in the developing world have been inconclusive.[1,93]

Pregnancy, Breastfeeding, and Inflammatory Bowel Disease

Mode of childbirth (studied because of its influence on the gut microbiota in infancy) has not been found to be significant associated with development of IBD.[94] Studies have also shown that breastfeeding may protect against development of IBD later in life, especially for UC.[1]

Role of Stress and Lifestyle in Inflammatory Bowel Disease

There is observational evidence for the association between stress, anxiety, and depression with a high risk of development of IBD.[95] Depression and anxiety have also been associated with a more severe course of disease, higher rate of surgery, decreased quality of life, as well as reduced responsiveness to immunosuppression.[1,95]

With regard to lifestyle, there seems to be a higher incidence of IBD among people who are in professions that lead them to be more sedentary compared with those whose profession requires increased activity.[96] Moreover, observational evidence suggests that there is an increased incidence of IBD among people with disruptive sleep pattern.[1,97]

Inflammatory Bowel Disease and Surgery

Recently, risk of surgery has decreased in patients with CD and UC.[2] This phenomenon has largely been attributed to the more aggressive medical therapy being used now compared with what was the case just a decade ago, but long-term results are not known.[1,2,34,98–100]

Although, traditionally, the cumulative probability of patients with CD undergoing surgery was 35%, 61%, and 82% after 1, 10, and 20 years respectively, there has been significant reduction in these probabilities in recent studies, with recent estimates of rates of surgery being approximately 10% to 14% and 18% to 35% after 1 and 5 years respectively.[34,98,101–104] With regard to age, location, and behavior of CD, the greatest risk of surgery is with ileocecal location and stricturing or penetrating/fistulizing behavior.[2,102,103] Permanent fecal diversion in the form of a stoma is eventually required in about 10% of patients with CD.[3,64] The risk factors for permanent fecal diversion include colonic and perianal CD.[3,105]

The traditional likelihood of colectomy in UC was slightly less than 10% at 1 year and slightly less than 25% at 10 years after diagnosis.[2,34,102,106] However, even lower rates of colectomy have recently been reported, with rates of 6% and 10% after 1 and 5 years respectively.[27,34,106–108] With regard to age and extent of UC among patients who undergo colectomy, most of these patients have had fairly recent diagnosis and have pancolitis.[2]

Also, more severe disease leads to earlier colectomy.[3] The likelihood of colectomy has been reported generally to be higher in studies on populations emanating from tertiary referral centers.[28,109,110] Medications used for medical management of severe fulminant UC, such as infliximab and cyclosporine, may delay or, less commonly, prevent colectomy.[3,111,112] Among patients with UC, definitive surgery is usually represented by total proctocolectomy and formation of ileal pouch–anal anastomoses. The most frequent form of ileal pouch–anal anastomoses used at present is the J pouch. The risk of acute pouchitis in these patients is about 50%, whereas, in about 5% to 10% of patients, pouchitis becomes chronic.[113]

Inflammatory Bowel Disease and Cancer

With regard to risk factors for colorectal cancer (CRC) in IBD, the primary drivers of risk are persistent active inflammation and immunosuppression followed by long-standing disease, extensive disease, young age at diagnosis, family history of CRC, and coexisting primary sclerosing cholangitis.[2,114]

Of all CRCs, CRCs that occur in UC and, by extension, in Crohn colitis account for about 1% of all CRCs, which means that in patients with UC or Crohn colitis there is a 10 to 25 times higher risk of CRC compared with the general population. Most commonly, CRC occurs in patients with UC or Crohn colitis in their 40s.[115–117]

Risk factors for CRC in patients with UC/Crohn colitis include extent of disease, duration of disease longer than 8 years, and younger age at diagnosis.[117] Other risk factors for CRC in UC include family history of CRC, concomitant primary sclerosing cholangitis, active histologic inflammation, and presence of colonic pseudopolyps.[115,117]

Because of this increased risk of CRC in UC, surveillance colonoscopies are recommended yearly in patients with UC (other than UC proctitis/proctosigmoiditis) after 8 years of disease. In Crohn colitis, this can be done at about 10 to 12 years after diagnosis. It is estimated that the risk of CRC after 10 years of UC or Crohn colitis is about 1%, at 20 years it is about 8%, and at 30 years it is approximately 18%.[115–117] Moreover, any colonic stricture in UC should raise suspicion for cancer because up to one-third of these may be harboring a malignancy. The pathogenesis of carcinogenesis in UC involves sequential somatic gene mutations and clonal expansion. These gene alterations include aneuploidy, mutations of oncogenes, tumor suppressor genes, and DNA repair genes.[116,117]

The risk of extraintestinal cancers, including lymphoproliferative as well as skin cancers, is significantly higher among patients with IBD compared with the general population.[2,118–120]

Inflammatory Bowel Disease and Mortality

Increased mortality is a concern in patients with CD based on most, but not all, data compared with the general population.[121–125] In patients with CD, surgical complications and malnourishment are prominent causes of direct CD-related mortality compared with other factors, including small bowel neoplasm.[121,126,127] As smoking is more common among patients with CD, sequelae related to smoking in the form of respiratory infection and diseases are additional causes of death among patients with CD.[127]

There is no definitive evidence to suggest a higher mortality among patients with UC compared with the general population.[124,125,128–130] Among patients with UC, colorectal neoplasia accounts for most of the mortality compared with surgical or other complications.[126,129] A population-based cohort from Copenhagen County comprising 1160 patients with UC noted that there was increased mortality within the first 2 years of diagnosis among patients who were older than 50 years of age at diagnosis and who had extensive colitis. The increased mortality was associated with postoperative pulmonary embolism and development of pneumonia.[129]

CONCLUDING REMARKS

A lot of information continues to emanate from epidemiologic studies, providing expanded insight into the occurrence, distribution, determinants, and mechanisms of IBD. This knowledge should be used to identify new approaches to management and therapeutics that move away from merely immunosuppressing patients with

IBD and advance their health using methods that involve prevention, preemption, and immunomodulation.

REFERENCES

1. Ananthakrishnan AN. Epidemiology and risk factors for IBD. Nat Rev Gastroenterol Hepatol 2015;12:205–17.
2. Burisch J, Munkholm P. The epidemiology of inflammatory bowel disease. Scand J Gastroenterol 2015;50(8):942–51.
3. Cosnes J, Gower-Rousseau C, Seksik P, et al. Epidemiology and natural history of inflammatory bowel diseases. Gastroenterology 2011;140(6):1785–94.
4. Abraham C, Cho JH. Inflammatory bowel disease. N Engl J Med 2009;361(21): 2066–78.
5. Loftus EV Jr. Clinical epidemiology of inflammatory bowel disease: incidence, prevalence, and environmental influences. Gastroenterology 2004;126(6): 1504–17.
6. Malik T, Mannon P. Inflammatory bowel diseases: emerging therapies and promising molecular targets. Front Biosci 2012;4:1172–89.
7. Kirsner JB. Historical aspects of inflammatory bowel disease. J Clin Gastroenterol 1988;10(3):286–97.
8. Kirsner JB. Historical origins of current IBD concepts. World J Gastroenterol 2001;7(2):175–84.
9. Crohn BB, Ginzburg L, Oppenheimer GD. Landmark article Oct 15, 1932. Regional ileitis. A pathological and clinical entity. By Burril B. Crohn, Leon Ginzburg, and Gordon D. Oppenheimer. JAMA 1984;251(1):73–9.
10. Ginzburg L. X-ray diagnosis of acute intestinal obstruction without the use of contrast media. Ann Surg 1932;96(3):368–80.
11. Targan SR, Hanauer SB, van Deventer SJ, et al. A short-term study of chimeric monoclonal antibody cA2 to tumor necrosis factor alpha for Crohn's disease. Crohn's Disease cA2 Study Group. N Engl J Med 1997;337(15):1029–35.
12. Present DH, Rutgeerts P, Targan S, et al. Infliximab for the treatment of fistulas in patients with Crohn's disease. N Engl J Med 1999;340(18):1398–405.
13. Hanauer SB, Feagan BG, Lichtenstein GR, et al. Maintenance infliximab for Crohn's disease: the ACCENT I randomised trial. Lancet 2002;359(9317): 1541–9.
14. Sands BE, Anderson FH, Bernstein CN, et al. Infliximab maintenance therapy for fistulizing Crohn's disease. N Engl J Med 2004;350(9):876–85.
15. Rutgeerts P, Sandborn WJ, Feagan BG, et al. Infliximab for induction and maintenance therapy for ulcerative colitis. N Engl J Med 2005;353(23):2462–76.
16. Sandborn WJ, Feagan BG, Stoinov S, et al. Certolizumab pegol for the treatment of Crohn's disease. N Engl J Med 2007;357(3):228–38.
17. Podolsky DK. Inflammatory bowel disease. N Engl J Med 2002;347(6):417–29.
18. Sood A, Midha V. Epidemiology of inflammatory bowel disease in Asia. Indian J Gastroenterol 2007;26(6):285–9.
19. Archampong TN, Nkrumah KN. Inflammatory bowel disease in Accra: what new trends. West Afr J Med 2013;32(1):40–4.
20. Ukwenya AY, Ahmed A, Odigie VI, et al. Inflammatory bowel disease in Nigerians: still a rare diagnosis? Ann Afr Med 2011;10(2):175–9.
21. Gasche C, Scholmerich J, Brynskov J, et al. A simple classification of Crohn's disease: report of the Working Party for the World Congresses of Gastroenterology, Vienna 1998. Inflamm Bowel Dis 2000;6(1):8–15.

22. Silverberg MS, Satsangi J, Ahmad T, et al. Toward an integrated clinical, molecular and serological classification of inflammatory bowel disease: report of a Working Party of the 2005 Montreal World Congress of Gastroenterology. Can J Gastroenterol 2005;19(Suppl A):5A–36A.

23. Dressel U, Allen TL, Pippal JB, et al. The peroxisome proliferator-activated receptor beta/delta agonist, GW501516, regulates the expression of genes involved in lipid catabolism and energy uncoupling in skeletal muscle cells. Mol Endocrinol 2003;17(12):2477–93.

24. Thia KT, Sandborn WJ, Harmsen WS, et al. Risk factors associated with progression to intestinal complications of Crohn's disease in a population-based cohort. Gastroenterology 2010;139(4):1147–55.

25. Munkholm P, Langholz E, Davidsen M, et al. Disease activity courses in a regional cohort of Crohn's disease patients. Scand J Gastroenterol 1995; 30(7):699–706.

26. Bengtson MB, Solberg C, Aamodt G, et al. Clustering in time of familial IBD separates ulcerative colitis from Crohn's disease. Inflamm Bowel Dis 2009;15(12): 1867–74.

27. Solberg IC, Lygren I, Jahnsen J, et al. Clinical course during the first 10 years of ulcerative colitis: results from a population-based inception cohort (IBSEN Study). Scand J Gastroenterol 2009;44(4):431–40.

28. Langholz E, Munkholm P, Davidsen M, et al. Course of ulcerative colitis: analysis of changes in disease activity over years. Gastroenterology 1994;107(1):3–11.

29. Sands BE. Inflammatory bowel disease: past, present, and future. J Gastroenterol 2007;42(1):16–25.

30. Molodecky NA, Soon IS, Rabi DM, et al. Increasing incidence and prevalence of the inflammatory bowel diseases with time, based on systematic review. Gastroenterology 2012;142(1):46–54.e42 [quiz: e30].

31. Kurata JH, Kantor-Fish S, Frankl H, et al. Crohn's disease among ethnic groups in a large health maintenance organization. Gastroenterology 1992;102:1940–8.

32. Bernstein CN, Wajda A, Svenson LW, et al. The epidemiology of inflammatory bowel disease in Canada: a population-based study. Am J Gastroenterol 2006;101(7):1559–68.

33. Pinchbeck BR, Kirdeikis J, Thomson AB. Inflammatory bowel disease in northern Alberta. An epidemiologic study. J Clin Gastroenterol 1988;10(5):505–15.

34. Vind I, Riis L, Jess T, et al. Increasing incidences of inflammatory bowel disease and decreasing surgery rates in Copenhagen City and County, 2003-2005: a population-based study from the Danish Crohn colitis database. Am J Gastroenterol 2006;101(6):1274–82.

35. Langholz E, Munkholm P, Nielsen OH, et al. Incidence and prevalence of ulcerative colitis in Copenhagen county from 1962 to 1987. Scand J Gastroenterol 1991;26(12):1247–56.

36. Moum B, Vatn MH, Ekbom A, et al. Incidence of ulcerative colitis and indeterminate colitis in four counties of southeastern Norway, 1990-93. A prospective population-based study. The Inflammatory Bowel South-Eastern Norway (IBSEN) Study Group of Gastroenterologists. Scand J Gastroenterol 1996;31(4):362–6.

37. Loftus EV Jr, Silverstein MD, Sandborn WJ, et al. Crohn's disease in Olmsted County, Minnesota, 1940-1993: incidence, prevalence, and survival. Gastroenterology 1998;114(6):1161–8.

38. Loftus EV Jr, Silverstein MD, Sandborn WJ, et al. Ulcerative colitis in Olmsted County, Minnesota, 1940-1993: incidence, prevalence, and survival. Gut 2000; 46(3):336–43.

39. Bernstein CN, Rawsthorne P, Cheang M, et al. A population-based case control study of potential risk factors for IBD. Am J Gastroenterol 2006;101(5): 993–1002.

40. Devlin HB, Datta D, Dellipiani AW. The incidence and prevalence of inflammatory bowel disease in North Tees Health District. World J Surg 1980;4(2): 183–93.

41. Auvin S, Molinie F, Gower-Rousseau C, et al. Incidence, clinical presentation and location at diagnosis of pediatric inflammatory bowel disease: a prospective population-based study in northern France (1988-1999). J Pediatr Gastroenterol Nutr 2005;41(1):49–55.

42. Mendeloff AI, Monk M, Siegel CI, et al. Some epidemiological features of ulcerative colitis and regional enteritis. A preliminary report. Gastroenterology 1966; 51(5):748–56.

43. Ogunbi SO, Ransom JA, Sullivan K, et al. Inflammatory bowel disease in African-American children living in Georgia. J Pediatr 1998;133:103–7.

44. Goldman CD, Kodner IJ, Fry RD, et al. Clinical and operative experience with non-Caucasian patients with Crohn's disease. Dis Colon Rectum 1986;29(5): 317–21.

45. Straus WL, Eisen GM, Sandler RS, et al. Crohn's disease: does race matter? The Mid-Atlantic Crohn's Disease Study Group. Am J Gastroenterol 2000;95(2): 479–83.

46. Mahid SS, Mulhall AM, Gholson RD, et al. Inflammatory bowel disease and African Americans: a systematic review. Inflamm Bowel Dis 2008;14(7):960–7.

47. Karban A, Waterman M, Panhuysen CI, et al. NOD2/CARD15 genotype and phenotype differences between Ashkenazi and Sephardic Jews with Crohn's disease. Am J Gastroenterol 2004;99(6):1134–40.

48. Yang H, McElree C, Roth MP, et al. Familial empirical risks for inflammatory bowel disease: differences between Jews and non-Jews. Gut 1993;34(4): 517–24.

49. Halme L, Paavola-Sakki P, Turunen U, et al. Family and twin studies in inflammatory bowel disease. World J Gastroenterol 2006;12(23):3668–72.

50. Kostic AD, Xavier RJ, Gevers D. The microbiome in inflammatory bowel disease: current status and the future ahead. Gastroenterology 2014;146(6):1489–99.

51. Jostins L, Ripke S, Weersma RK, et al. Host-microbe interactions have shaped the genetic architecture of inflammatory bowel disease. Nature 2012;491(7422): 119–24.

52. Nagalingam NA, Lynch SV. Role of the microbiota in inflammatory bowel diseases. Inflamm Bowel Dis 2012;18(5):968–84.

53. Darfeuille-Michaud A, Boudeau J, Bulois P, et al. High prevalence of adherent-invasive *Escherichia coli* associated with ileal mucosa in Crohn's disease. Gastroenterology 2004;127(2):412–21.

54. Martini GA, Brandes JW. Increased consumption of refined carbohydrates in patients with Crohn's disease. Klin Wochenschr 1976;54(8):367–71.

55. Thornton JR, Emmett PM, Heaton KW. Diet and Crohn's disease: characteristics of the pre-illness diet. Br Med J 1979;2(6193):762–4.

56. Asakura H, Suzuki K, Kitahora T, et al. Is there a link between food and intestinal microbes and the occurrence of Crohn's disease and ulcerative colitis? J Gastroenterol Hepatol 2008;23(12):1794–801.

57. Bedford PA, Todorovic V, Westcott ED, et al. Adipose tissue of human omentum is a major source of dendritic cells, which lose MHC Class II and stimulatory function in Crohn's disease. J Leukoc Biol 2006;80(3):546–54.

58. Geerling BJ, v Houwelingen AC, Badart-Smook A, et al. Fat intake and fatty acid profile in plasma phospholipids and adipose tissue in patients with Crohn's disease, compared with controls. Am J Gastroenterol 1999;94(2):410–7.

59. Karmiris K, Koutroubakis IE, Kouroumalis EA. Leptin, adiponectin, resistin, and ghrelin–implications for inflammatory bowel disease. Mol Nutr Food Res 2008; 52(8):855–66.

60. Yamamoto K, Kiyohara T, Murayama Y, et al. Production of adiponectin, an anti-inflammatory protein, in mesenteric adipose tissue in Crohn's disease. Gut 2005; 54(6):789–96.

61. Blain A, Cattan S, Beaugerie L, et al. Crohn's disease clinical course and severity in obese patients. Clin Nutr 2002;21(1):51–7.

62. Hass DJ, Brensinger CM, Lewis JD, et al. The impact of increased body mass index on the clinical course of Crohn's disease. Clin Gastroenterol Hepatol 2006; 4(4):482–8.

63. Harries AD, Baird A, Rhodes J. Non-smoking: a feature of ulcerative colitis. Br Med J 1982;284(6317):706.

64. Cosnes J. Crohn's disease phenotype, prognosis, and long-term complications: what to expect? Acta Gastroenterol Belg 2008;71(3):303–7.

65. Cosnes J, Nion-Larmurier I, Afchain P, et al. Gender differences in the response of colitis to smoking. Clin Gastroenterol Hepatol 2004;2(1):41–8.

66. Lakatos PL, Szamosi T, Lakatos L. Smoking in inflammatory bowel diseases: good, bad or ugly? World J Gastroenterol 2007;13(46):6134–9.

67. Higuchi LM, Khalili H, Chan AT, et al. A prospective study of cigarette smoking and the risk of inflammatory bowel disease in women. Am J Gastroenterol 2012; 107(9):1399–406.

68. Cosnes J, Carbonnel F, Beaugerie L, et al. Effects of cigarette smoking on the long-term course of Crohn's disease. Gastroenterology 1996;110(2): 424–31.

69. Cosnes J, Carbonnel F, Carrat F, et al. Effects of current and former cigarette smoking on the clinical course of Crohn's disease. Aliment Pharmacol Ther 1999;13(11):1403–11.

70. Biedermann L, Brulisauer K, Zeitz J, et al. Smoking cessation alters intestinal microbiota: insights from quantitative investigations on human fecal samples using FISH. Inflamm Bowel Dis 2014;20(9):1496–501.

71. Persson PG, Hellers G, Ahlbom A. Use of oral moist snuff and inflammatory bowel disease. Int J Epidemiol 1993;22(6):1101–3.

72. Shaw SY, Blanchard JF, Bernstein CN. Association between the use of antibiotics in the first year of life and pediatric inflammatory bowel disease. Am J Gastroenterol 2010;105(12):2687–92.

73. Chan SS, Luben R, Bergmann MM, et al. Aspirin in the aetiology of Crohn's disease and ulcerative colitis: a European prospective cohort study. Aliment Pharmacol Ther 2011;34(6):649–55.

74. Ananthakrishnan AN, Higuchi LM, Huang ES, et al. Aspirin, nonsteroidal anti-inflammatory drug use, and risk for Crohn disease and ulcerative colitis: a cohort study. Ann Intern Med 2012;156(5):350–9.

75. Cornish JA, Tan E, Simillis C, et al. The risk of oral contraceptives in the etiology of inflammatory bowel disease: a meta-analysis. Am J Gastroenterol 2008; 103(9):2394–400.

76. Khalili H, Higuchi LM, Ananthakrishnan AN, et al. Hormone therapy increases risk of ulcerative colitis but not Crohn's disease. Gastroenterology 2012; 143(5):1199–206.

77. Khalili H, Higuchi LM, Ananthakrishnan AN, et al. Oral contraceptives, reproductive factors and risk of inflammatory bowel disease. Gut 2013;62(8): 1153–9.
78. Aamodt G, Bukholm G, Jahnsen J, et al. The association between water supply and inflammatory bowel disease based on a 1990-1993 cohort study in southeastern Norway. Am J Epidemiol 2008;168(9):1065–72.
79. Bernstein CN, Blanchard JF, Rawsthorne P, et al. Population-based case control study of seroprevalence of *Mycobacterium paratuberculosis* in patients with Crohn's disease and ulcerative colitis. J Clin Microbiol 2004; 42(3):1129–35.
80. Selby W, Pavli P, Crotty B, et al. Two-year combination antibiotic therapy with clarithromycin, rifabutin, and clofazimine for Crohn's disease. Gastroenterology 2007;132(7):2313–9.
81. Gradel KO, Nielsen HL, Schonheyder HC, et al. Increased short- and long-term risk of inflammatory bowel disease after salmonella or campylobacter gastroenteritis. Gastroenterology 2009;137(2):495–501.
82. Thompson NP, Montgomery SM, Pounder RE, et al. Is measles vaccination a risk factor for inflammatory bowel disease? Lancet 1995;345(8957):1071–4.
83. Bernstein CN, Rawsthorne P, Blanchard JF. Population-based case-control study of measles, mumps, and rubella and inflammatory bowel disease. Inflamm Bowel Dis 2007;13(6):759–62.
84. Davis RL, Kramarz P, Bohlke K, et al. Measles-mumps-rubella and other measles-containing vaccines do not increase the risk for inflammatory bowel disease: a case-control study from the Vaccine Safety Datalink project. Arch Pediatr Adolesc Med 2001;155(3):354–9.
85. Ananthakrishnan AN, Issa M, Binion DG. *Clostridium difficile* and inflammatory bowel disease. Gastroenterol Clin North Am 2009;38(4):711–28.
86. Singh S, Graff LA, Bernstein CN. Do NSAIDs, antibiotics, infections, or stress trigger flares in IBD? Am J Gastroenterol 2009;104(5):1298–313 [quiz: 1314].
87. Feeney M, Ciegg A, Winwood P, et al. A case-control study of measles vaccination and inflammatory bowel disease. The East Dorset Gastroenterology Group. Lancet 1997;350(9080):764–6.
88. Morris DL, Montgomery SM, Thompson NP, et al. Measles vaccination and inflammatory bowel disease: a national British Cohort Study. Am J Gastroenterol 2000;95(12):3507–12.
89. Strachan DP. Hay fever, hygiene, and household size. BMJ 1989;299(6710): 1259–60.
90. Timm S, Svanes C, Janson C, et al. Place of upbringing in early childhood as related to inflammatory bowel diseases in adulthood: a population-based cohort study in Northern Europe. Eur J Epidemiol 2014;29(6):429–37.
91. Radon K, Windstetter D, Poluda AL, et al. Contact with farm animals in early life and juvenile inflammatory bowel disease: a case-control study. Pediatrics 2007; 120(2):354–61.
92. Van Kruiningen HJ, Joossens M, Vermeire S, et al. Environmental factors in familial Crohn's disease in Belgium. Inflamm Bowel Dis 2005;11(4):360–5.
93. Sood A, Amre D, Midha V, et al. Low hygiene and exposure to infections may be associated with increased risk for ulcerative colitis in a North Indian population. Ann Gastroenterol 2014;27(3):219–23.
94. Bager P, Simonsen J, Nielsen NM, et al. Cesarean section and offspring's risk of inflammatory bowel disease: a national cohort study. Inflamm Bowel Dis 2012; 18(5):857–62.

95. Bernstein CN, Singh S, Graff LA, et al. A prospective population-based study of triggers of symptomatic flares in IBD. Am J Gastroenterol 2010;105(9): 1994–2002.

96. Sonnenberg A. Occupational distribution of inflammatory bowel disease among German employees. Gut 1990;31(9):1037–40.

97. Ananthakrishnan AN, Long MD, Martin CF, et al. Sleep disturbance and risk of active disease in patients with Crohn's disease and ulcerative colitis. Clin Gastroenterol Hepatol 2013;11(8):965–71.

98. Nguyen GC, Nugent Z, Shaw S, et al. Outcomes of patients with Crohn's disease improved from 1988 to 2008 and were associated with increased specialist care. Gastroenterology 2011;141(1):90–7.

99. Ramadas AV, Gunesh S, Thomas GA, et al. Natural history of Crohn's disease in a population-based cohort from Cardiff (1986-2003): a study of changes in medical treatment and surgical resection rates. Gut 2010; 59(9):1200–6.

100. Lakatos PL, Golovics PA, David G, et al. Has there been a change in the natural history of Crohn's disease? Surgical rates and medical management in a population-based inception cohort from Western Hungary between 1977-2009. Am J Gastroenterol 2012;107(4):579–88.

101. Lakatos L, Kiss LS, David G, et al. Incidence, disease phenotype at diagnosis, and early disease course in inflammatory bowel diseases in Western Hungary, 2002-2006. Inflamm Bowel Dis 2011;17(12):2558–65.

102. Burisch J, Pedersen N, Cukovic-Cavka S, et al. Initial disease course and treatment in an inflammatory bowel disease inception cohort in Europe: the ECCO-EpiCom cohort. Inflamm Bowel Dis 2014;20(1):36–46.

103. Solberg IC, Vatn MH, Hoie O, et al. Clinical course in Crohn's disease: results of a Norwegian population-based ten-year follow-up study. Clin Gastroenterol Hepatol 2007;5(12):1430–8.

104. Sands BE, Arsenault JE, Rosen MJ, et al. Risk of early surgery for Crohn's disease: implications for early treatment strategies. Am J Gastroenterol 2003; 98(12):2712–8.

105. Galandiuk S, Kimberling J, Al-Mishlab TG, et al. Perianal Crohn disease: predictors of need for permanent diversion. Ann Surg 2005;241(5):796–801 [discussion: 801–2].

106. Hoie O, Wolters F, Riis L, et al. Ulcerative colitis: patient characteristics may predict 10-yr disease recurrence in a European-wide population-based cohort. Am J Gastroenterol 2007;102(8):1692–701.

107. Vester-Andersen MK, Prosberg MV, Jess T, et al. Disease course and surgery rates in inflammatory bowel disease: a population-based, 7-year follow-up study in the era of immunomodulating therapy. Am J Gastroenterol 2014;109(5): 705–14.

108. Vester-Andersen MK, Vind I, Prosberg MV, et al. Hospitalisation, surgical and medical recurrence rates in inflammatory bowel disease 2003–2011—a Danish population-based cohort study. J Crohns Colitis 2014; 8(12):1675–83.

109. Hoie O, Wolters FL, Riis L, et al. Low colectomy rates in ulcerative colitis in an unselected European cohort followed for 10 years. Gastroenterology 2007; 132(2):507–15.

110. Henriksen M, Jahnsen J, Lygren I, et al. Ulcerative colitis and clinical course: results of a 5-year population-based follow-up study (the IBSEN study). Inflamm Bowel Dis 2006;12(7):543–50.

111. Campbell S, Travis S, Jewell D. Ciclosporin use in acute ulcerative colitis: a long-term experience. Eur J Gastroenterol Hepatol 2005;17(1):79–84.
112. Jarnerot G, Hertervig E, Friis-Liby I, et al. Infliximab as rescue therapy in severe to moderately severe ulcerative colitis: a randomized, placebo-controlled study. Gastroenterology 2005;128(7):1805–11.
113. Shen B, Fazio VW, Remzi FH, et al. Comprehensive evaluation of inflammatory and noninflammatory sequelae of ileal pouch-anal anastomoses. Am J Gastroenterol 2005;100(1):93–101.
114. Beaugerie L. Inflammatory bowel disease therapies and cancer risk: where are we and where are we going? Gut 2012;61(4):476–83.
115. Eaden JA, Abrams KR, Mayberry JF. The risk of colorectal cancer in ulcerative colitis: a meta-analysis. Gut 2001;48(4):526–35.
116. Basseri RJ, Basseri B, Papadakis KA. Dysplasia and cancer in inflammatory bowel disease. Expert Rev Gastroenterol Hepatol 2011;5(1):59–66.
117. Farraye FA, Odze RD, Eaden J, et al. AGA medical position statement on the diagnosis and management of colorectal neoplasia in inflammatory bowel disease. Gastroenterology 2010;138(2):738–45.
118. Pedersen N, Duricova D, Elkjaer M, et al. Risk of extra-intestinal cancer in inflammatory bowel disease: meta-analysis of population-based cohort studies. Am J Gastroenterol 2010;105(7):1480–7.
119. Kandiel A, Fraser AG, Korelitz BI, et al. Increased risk of lymphoma among inflammatory bowel disease patients treated with azathioprine and 6-mercaptopurine. Gut 2005;54(8):1121–5.
120. Long MD, Herfarth HH, Pipkin CA, et al. Increased risk for non-melanoma skin cancer in patients with inflammatory bowel disease. Clin Gastroenterol Hepatol 2010;8(3):268–74.
121. Jess T, Frisch M, Simonsen J. Trends in overall and cause-specific mortality among patients with inflammatory bowel disease from 1982 to 2010. Clin Gastroenterol Hepatol 2013;11(1):43–8.
122. Wolters FL, Russel MG, Sijbrandij J, et al. Crohn's disease: increased mortality 10 years after diagnosis in a Europe-wide population based cohort. Gut 2006; 55(4):510–8.
123. Hovde O, Kempski-Monstad I, Smastuen MC, et al. Mortality and causes of death in Crohn's disease: results from 20 years of follow-up in the IBSEN study. Gut 2014;63(5):771–5.
124. Romberg-Camps M, Kuiper E, Schouten L, et al. Mortality in inflammatory bowel disease in the Netherlands 1991-2002: results of a population-based study: the IBD South-Limburg cohort. Inflamm Bowel Dis 2010; 16(8):1397–410.
125. Manninen P, Karvonen AL, Huhtala H, et al. Mortality in ulcerative colitis and Crohn's disease. A population-based study in Finland. J Crohns Colitis 2012; 6(5):524–8.
126. Jess T, Gamborg M, Munkholm P, et al. Overall and cause-specific mortality in ulcerative colitis: meta-analysis of population-based inception cohort studies. Am J Gastroenterol 2007;102(3):609–17.
127. Bewtra M, Kaiser LM, TenHave T, et al. Crohn's disease and ulcerative colitis are associated with elevated standardized mortality ratios: a meta-analysis. Inflamm Bowel Dis 2013;19(3):599–613.
128. Jess T, Loftus EV Jr, Harmsen WS, et al. Survival and cause specific mortality in patients with inflammatory bowel disease: a long term outcome study in Olmsted County, Minnesota, 1940-2004. Gut 2006;55(9):1248–54.

129. Winther KV, Jess T, Langholz E, et al. Survival and cause-specific mortality in ulcerative colitis: follow-up of a population-based cohort in Copenhagen County.
Gastroenterology 2003;125(6):1576–82.
130. Hoie O, Schouten LJ, Wolters FL, et al. Ulcerative colitis: no rise in mortality in a
European-wide population based cohort 10 years after diagnosis. Gut 2007;
56(4):497–503.

Diagnostic Modalities for Inflammatory Bowel Disease: Serologic Markers and Endoscopy

Clarence Clark, MD, Jacquelyn Turner, MD*

KEYWORDS

• Serologic markers • Endoscopy • Inflammatory bowel disease

KEY POINTS

• Perinuclear antineutrophil cytoplasmic antibody is associated with ulcerative colitis; anti-*Saccharomyces cerevisiae* mannan antibodies are more commonly detected in patients with Crohn's disease (CD).
• Deep endoscopy is a useful tool for detection and surveillance of small bowel CD.
• Video capsule endoscopy and colon capsule endoscopy are promising modalities for gastrointestinal evaluation.
• Chromoendoscopy and confocal laser endomicroscopy allow for targeted biopsies which have shown to detect more intraepithelial neoplasms with fewer biopsy specimens.
• Endoscopic scoring systems help to increase intraobserver agreement of disease activity and severity among endoscopists.

INTRODUCTION

As endoscopic technology and advances in laboratory assays have evolved in the past two decades, better understanding of the pathogenesis and natural history of inflammatory bowel disease (IBD) has emerged. Central to these medical advances is the ability to discriminate between the subtypes of IBD (Crohn's disease [CD], ulcerative colitis [UC], and indeterminate colitis) especially when limited to the colon. Gross endoscopic and histologic findings in concert with serologic markers are critical to medicine and surgical specialties treating persons with these conditions. Herein, we examine the current literature as it pertains to endoscopy and serology as diagnostic tools for IBD.

The authors have nothing to disclose.
Department of Surgery, Division of Colon and Rectal Surgery, Morehouse School of Medicine, 720 Westview Drive Southwest, Atlanta, GA 30310, USA
* Corresponding author.
E-mail address: jturner@msm.edu

Surg Clin N Am 95 (2015) 1123–1141
http://dx.doi.org/10.1016/j.suc.2015.07.008
0039-6109/15/$ – see front matter © 2015 Elsevier Inc. All rights reserved.

RELEVANT ANATOMY AND PATHOPHYSIOLOGY

Essential to the pathogenesis of IBD is the epithelial barrier of the gastrointestinal tract. This first line of defense is composed of a mucinous layer coupled with an epithelium that produces antimicrobial peptides that limit bacterial invasion.[1] Damage to the epithelial barrier leads to increased permeability and an increased uptake of luminal antigens. This process is often regarded as a key stage in the pathogenesis of IBD.

Pathologic features of UC include mucin depletion, erosion, and ulceration. Crypt architecture in UC is often distorted in addition to crypt branching, decreased crypt density, and crypt abscesses. Crypt architecture abnormalities are more common in UC than CD (57%–100% of cases compared with 21%–71% of cases, respectively).[2] At the level of the laminal propria, UC is notable for transmucosal inflammation and basal plasmacytosis.[1,2] In contrast, granulomas are characteristic of CD and be present in 21% to 37% of specimens taken.[2] Crypt architecture in CD includes segmental crypt atrophy and distortion. Both CD and UC have increased basal lamina propria cellularity and basal plasmacytosis.

CLINICAL PRESENTATION

Tables 1 and **2** and **Figs. 1–5** detail the clinical presentation of IBD.

SEROLOGIC MARKERS AS DIAGNOSTIC MODALITIES FOR INFLAMMATORY BOWEL DISEASE

Increased exposure to environmental microbiota and inflammatory response to common environmental pathogens have been implicated in the pathogenesis of IBD.[2–7] This association has led to a host of studies identifying serologic markers to these antigens for diagnosis and differentiation of the various subtypes of IBD. In this section, we review these serologic markers and the evidence for their use in the diagnosis and management of IBD.

Atypical Perinuclear Antineutrophil Cytoplasmic Antibody

Atypical perinuclear antineutrophil cytoplasmic antibody (pANCA) is a type of antibody that targets antigens present on azurophilic granules of polymorphonuclear leukocytes with a perinuclear staining pattern.[8] A number of studies have demonstrated

Table 1	
Signs and symptoms of inflammatory bowel disease	
Ulcerative Colitis	**Crohn's Disease**
• Disease confined to the colon; colonic involvement is usually left sided	• Small bowel is involved in 80% of cases; right sided colonic involvement
• Rectosigmoid colon is invariably involved	• Rectosigmoid junction is often spared
• Chronic, episodic	• Chronic, episodic
• Increased risk of colon cancer	• Perianal disease
• Bloody stools	• Fistulizing
• Tenesmus/fecal urgency	• Bowel obstruction
• Abdominal pain	• Increased risk of colon cancer
• Fever	• Nausea/vomiting
• Nocturnal diarrhea	• Weight loss
• Frequent small bowel movements	• Severe malabsorption
	• Bloody stools
	• Abdominal pain

Table 2
Endoscopic characteristics of inflammatory bowel disease

Ulcerative Colitis	Crohn's Disease
• Erythema	• Erythema
• Friability	• Friability
• Pseudopolyps	• Pathos ulcers
• Rectal involvement	• Linear/serpiginous ulcers
• Continuous involvement	• Rectal involvement (fairly common)
• Mucosa erythema	• Pseudopolyps (fairly common)
• Loss of colon architecture	• Segmental inflammation
• loss of vascular pattern	• Strictures
• Erosions	• Mucosal erythema
• Ulcerations	• Loss of villi
• Spontaneous bleeding	• Mucosal fissures
• Granularity	• Fistula scaring
	• Cobblestone appearance

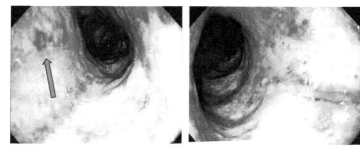

Fig. 1. Endoscopic findings of a Crohn's patient with loss of colonic architecture, friability, erythema, and aphthous ulceration (*blue arrow*).

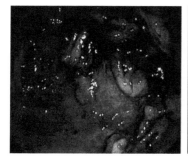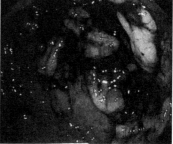

Fig. 2. Endoscopic findings from a patient with Crohn's disease with friability, erythema, and severe cobblestone appearance of the mucosa.

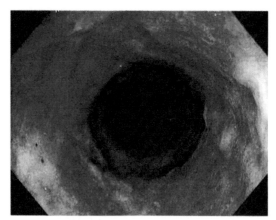

Fig. 3. A patient with Crohn's disease misdiagnosed as ulcerative colitis. Endoscopy shows loss of colon architecture, erythema, and friability.

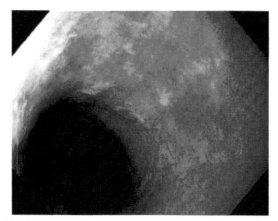

Fig. 4. Patient with ulcerative colitis showing mild left-sided colitis with loss of mucosal architecture.

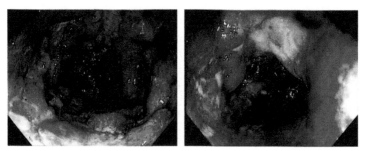

Fig. 5. Endoscopic findings of a patient with ulcerative colitis with pseudopolyps, erythema, friability, loss of vascular pattern, and fibrinous exudate.

the presence of these antibodies in the sera of patients with idiopathic inflammatory disorders, including but not limited to idiopathic rapidly progressive glomerulonephritis, microscopic polyangiitis, primary sclerosing cholangitis, and IBD.[9–11]

The prevalence of pANCA ranges from 40% to 80% in UC and from 0% to 20% in CD.[12–16] Peeters and colleagues[17] used indirect immunofluorescence for the detection of pANCA and showed a sensitivity, specificity, positive predictive value, and negative predictive value in differentiating IBD from controls of 50%, 95%, 69%, and 89%, respectively. This pattern of low sensitivity and high specificity for pANCA is also seen in patients with UC in various cohort studies.[18–22] In addition, Sandborn and colleagues[20] showed that the low sensitivity was seen across several laboratories with a range of 0% to 60% in patients with UC. In a metaanalysis of 60 studies composed of 3841 UC and 4019 CD patients, Reese and colleagues[21] reported a sensitivity and specificity of 55.3% and 88.5%, respectively, in UC patients positive for pANCA. Furthermore, the authors found an increased sensitivity and specificity (70.3% and 93.4%, respectively) in their pediatric subgroup when combined with a negative anti-*Saccharomyces cerevisiae* mannan antibodies (ASCA) tests. The use of pANCA alone, therefore, has utility in ruling out the presence of UC if this serology test is negative. Its use in combination with ASCA serologic testing, however, may offer improved diagnostic accuracy when differentiating patients with UC and CD.

Anti-Saccharimyces cerevisiae Antibody

In 1988, Main and colleagues[22] published one of the earliest reports of significantly elevated immunoglobulin (Ig)G and IgA blood titers to ASCA in 55 patients with Crohn's disease when compared with 30 controls. Since this study, numerous reports have been published examining this yeast found in dietary products and serologic markers associated with this organism.

Annese and colleagues[23] examined the presence of ASCA using standard enzyme-linked immunosorbent assay of patients with sporadic and familial CD or UC and their unaffected relatives. They found ASCAs were detected in 35% of patients with sporadic CD, 12% with sporadic UC, and 4% of controls. In addition, the presence of ASCA was significantly more frequent in patients with familial CD and familial UC than in sporadic cases. Accuracy data reported by Peeters and colleagues[17] revealed a sensitivity, specificity, positive predictive value, and negative predictive value rates for differentiating IBD from controls, using ASCA as a marker, of 60%, 91%, 88%, and 68%, respectively. Specifically in patients with CD, a similar sensitivity rate, ranging from 39% to 76%, has been reported in the literature.[20,24] However, with regard to CD limited to the colon, studies have shown a decrease in sensitivity of this serologic marker.[21]

When combined with a negative pANCA, a positive ASCA test has shown to have a higher sensitivity for CD at 54.6% with a 92.8% specificity in a recent metaanalysis.[21] Ruemmele and colleagues[18] showed that ASCA titers decreased toward normal values after resection in patients with CD. In summary, the presence of ASCA is most useful in confirming the diagnosis of CD and maybe a useful marker to trend after surgical resection for complicated CD.

Antibodies to Escherichia coli Outer Membrane Porin

Gram-negative bacteria cells are surrounded by an outer membrane layer with various transport proteins such as *Escherichia coli* outer membrane porin C (OmpC).[25] Serum antibodies to OmpC (anti-OmpC) have been used in the evaluation of IBD. Conflicting data exist regarding the utility of this serologic marker for the assessment of IBD. Mei and colleagues[26] showed, in their cohort study of CD patients from CD-only families and from families with both UC and CD, a prevalence rate of 37.8% and 43.8%, respectively. A similar rate was seen by Arnott and colleagues[27] in CD patients, suggesting a possible role for this marker in the evaluation of IBD patients, specifically those with likely CD. To further define the role of this marker, anti-OmpC was assessed in various phenotypes of CD and was independently associated with internal perforations in patients with complicated small bowel CD.[28]

Several studies did not show, however, any benefit or diagnostic value of this assay.[29,30] In a retrospective review of 81 children with CD, 54 with UC, and 63 controls, Zholudev and colleagues[31] showed a sensitivity rate for CD and UC of 24% and 11%, respectively, for the anti-OmpC assay. The utility of this serologic marker alone in the management of IBD, therefore, has yet to be clearly elucidated thus far.

Pseudomonas fluorescens–Associated Sequence I2

The emergence of P fluorescens-associated sequence I2 began at the turn of the millennium. Sutton and colleagues[32] in 2000 identified I2 DNA in 43% of colonic specimens of CD patients compared with only 9% of UC and 5% of non-IBD tissue. The authors found this DNA to be prevalent in CD specimens, especially those originating from the ileum. Subsequently, P fluorescens was found to be the microorganism that encoded this DNA sequence.[33] To better understand the clinical utility of this marker, Arnott and colleagues,[27] in an observational study, showed anti-I2 was present in 52% of the sera from of CD patients. This pattern was also seen in pediatric patients with CD by Iltanen and colleagues.[34] This serologic marker thus has some promise when attempting to distinguish the various subtypes of IBD with a predilection to CD.

Flagellin CBir1/Fla-X/A4-Fla2

In 2004, Lodes and colleagues[35] showed elevated serum anti–flagellin IcG2a in an IBD mouse model and flagellin-specific CD4$^+$ T-cell induction of severe colitis in immunodeficient mice. From this observation, they were able to show the presence of serum IgG to these flagellins in patients with CD but not in patients with UC or controls. Specifically, significantly higher levels of serum anti–CBir1 and anti–Fla-X were found in CD patients. These findings suggest that CBir1 responses may be valuable in the diagnosis of IBD and discrimination between IBD subtypes.

After this study, further evidence was published to further define the role of CBir1 in the diagnosis of IBD. Enzyme-linked immunosorbent assay analysis of anti-CBir1 by Targan and colleagues[36] of 40 normal controls, 21 disease controls, 50 UC patients, and 373 CD patients previously typed for ASCA, anti-I2, anti-OmpC, and pANCA further defined the value of this marker. The authors showed IgG anti-CBir1 was associated with CD independently, especially in pANCA-positive patients with CD. In addition, anti-CBir1 expression was found to be associated with small bowel, internal-penetrating, and fibrostenosing disease.

With regard to the role of Fla-X flagellin, further studies by Schoepfer and colleagues[37] have defined the seroreactivity to Fla-X as well as similar flagellin strain, A4-Fla2, in a population of CD, UC, and healthy controls. Seropositivity to A4-Fla2 and Fla-X was found in 59% and 57% of patients with CD, respectively, whereas only 6% each in patients with UC, and 0% and 2% of healthy controls, respectively, were noted. These data along with prior studies demonstrate anti-CBir1, anti-Fla-X, and anti-A4-Fla2 may play a role in the diagnosis and discrimination between IBD subtypes favoring the CD subtype when present. A summary of serologic markers is presented in **Table 3**.

Serologic Panels

Various combinations of ASCA, pANCA, anti-OmpC, anti-CBir1, and anti-I2 have been studied starting with pANCA and ASCA combined compared with more complex panels.[17,18,21,36–39] Although patterns of these markers may discriminate between CD and UC, the utility of such panels has recently come into question, more specifically as it compares with inexpensive, conventional laboratory blood tests such as complete blood count and/or erythrocyte sedimentation rate (ESR).

Sabery and colleagues[38] demonstrated in a pediatric observational study that serologic testing for IBD had 60% sensitivity, 92% specificity, and 60% positive predictive value. The authors found these rates were much lower compared with those seen in tests for anemia and ESR, especially in a subgroup of patients who do not have rectal bleeding. Similar findings were seen by Benor and colleagues,[39] who reported a sensitivity, specificity, positive predictive value, and negative predictive value for the serologic panel of 67%, 76%, 63%, 79%, and 42%, respectively. Higher values were seen in abnormal routine laboratory tests (age-adjusted hemoglobin, platelet count, and ESR) which were 72%, 94%, 85%, 79%, and 47%, respectively. The authors also reported a lower cost for complete blood count and ESR testing (<$100) compared with the cost of the IBD serology 7 panel (approximately $450). The use of combination serology panels, therefore, has promise but, given the cost and diagnostic value compared with conventional blood tests, the routine use of these panels is still being elucidated.

Table 3
Summary of serologic markers used for inflammatory bowel disease

Serologic Marker	Target	Disease Association
Perinuclear antineutrophil cytoplasmic antibody (pANCA)	Targets antigen on azurophilic granules of polymorphonuclear leukocytes	More commonly detected in UC
Anti-*Saccharomyces cerevisiae* mannan antibodies (ASCA)	Targets *Saccharimyces cerevisiae* antibody	More commonly detected in CD
Anti-outer membrane porin C (OmpC)	Targets the outer membrane transport protein found on *E coli*	More commonly detected in CD; specifically associated with perforated CD
Anti-I2	Antibodies to DNA sequence I2 encoded by *Pseudomonas flourescens*	More commonly detected in CD
Anti-CBir1	Antibodies to flagellin CBir1	More commonly detected in CD; specifically associated with small bowel, internal-penetrating, fibrostenosing disease
Anti-Fla-X/anti –A4-Fla2	Antibodies to flagellin Fla-X and similar flagellin strain A4-Fla2	More commonly detected in CD

Abbreviations: CD, Crohn's disease; UC, ulcerative colitis.

ENDOSCOPIC DIAGNOSTIC MODALITIES
Deep Enteroscopy

Deep enteroscopy is a useful way to assess the small bowel that in the past was inaccessible by routine endoscopy. The technique of deep enteroscopy was described in 2002.[40] The typical endoscope used for this procedure has a total working length ranging between 200 and 250 cm. With various maneuvers, this length allows the endoscopist to examine approximately 430 cm of small bowel via an oral antegrade approach or a retrograde approach through the rectum.[40,41]

There are 4 different deep enteroscopy systems currently available: balloon-assisted enteroscopy, single-balloon enteroscopy (SBE), double-balloon enteroscopy (DBE), and spiral enteroscopy (SE).[42] Herein, we examine these systems closely and the literature to support their use.

Balloon-assisted enteroscopy

Balloon-assisted enteroscopy uses a standard endoscope and an overtube with a balloon at its distal end. The purpose of the balloon is to stabilize the endoscope while in the small intestine.[43] The overtube, on the other hand, increases the stiffness of the scope, which can reduce excess looping in the stomach.[41] The overtube has been found to increase the depth of insertion significantly, although few clinical data exist supporting this added benefit.[43,44]

Single-balloon enteroscopy

The SBE is a push–pull technique using a standard endoscope with a flexible overtube. A latex-free balloon is attached at the tip of the overtube. The inflation and deflation of the balloon is controlled by a pressure-controlled pump system. The technique of SBE is described below.[45]

1. The endoscope with an overtube is introduced orally and advanced into the stomach.
2. The balloon on the overtube remains deflated until the duodenum is reached.
3. Once in the duodenum, the balloon is inflated to stabilize the enteroscope while it is advanced to a maximum distance.
4. The overtube balloon is then deflated and advanced along the enteroscope until the tip is reached.
5. The overtube balloon is then reinflated and the process is repeated.

The tip of the enteroscope can be angled to enable hooking behind a fold for stabilization. For further advancement, the enteroscope and the overtube can be pulled back simultaneously while the balloon is inflated to compress the bowel. An alternative for advancement is to pull back the overtube with the balloon inflated while simultaneously advancing the enteroscope.

Double-balloon enteroscopy

The DBE is also a push–pull technique that consist of a 2-balloon system (prototype: Fujinon, Inc, Saitman, Japan)[42]: 1 balloon is attached to a semiflexible overtube and the second balloon is attached to the enteroscope. The balloon inflation and deflation is controlled by a pressure-controlled pump system. The technique of DBE is described below.[40]

1. The endoscope with an overtube is introduced orally and advanced into the stomach.
2. The balloons remain deflated until the duodenum is reached.

3. Once in the duodenum, the balloon on the overtube is inflated to stabilize it in the intestine while the enteroscope is inserted to a maximum distance.
4. After the enteroscope is inserted at its maximum distance, the balloon on the enteroscope is inflated.
5. The balloon on the overtube is deflated and advanced over the endoscope until the tip of the scope is reached.
6. The balloon on the overtube is now reinflated to stabilize the bowel at a second point. The overtube is withdrawn to compress the bowel. The sequence is then repeated until the full length of the small bowel is reached.

Spiral enteroscopy

Spiral enteroscopy incorporates a rotational technique by using a special overtube with a helical thread at its distal segment (prototype: Spirus Medical INC, Stoughton, MA).[46] The overtube used for SE is slightly larger than the largest overtube used for DBE (16-mm vs 13.2-mm diameter, respectively).[42] The technique of SE is described below.[46]

1. The endoscope with an overtube is introduced orally and advanced into the stomach.
2. The endoscope is passed through the overtube and locked at the proximal end.
3. The scope and overtube are advanced beyond the ligament of Treitz.
4. The scope is then unlocked from the overtube and further advanced.
5. The overtube is then advanced over the scope in a clockwise rotation until it is just proximal to the tip of the scope (about 12 cm).
6. The overtube is relocked. The bowel becomes pleated with the advancement of the overtube. The steps are repeated until the rotation is no longer effective.
7. After the scope has reached its maximum distance, the scope and overtube are withdrawn. During withdrawal, the overtube is turned counterclockwise while examining the mucosa.

Outcomes of Deep Enteroscopy

When comparing the different techniques, DBE, SBE, and SE have similar diagnostic yields. Lenz and colleagues[43] evaluated several studies comparing DBE, SBE, and SE. Oral intubation depth was comparable between DBE (239 ± 24.3 cm), SBE (233 ± 31 cm), and SE (236 ± 23 cm). However, anal intubation depth was much lower in the SE group (88 ± 25 cm) compared with the depth obtained by DBE (130 ± 18 cm) and SBE (123 ± 34 cm). Complete enteroscopy was more likely to be achieved in the DBE group ($33.9\% \pm 10.1\%$) compared with the SBE ($12.4\% \pm 9.8\%$) and SE ($2.9\% \pm 4.3\%$).[43] When comparing SBE with SE, there are no differences in procedure time despite the shorter depth of insertion seen in the SBE group.[47] Messer and colleagues[42] compared DBE with SE and found a significantly higher complete enteroscopy rate with DBE (92%) compared with SE (8%). However, DBE is more time consuming with an average examination time of 59.62 ± 12.5 minutes, whereas SE has an average examination time of 43.43 ± 10.19 minutes. There was no difference in diagnostic or therapeutic yields when DBE was compared with SE (69% vs 46%, respectively; $P = 0.428$).

The most common site for CD is the terminal ileum, which may be difficult to evaluate in its entirety. Observation of about 100 cm of bowel from the terminal ileum is usually significant.[48] A combination of small bowel follow through, DBE, and ileal intubation during colonoscopy can provide adequate assessment of the ileum.

With regard to postprocedure outcomes, deep enteroscopy has a low complication rate. Specifically, DBE has a complication rate of 1%.[42] Pancreatitis is a commonly reported complication of deep enteroscopy. Pancreatitis can be avoided by inflating the balloons after passing the ligament of Treitz.[43] Significant abdominal pain and perforation (likely caused by the overtube or at the site of ulcerative pathology) has also been reported.[42,48]

Video Capsule Endoscopy

Video capsule endoscopy (VCE; prototype: Given Imaging; Yoqneam, Israel) has been available in the United States since 2001.[49] The VCE is a wireless video-containing capsule. Within the capsule is a sensing system that includes a sensing belt, data recorder unit, battery pack, and real-time viewer. Contraindications of VCE include known strictures, obstruction, fistulas, and pregnancy. Implanted electromedical devices, such as a cardiac pacemaker, are a relative contraindication owing to a potential risk of magnetic interference. MRI or computed tomographic enterography is needed in patients with suspected CD to evaluate for strictures before VCE. Optionally, a patency capsule, made up of lactose and barium sulfate surrounded by cellophane walls, has been used to determine patency of the gastrointestinal tract before VCE. If the capsule is retained, the components of the capsule dissolve after 30 hours. The nondissolvable components are usually able to pass through strictures. VCE is then performed if the capsule passes intact or if the radiofrequency tag inside the capsule is not detected by the radiofrequency scanner after 30 hours.

VCE has been compared with push enteroscopy and enteroclysis. VCE has a higher yield of detecting small bowel disease.[50,51] A metaanalysis comparing VCE with push enteroscopy for obscure gastrointestinal bleeding found that VCE had a higher diagnostic yield than push enteroscopy (63% vs 28%, respectively; $P<0.00001$).[51] Chong and colleagues[50] detected small bowel disease in 3 of 22 patients with known CD who underwent push enteroscopy, 4 of 21 patients who underwent enteroclysis, and 17 of 22 patients who underwent VCE ($P<0.001$). However, disadvantages of VCE include the inability to definitively localize and/or sample pathology.[48] In addition, incomplete examinations can occur in up to 80% of patients. Inpatient status, delayed gastric emptying, and prior abdominal surgery have been associated with incomplete examinations. Chong and colleagues[50] reported battery life as a problem with capsule endoscopy and that 6 of 43 patients had incomplete examinations owing to a limited battery life. Complications include capsule retention with 1.4% needing surgical or endoscopic removal of the retained capsule.[49] A summary of deep endoscopy modalities and VCE is presented in **Table 4**.

Magnification Endoscopy and Chromoendoscopy (Dye-Based and Dyeless Chromoendoscopy)

Several techniques have emerged to enhance the visualization of mucosal surfaces in IBD patients. Detailed characterization of mucosal surfaces and pit patterns can aid in targeted biopsies for more effective surveillance of IBD patients. Enhancing the mucosal surface features can be accomplished with magnification, dye agents, and optical or digital enhancement.[52–54]

Magnification endoscopy allows for detailed inspection of the mucosa through a movable lens with 1.5- to 150-fold magnification.[52,53] This technology is often used in conjunction with chromoendoscopy. Chromoendoscopy uses dyes to stain the mucosa surface, resulting in improved pattern recognition and clarify borders of neoplastic lesion.[53,54] The dyes are sprayed by a catheter through the working channel of the endoscope. Such dyes include absorptive agents (Lugol solution, methylene blue, toluidine blue, and cresyl violet), contrast agents (indigo carmine and acetic acid), and reactive staining agents (Congo red and phenol red). The enhancement

Table 4
Summary of deep endoscopy modalities and video capsule endoscopy

	Advantages	Disadvantages
Balloon-assisted enteroscopy	Push–pull technique	• Risk of perforation, postprocedural pancreatitis, and postprocedural abdominal pain • Associated learning curve
Single-balloon enteroscopy	Push–pull technique	• Risk of perforation, postprocedural pancreatitis, and postprocedural abdominal pain • Associated learning curve
Double-balloon enteroscopy	• Push–pull technique • More likely to perform complete enteroscopy	• More time consuming • Risk of perforation, postprocedural pancreatitis, and postprocedural abdominal pain • Associated learning curve
Spiral enteroscopy	• Rotational technique • Less time consuming	• Shorter depth of intubation with anal approach • Risk of perforation, postprocedural pancreatitis, and postprocedural abdominal pain • Associated learning curve
Video capsule endoscopy	• Video capsule technique • Less invasive • High negative predictive value for Crohn's disease • Higher diagnostic yield for detecting small bowel disease	• Contraindicated with known strictures, obstruction, fistulas and pregnancy • Need preprocedural evaluation with computed tomography enterography, MRI, or patency capsule to evaluate for strictures • Relatively contraindicated with implanted electromedical devices • Inability to definitively localize lesion • Inability to sample tissue • Capsule retention may occur needing endoscopic removal of retained capsule

of mucosal detail has allowed for categorization of the different staining patterns of the colon.[52,53]

Dyeless chromoendoscopy uses either optical imaging or computer based imaging. Narrow band imaging (Olympus, Tokyo, Japan) or compound band imaging (Aohua, Shanghai, China) are 2 common optical chromoendoscopy enhancement systems that alter the bandwidth of transmitted light through filters within the light source of the endoscope. I-scan (Pentax, Tokyo, Japan) and Fujinon intelligent color enhancement (Fujinon, Tokyo, Japan) are 2 digital chromoendoscopy enhancement systems.[52]

Colonic chromoendoscopy and targeted biopsies of suspicious lesions are more effective in surveying IBD patients for intraepithelial neoplasia than previous methods of taking multiple, random biopsies.[52,53] In addition, chromoendoscopy has been shown to provide more accurate diagnosis of disease activity when compared with white light endoscopy.[55,56] Neumann and colleagues[56] demonstrated that there is an increased agreement between histology and dyeless chromoendoscopy compared with high-definition white light colonoscopy with regard to disease extent (48.71% and 92.31%, respectively) and disease activity (53.85% and 89.74%) of UC.

There are several limitations to magnification and chromoendoscopy. The high magnification setting can make screening impractical in this mode and examination difficult with peristalsis and respiratory movements. In addition, inflammation can disturb the image and produce false-positive results. Last, there is a learning curve to this technique that can increase the procedure time initially.[53]

Confocal Laser Endomicroscopy

Endomicroscopy is relatively new technology that allows for imaging of the cellular and subcellular level of the mucosa during colonoscopy.[54] It is being used for IBD patients to improve dysplasia detection and differentiation of lesions, such as colitis-associated neoplasia, sporadic neoplasia, and nonneoplastic lesions. These lesions can easily be missed with standard endoscopy owing to their flat appearance in colitis patients.[57] The technique of confocal laser endomicroscopy (CLE) involves using a low-power laser to focus on a single point in a microscopic field of view. The lens used for CLE allows for both illumination and detection systems to align in the same focal plane, thus the term confocal.

Currently, there are 2 CLE-based systems: the Pentax Endomicroscopy System from Japan, which uses an integrated confocal scanner at the tip of a flexible endoscope, and the Cellvizio Endomicroscopy System (Mauna Kea Technologies, Paris, France), which uses a flexible miniprobe inserted through the working channel of an endoscope.[54] CLE can be further guided using contrast agents, such as intravenous fluorescein and topical acriflavine and cresyl violet, to enhance the image.

CLE is useful in predicting inflammatory and neoplastic activity. Kiesslich and colleagues[57] found overall concordance between CLE and histology in determining UC disease activity to be 92.5% compared with 58.9% concordance with standard endoscopy. Moreover, this study revealed more intraepithelial neoplastic lesions are identified with CLE (19 of 80) compared with standard endoscopy (4 of 73; $P = 0.005$). Neumann and colleagues[58] determined that CLE could identify architectural changes (such as crypt tortuosity, crypt dilation, microerosion, vascularity, number of goblet cells, and cellular infiltrate in the laminal propria) in patients with active CD similar to established histopathologic criteria.

Similar to chromoendoscopy, CLE allows for targeted biopsies thus reducing the number of random biopsies.[54,57] Overall, 4.75-fold more intraepithelial neoplasms could be detected with 50% fewer biopsy specimens using CLE when compared with standard endoscopy.[57] One limitation, as seen with chromoendoscopy, is the lengthy time required to examine large surface areas.

Colon Capsule Endoscopy

Recently, a VCE device, referred to as colon capsule endoscopy (CCE), was developed specifically to target colonic mucosal evaluation. One such device is PillCam Colon (Given Imaging).[49,59] In a study by Herrerias-Gutierrez et al,[60] 144 patients were evaluated with the aim of comparing outcomes of CCE with colonoscopy. These authors found a rate of agreement between CCE and colonoscopy to be 75.6%. There are few studies evaluating CCE as a diagnostic modality for IBD to date. Sung and colleagues[61] have published the largest prospective trial evaluating the PillCam Colon in UC patients. One hundred patients were evaluated with 4 patients excluded owing to technical failure or slow transit time of the capsule. Nine patients had transit times of greater than 8.5 hours requiring endoscopic removal of the capsule. The specificity and sensitivity to detect mucosal inflammation was 89% and 75%, respectively. The authors concluded that CCE is a safe procedure and can be used to monitor mucosal healing in UC. A summary of colonoscopy imaging modalities is provided in **Table 5**.

Table 5
Summary of colonoscopic imaging techniques

	Advantages	Disadvantages
Magnification endoscopy	• Enhances mucosal surfaces through a magnification lens • Can be used for targeted biopsies • Can be used in conjunction with chromoendoscopy	• Not practical for screening endoscopy • Inflammation in colitis can produce false positives • Associated learning curve
Chromoendoscopy	• Enhances mucosal surfaces through spray dyes • Can be used for targeted biopsies • Can be used in conjunction with chromoendoscopy and confocal laser endomicroscopy • More accurate diagnosis of disease activity than white light endoscopy	• Inflammation in colitis can produce false positives • Associated learning curve
Confocal laser endomicroscopy	• Images the cellular and subcellular level of the mucosa • Improves the detection of dysplasia, colitis-associated neoplasia, sporadic neoplasia, and nonneoplastic lesions • Can be used in conjunction with chromoendoscopy • Can be used for targeted biopsies	• Time consuming • Not practical for screening endoscopy
Colon capsule endoscopy	• Video capsule technique • Less invasive	• Capsule retention may occur which may limit examination • Limited studies

ENDOSCOPIC MONITORING OF DISEASE ACTIVITY

Endoscopic monitoring and determining severity of disease activity can be interpreted differently by clinicians. Scoring systems have been developed to increase intraobserver agreement of disease activity and severity. There are many scoring systems for endoscopic monitoring of disease activity in both CD and UC. The commonly used scoring systems for UC and CD are presented in **Tables 6–8.**

Currently, the Mayo endoscopic subscore is the most used to describe endoscopic activity in clinical trials.[2] A Mayo subscore of 0 or 1 is commonly accepted as criteria for mucosal healing with a decreased likelihood of needed a colectomy.[2,62] In addition

Table 6
Mayo endoscopic subscore

Subscore	Disease Activity	Endoscopic Feature
0	Normal or inactive disease	—
1	Mild disease	Erythema, decreased vascular pattern, mild friability
2	Moderate disease	Marked erythema, absent vascular patter, friability, erosions
3	Severe disease	Spontaneous bleeding, ulceration

Adapted from Mazzouli S, Guglielmi F, Antonelli E, et al. Definition and evaluation of mucosal healing in clinical practice. Dig Liver Dis 2013;45:969–77; and Schroeder K, Tremaine W, Ilstrup D. Coated oral 5-aminosalicylic acid therapy for mildly to moderately active ulcerative colitis. A randomized study. N Engl J Med 1987;317(1987):1625–9.

Table 7
Ulcerative Colitis Colonoscopic Index of Severity (UCCIS)

Lesion	Score	Endoscopic Feature
Vascular pattern	0	Normal, clear vascular pattern
	1	Partially visible vascular pattern
	2	Complete loss of vascular patter
Granularity	0	Normal, smooth and glistening
	1	Fine
	2	Coarse
Ulceration	0	Normal, no erosion or ulcer
	1	Erosions or pinpoint ulcerations
	2	Numerous shallow ulcers with mucopus
	3	Deep, excavated ulcerations
	4	Diffusely ulcerated with >30% involvement
Bleeding/friability	0	Normal, no bleeding, no friability
	1	Friable, bleeding to light touch
	2	Spontaneous bleeding
Grading of global assessment of endoscopic severity and segmental assessment of endoscopic severity	0	Normal/quiescent: visible vascular pattern with no bleeding, erosions, ulcers, or friability
	1	Mild: erythema, decreased or loss of vascular pattern, fine granularity, but no friability or spontaneous bleeding
	2	Moderate: friability with bleeding to light touch, coarse granularity, erosions, or pinpoint ulcerations
	3	Severe: spontaneous bleeding or gross ulcers

From Samuel S, Bruining D, Loftus E, et al. Validation of the ulcerative colitis colonoscopic index of severity and its correlation with disease activity measures. Clin Gastroenterol Hepatol 2013;11:50; with permission.

to the Mayo endoscopic subscore, the Mayo score consist of evaluating stool frequency, rectal bleeding, endoscopic findings, and physician global assessment on a scale of 0 to 3 for a total possible score between 0 and 12. A score of less than 2 indicates remission, whereas a score of 11 or 12 indicates severe disease. Several studies have reported fair intraobserver agreement for the Mayo scale.[63–65]

Table 8
Sample of Crohn's Disease Endoscopic Index of Severity (CDEIS) score sheet

Parameter	Rectum	Sigmoid and Left Colon	Transverse Colon	Right Colon	Ileum	Total
Deep ulceration (12 if present, 0 if absent)	—	—	—	—	—	Total 1
Superficial ulceration (6 if present, 0 if absent)	—	—	—	—	—	Total 2
Surface involved by disease (in cm)	—	—	—	—	—	Total 3
Ulcerated surface (in cm)	—	—	—	—	—	Total 4

Total 1 + 2 + 3 + 4 = Total A.
  Number of segments totally or partially explored (1–5) = n.
  Total A/n = Total B.
  If ulcerated stenosis is present, Total C = 3. If no ulcerated stenosis is present Total C = 0.
  If nonulcerated stenosis is present, Total D = 3, If no ulcerated stenosis is present Total D = 0.
  Total B + Total C + Total D = CDEIS.
  From Cohen R. Should mucosal healing be used instead? AGA Perspectives 2013;9(2):7.

The Mayo scoring system was created based on sigmoidoscopy examinations. In contrast, the Ulcerative Colitis Colonoscopic Index of Severity is a scoring system created from full, high-definition colonoscopic findings.[49] The Ulcerative Colitis Colonoscopic Index of Severity significantly correlates with clinical indexes of disease activity and laboratory parameters of active inflammation (hemoglobin, albumin, and C-reactive protein).[64]

The Crohn's Disease Endoscopic Index of Severity, which was developed in 1989, is the first endoscopic scoring system for evaluating CD.[2] This scoring system is not only used to guide treatment strategies, it has shown to predict corticosteroid-free clinical remission.[66]

SUMMARY

A thorough history and physical examination are essential to diagnose IBD clinically. Endoscopic, serologic, and histologic evaluation is needed to confirm the diagnosis of IBD. Distinguishing between UC and CD can be a challenge. Serologic studies can aid in this process. ASCA, anti-OmpC, anti-CBir1, and anti–Fla-X-flagellin are detected more commonly in CD, whereas pANCA is more commonly detected in UC.

The visual assessment and monitoring of small bowel CD can be particularly difficult for the clinician. Deep enteroscopy and ileal intubation during colonoscopy can provide adequate assessment of the entire small bowel. VCE has a higher yield of detecting small bowel disease when compared with enteroscopy. Conversely, the inability to definitively localize lesions and obtain tissue samples is a disadvantage of VCE.

The emergence of novel imaging technology for the evaluation of the colon and rectum has shown promise in the management of IBD. Chromoendoscopy has shown to increase agreement between endoscopy and histology when compared with high-definition white light colonoscopy. Both chromoendoscopy and CLE allow for targeted biopsies, thus decreasing the number of random biopsies. However, the lengthy time required to examine large surface areas currently limits this technique when surveying the entire colon. CCE is still being developed as a diagnostic tool for IBD as well as the use of scoring systems to improve observer agreement among clinicians.

REFERENCES

1. Ordas I, Eckmann L, Talamini M, et al. Ulcerative colitis. Lancet 2012;380: 1606–19.
2. Mazzouli S, Guglielmi F, Antonelli E, et al. Definition and evaluation of mucosal healing in clinical practice. Dig Liver Dis 2013;45:969–77.
3. Wayne LG, Hollander D, Anderson B, et al. Immunoglobulin A (IgA) and IgG serum antibodies to mycobacterial antigens in patients with Crohn's disease and their relatives. J Clin Microbiol 1992;30:2013–8.
4. Blaser MJ, Miller RA, Lacher J, et al. Patients with active Crohn's disease have elevated serum antibodies to antigens of seven enteric bacterial pathogens. Gastroenterology 1984;87:888–94.
5. Liu Y, Van Kruiningen HJ, West AB, et al. Immunocytochemical evidence of Listeria, *Escherichia coli*, and Streptococcus antigens in Crohn's disease. Gastroenterology 1995;108:1396–404.
6. De Hertogh G, Aerssens J, Geboes KP, et al. Evidence for the involvement of infectious agents in the pathogenesis of Crohn's disease. World J Gastroenterol 2008;14(6):845–52.

7. Chen S-J, Liu X-W, Liu J-P, et al. Ulcerative colitis as a polymicrobial infection characterized by sustained broken mucus barrier. World J Gastroenterol 2014; 20(28):9468–75.

8. Hartman C, Eliakim R, Shamir R. Perinuclear antineutrophil cytoplasmic autoantibodies and anti-Saccharomyces cerevisiae antibodies: serologic markers in inflammatory bowel disease. Isr Med Assoc J 2004;6(4):221–6.

9. Morgan MD, Harper L, Williams J, et al. Anti-neutrophil cytoplasm-associated glomerulonephritis. J Am Soc Nephrol 2006;17(5):1224–34.

10. Stone JH, Talor M, Stebbing J, et al. Test characteristics of immunofluorescence and ELISA tests in 856 consecutive patients with possible ANCA-associated conditions. Arthritis Care Res 2000;13:424–34.

11. Seibold F, Weber P, Schöning A, et al. Neutrophil antibodies (pANCA) in chronic liver disease and inflammatory bowel disease: do they react with different antigens? Eur J Gastroenterol Hepatol 1996;8:1095–100.

12. Saxon A, Shanahan F, Landers C, et al. A distinct subset of antineutrophil cytoplasmic antibodies is associated with inflammatory bowel disease. J Allergy Clin Immunol 1990;86:202.

13. Rump JA, Schölmerich J, Gross V, et al. A new type of perinuclear antineutrophil cytoplasmic antibody (p-ANCA) in active ulcerative colitis but not in Crohn's disease. Immunobiology 1990;181:406–13.

14. Duerr RH, Targan SR, Landers CJ, et al. Anti-neutrophil cytoplasmic antibodies in ulcerative colitis: comparison with other colitides/diarrheal illnesses. Gastroenterology 1991;100:1590–6.

15. Colombel JF, Reumaux D, Duthilleul P, et al. Antineutrophil cytoplasmic autoantibodies in inflammatory bowel diseases. Gastroenterol Clin Biol 1992;16:656–60, 7 Cambridge G.

16. Rampton DS, Stevens TRJ, Reumaux D, et al. Antineutrophil antibodies in inflammatory bowel disease: prevalence and diagnostic role. Gut 1992;33:668–74.

17. Peeters M, Joossens S, Vermeire S, et al. Diagnostic value of anti-Saccharomyces cerevisiae and antineutrophil cytoplasmic autoantibodies in inflammatory bowel disease. Am J Gastroenterol 2001;96(3):730–4.

18. Ruemmele FM, Targan SR, Levy G, et al. Diagnostic accuracy of serological assays in pediatric inflammatory bowel disease. Gastroenterology 1998;115:822–9.

19. Vermeire S, Peeters M, Vlietinck R, et al. Anti-Saccharomyces cerevisiae antibodies (ASCA), phenotypes of IBD, and intestinal permeability: a study in IBD families. Inflamm Bowel Dis 2001;7(1):8–15.

20. Sandborn WJ, Loftus EV Jr, Colombel JF, et al. Evaluation of serologic disease markers in a population-based cohort of patients with ulcerative colitis and Crohn's disease. Inflamm Bowel Dis 2001;7(3):192–201.

21. Reese GE, Constantinides VA, Simillis C, et al. Diagnostic precision of anti-Saccharomyces cerevisiae antibodies and perinuclear antineutrophil cytoplasmic antibodies in inflammatory bowel disease. Am J Gastroenterol 2006; 101(10):2410–22.

22. Main J, McKenzie H, Yeaman GR, et al. Antibody to Saccharomyces cerevisiae (bakers' yeast) in Crohn's disease. BMJ 1988;297(6656):1105–6.

23. Annese V, Andreoli A, Andriulli A, et al. Familial expression of anti-Saccharomyces cerevisiae Mannan antibodies in Crohn's disease and ulcerative colitis: a GISC study. Am J Gastroenterol 2001;96(8):2407–12.

24. Vermeire S, Joossens S, Peeters M, et al. Comparative study of ASCA (Anti-Saccharomyces cerevisiae antibody) assays in inflammatory bowel disease. Gastroenterology 2001;120(4):827–33.

25. Nikaido H. Porins and specific channels of bacterial outer membranes. Mol Microbiol 1992;6(4):435–42.

26. Mei L, Targan SR, Landers CJ, et al. Familial expression of anti-*Escherichia coli* outer membrane porin C in relatives of patients with Crohn's disease. Gastroenterology 2006;130(4):1078–85.

27. Arnott ID, Landers CJ, Nimmo EJ, et al. Sero-reactivity to microbial components in Crohn's disease is associated with disease severity and progression, but not NOD2/CARD15 genotype. Am J Gastroenterol 2004;99(12):2376–84.

28. Mow WS, Vasiliauskas EA, Lin YC, et al. Association of antibody responses to microbial antigens and complications of small bowel Crohn's disease. Gastroenterology 2004;126(2):414–24.

29. Davis MK, Andres JM, Jolley CD, et al. Antibodies to *Escherichia coli* outer membrane porin C in the absence of anti-Saccharomyces cerevisiae antibodies and anti-neutrophil cytoplasmic antibodies are an unreliable marker of Crohn disease and ulcerative colitis. J Pediatr Gastroenterol Nutr 2007;45(4):409–13.

30. Petersen AM, Schou C, Mirsepasi H, et al. Seroreactivity to E. coli outer membrane protein C antibodiesin active inflammatory bowel disease; diagnostic value and correlation with phylogroup B2 E. coli infection. Scand J Gastroenterol 2012; 47(2):155–61.

31. Zholudev A, Zurakowski D, Young W, et al. Serologic testing with ANCA, ASCA, and anti-OmpC in children and young adults with Crohn's disease and ulcerative colitis: diagnostic value and correlation with disease phenotype. Am J Gastroenterol 2004;99(11):2235–41.

32. Sutton CL, Kim J, Yamane A, et al. Identification of a novel bacterial sequence associated with Crohn disease. Gastroenterology 2000;119(1):23–31.

33. Wei B, Huang T, Dalwadi H, et al. *Pseudomonas fluorescens* encodes the Crohn's disease-associated I2 sequence and T-cell superantigen. Infect Immun 2002; 70(12):6567–75.

34. Iltanen S, Tervo L, Halttunen T, et al. Elevated serum anti-I2 and anti-OmpW antibody levels in children with IBD. Inflamm Bowel Dis 2006;12(5):389–94.

35. Lodes MJ, Cong Y, Elson CO, et al. Bacterial flagellin is a dominant antigen in Crohn disease. J Clin Invest 2004;113(9):1296–306.

36. Targan SR, Landers CJ, Yang H, et al. Antibodies to CBir1 flagellin define a unique response that is associated independently with complicated Crohn's disease. Gastroenterology 2005;128(7):2020–8.

37. Schoepfer AM, Schaffer T, Mueller S, et al. Phenotypic associations of Crohn's disease with antibodies to flagellins A4-Fla2 and FlaX, ASCA, p-ANCA, PAB, and NOD2 mutations in a Swiss Cohort. Inflamm Bowel Dis 2009;15(9): 1358–67.

38. Sabery N, Bass D. Use of serologic markers as a screening tool in inflammatory bowel disease compared with elevated erythrocyte sedimentation rate and anemia. Pediatrics 2007;119(1):e193–9.

39. Benor S, Russell GH, Silver M, et al. Shortcomings of the inflammatory bowel disease Serology 7 panel. Pediatrics 2010;125(6):1230–6.

40. Yamamoto H, Sugano K. A new method of enteroscopy – the double-balloon method. Can J Gastroenterol 2003;17:273–4.

41. Tharian B, Caddy G, Tham T. Enteroscopy in small bowel Crohn's disease: a review. World J Gastrointest Endosc 2013;5(10):476–86.

42. Messer I, May A, Manner H, et al. Prospective, randomized, single-center trial comparing double balloon enteroscopy and spiral enteroscopy in patients with suspected small-bowel disorders. Gastrointest Endosc 2013;77(2):241–9.

43. Lenz P, Domagk D. Double- vs. single- balloon vs spiral enteroscopy. Best Pract Res Clin Gastroenterol 2012;26:303–13.
44. Benz C, Jakobs R, Rieman J. Do we need the overtube for push-enteroscopy? Endoscopy 2001;33(8):658–61.
45. Hartmann D, Eickhoff A, Tamm R, et al. Balloon-assisted enteroscopy using a single-balloon technique. Endoscopy 2007;39:E276.
46. Akerman P, Agrawal D, Chen W, et al. Spiral enteroscopy: a novel method of enteroscopy by using the Endo-Ease Discovery SB overtube and a pediatric colonoscope. Gastrointest Endosc 2009;69(2):327–32.
47. Khashab M, Helper D, Johnson C, et al. Predictors of depth of maximal insertion at double-balloon enteroscopy. Dig Dis Sci 2010;55(5):1391–5.
48. Sunada K, Yamamoto H, Yano T, et al. Advances in the diagnosis and treatment of small bowel lesions with Crohn's disease using double-balloon endoscopy. Therap Adv Gastroenterol 2009;2:357–66.
49. Bouchard S, Ibrahim M, Gossum A. Video capsule endoscopy: perspectives of a revolutionary technique. World J Gastroenterol 2014;20(46):17330–44.
50. Chong A, Taylor A, Miller A, et al. Capsule endoscopy vs. push enteroscopy and enteroclysis in suspected small-bowel Crohn's disease. Gastrointest Endosc 2005;61(2):255–61.
51. Triester S, Leighton J, Leontiadis G, et al. A meta-analysis of the yield of capsule endoscopy compared to other diagnostic modalities in patients with obscure gastrointestinal bleeding. Am J Gastroenterol 2005;100(11):2407–8.
52. Tontini G, Vecchi M, Neuraht M, et al. Advanced endoscopic imaging techniques in Crohn's disease. J Crohns Colitis 2014;8:261–9.
53. Kiesslich R, Jung M, DiSario J, et al. Perspectives of chromo and magnifying endoscopy- how, how much, when, whom should we stain? J Clin Gastroenterol 2004;38(1):7–13.
54. Teubner D, Kiesslich R, Matsumoto T, et al. Beyond standard image-enhanced endoscopy confocal endomicroscopy. Gastrointest Endosc Clin N Am 2014;24: 427–34.
55. Kiesslich R, Fritsch J, Holtmann M, et al. Methylene blue-aided chromoendoscopy for the detection of intraepithelial neoplasia and colon cancer in ulcerative colitis. Gastroenterology 2003;124:880–8.
56. Neumann H, Vieth M, Gunther C, et al. Virtual chromoendoscpy for prediction of severity and disease extent with inflammatory bowel disease: a randomized controlled study. Inflamm Bowel Dis 2013;19(9):1935–42.
57. Kiesslich R, Goetz M, Lammersdorf K, et al. Chromoscopy-guided endomicroscopy increases the diagnostic yield of intraepithelial neoplasia in ulcerative colitis. Gastroenterology 2007;132:874–82.
58. Neumann H, Vieth M, Atreya R, et al. Assessment of Crohn's disease activity by confocal laser endomicroscopy. Inflamm Bowel Dis 2012;18(12):2261–9.
59. Eliakam R, Fireman Z, Gralnek M, et al. Evaluation of the PillCam colon capsule in the detection of colonic pathology: results of the first multicenter, prospective comparative study. Endoscopy 2006;38(10):963–70.
60. Herrerias-Gutierrez J, Arguelles-Arias F, Caunedo-Alvarez A, et al. PillCamColon capsule for the study of colonic pathology in clinical practice. Study of agreement with colonoscopy. Rev Esp Enferm Dig 2011;103(2):69–75.
61. Sung J, Ho K, Chiu H, et al. The use of Pillcam colon in assessing mucosal inflammation in ulcerative colitis: a multicenter study. Endoscopy 2012;44(8): 754–8.

62. Schroeder K, Tremaine W, Ilstrup D. Coated oral 5-aminosalicylic acid therapy for mildly to moderately active ulcerative colitis. A randomized study. N Engl J Med 1987;317(26):1625–9.
63. Daperno M, Comberlato M, Bossa F, et al. Intra-observer agreement in endoscopic scoring systems: Preliminary report of an ongoing study from the Italian Group for Inflammatory Bowel Disease (IG-IBD). Dig Liver Dis 2014;46:969–73.
64. Samuel S, Bruining D, Loftus E, et al. Validation of the ulcerative colitis colonoscopic index of severity and its correlation with disease activity measures. Clin Gastroenterol Hepatol 2013;11:49–54.
65. Walsh A, Brain O, Keshav S, et al. How variable is the Mayo score between observers and might this affect trial recruitment or outcome? Gastroenterology 2009;136:A677.
66. Ferrante M, Colobel J, Sandborn W, et al. Validation of endoscopic activity scores in patients with Crohn's disease based on a post hoc analysis of data from SONIC. Gastroenterology 2013;145:978–86.

Imaging for Inflammatory Bowel Disease

Melanie S. Morris, MD*, Daniel I. Chu, MD

KEYWORDS

- Imaging • Inflammatory bowel disease • Crohn's disease • Ulcerative colitis
- CT enterography • MRI • MRE

KEY POINTS

- Plain abdominal radiographs can diagnose complications from inflammatory bowel disease and should be a first imaging study in critically ill patients to evaluate for free intraperitoneal air.
- Upper gastrointestinal series with small bowel follow through (SBFT) is useful in diagnosing stricturing Crohn's disease, and upper gastrointestinal series with SBFT may diagnose fistulas related to Crohn's disease.
- Abdominal computed tomographic (CT) scanning is usually the preferred initial radiographic imaging study in patients with inflammatory bowel disease; CT scans can evaluate the entire gastrointestinal tract and other intra-abdominal organs.
- MRI is a noninvasive, nonionizing imaging modality useful in evaluating intestinal and extraintestinal pathology, particularly in Crohn's disease.
- Capsule endoscopy (CE) provides state-of-the-art imaging of the mucosal lining of the intestines, particularly in the small bowel; CE is an expensive test but is outpatient, noninvasive, with no nonionizing radiation.

PLAIN RADIOGRAPHS

Introduction

Plain abdominal radiographs still play a role in imaging for inflammatory bowel disease (IBD) including diagnosing dilation, obstruction, bowel perforation, bowel wall thickening, or loss of haustral markings. Radiographs can be portable, are widely available, quick, painless, inexpensive, and have low radiation dose exposure making them a good initial diagnostic test in some scenarios (**Table 1**). However, plain radiographs do not give much detailed information and cannot make a definitive diagnosis of IBD.

Authors have nothing to disclose.
Department of Surgery, University of Alabama, KB 428, 1720 2nd Ave South, Birmingham, AL 35294-0016, USA
* Corresponding author.
E-mail address: morrisme@uab.edu

Table 1	
Clinical relevance of plain radiograph findings	
Plain Radiograph Findings	Clinical Relevance
Free air (pneumoperitoneum)	Perforated viscous
Thumbprinting	Colitis (ischemic, ulcerative, or infectious)
Megacolon	Colon dilated >6 cm, concern for perforation
Tubelike/lead-pipe/featureless	Chronic ulcerative colitis

Radiographs use invisible electromagnetic energy beams to produce images of internal tissues, bones, and organs on film. Standard radiographs are performed for many reasons. Abdominal radiographs may be taken with the patient in the upright position (erect abdominal view), lying flat with the exposure made from above the patient (supine abdominal view), or lying flat with the exposure made from the side of the patient (cross-table lateral view). The left side-lying position (left lateral decubitus view) may be used for patients who cannot stand erect.

A plain flat and upright abdominal radiograph should be the first imaging study in critically ill patients in whom a perforation is suspected. Perforation is identified by free air on an upright abdominal radiograph (**Fig. 1**) and should be ordered on any patient with acute onset abdominal pain. These images can be performed in most settings with portable radiograph machines and are widely available.

Patients with ulcerative colitis may exhibit "thumbprinting" on a plain abdominal radiograph. On radiograph the distance between loops of bowel is increased because of thickening of the bowel wall from inflammation (**Fig. 2**). Although classically described with ischemic colitis, this finding is also noted in other forms of colitis, including ulcerative and infectious colitis.[1]

Patients with fulminant colitis may be followed with serial abdominal radiographs to diagnose "toxic megacolon." Toxic megacolon is defined as dilation greater than 6 cm and is an indication for emergent surgical intervention to prevent perforation. Chronic

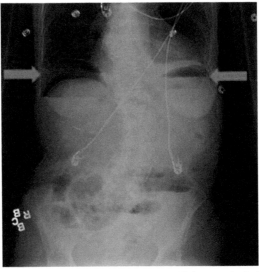

Fig. 1. An upright abdominal radiograph in a patient with known Crohn's disease and acute onset of abdominal pain. *Arrows* indicate pneumoperitoneum.

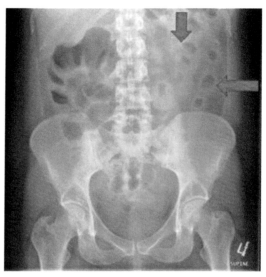

Fig. 2. Radiograph of ulcerative colitis "thumbprinting." *Arrows* show thickened colon wall.

ulcerative colitis may appear as a "tubelike" or "lead-pipe" colon with loss of haustral markings and a "featureless" colon on plain radiograph.

Contrast Radiologic Studies

Upper gastrointestinal series with small bowel follow through

Upper gastrointestinal series with small bowel follow through (SBFT) involves ingestion of a barium solution with subsequent radiologic imaging of the small intestine with fluoroscopy and radiograph. Features of Crohn's disease involving the small bowel include narrowing of the lumen with nodularity and ulceration, a "string" sign from advanced narrowing or with severe spasm, a cobblestone appearance, fistulas and abscess formation, and separation of bowel loops suggesting transmural inflammation with bowel wall thickening. Gastroduodenal Crohn's disease may manifest as gastric antral narrowing and stricturing of the duodenum.

Double-contrast barium enema

Double-contrast barium enema is performed by inserting a tube in the rectum, instilling barium to outline the colon and rectum, then passing air through the tube to enhance the detail. Finally, multiple radiographs are obtained from different views. Patients must take laxatives before the study. In patients with mild ulcerative colitis, findings on double-contrast barium enema may consist of a fine granular appearance of the colon as a result of mucosal edema and hyperemia, or a diffusely reticulated pattern with superimposed punctate collections of barium in microulcerations. In chronic or severe disease, there may be spiculated collar button ulcers, shortening of the colon, loss of haustral folds, narrowing of the luminal caliber, pseudopolyps, and filiform polyps. Barium enema should be avoided in patients who are severely ill because it may complicate toxic megacolon, and those with an obstruction because perforation may occur. Advantages include low-risk procedure, less expensive than other tests, and no sedation necessary as with colonoscopy. Disadvantages are preprocedure laxative preparation, discomfort from the test, and radiation exposure.

ABDOMINAL COMPUTED TOMOGRAPHIC AND COMPUTED TOMOGRAPHY ENTEROGRAPHY

Abdominal computed tomographic (CT) scanning is the preferred initial radiographic imaging study in patients with IBD. It allows detailed evaluation of the entire gastrointestinal tract and associated findings, such as abscesses and fistulas. In addition, it allows evaluation of other intra-abdominal organs that may exhibit extraintestinal manifestations of IBD, such as dilated hepatic ducts in the liver of patients with primary sclerosing cholangitis.

A CT scan is an imaging method that uses x-rays to create pictures of cross-sections of the body. The patient lies on a narrow table that slides into the center of the CT scanner. Modern "spiral" scanners can perform the examination by rotating the x-ray beam around the patient without stopping. A computer creates separate images of the body area, called slices. These images are stored, viewed on a monitor, or printed on film. Three-dimensional models of the body area are created by stacking the slices together in multiple configurations.

CT scanning is not a very sensitive test for detecting the mucosal abnormalities of mild or early ulcerative colitis. Inflammatory pseudopolyps may be seen in well-distended bowel. In areas of mucosal denudation, abnormal thinning of the bowel may also be evident. A cross-section of the inflamed and thickened bowel has a target appearance with concentric rings of varying attenuation, also known as mural stratification.[2] More advanced ulcerative colitis often has a hallmark finding of diffuse colonic wall thickening (>3 mm). Benefits of CT are the ability to evaluate intraluminal and extraluminal disease, guide and monitor response to treatment, and detect complications.

CT may suggest the diagnosis of Crohn's disease with thickening of small bowel, especially the terminal ileum. **Fig. 3** shows an axial-view CT scan of a patient with Crohn's disease. **Fig. 4** is a coronal-view CT scan of another patient with Crohn's disease.

CT enterography (CTE) uses oral contrast, intravenous contrast, and thin-cut multiplanar CT image acquisitions. Neutral oral contrast is used to distend the small bowel allowing for better evaluation of the wall of the small bowel, which is difficult to see with standard barium solutions. It is useful for the evaluation of suspected or known Crohn's disease and can detect dilation, obstruction, fistulas, and abscesses. **Fig. 5** shows thickening of the small bowel as seen in Crohn's disease. These studies should be used when clinically indicated because there is increasing concern for repeated exposure to radiation from CT scanning performed in patients with IBD.[3]

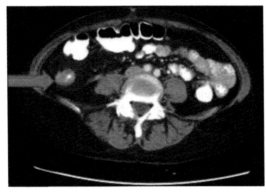

Fig. 3. Axial view CT scan of a patient with Crohn's disease. The *arrow* shows the thickened terminal ileum with contrast filling the narrowed lumen.

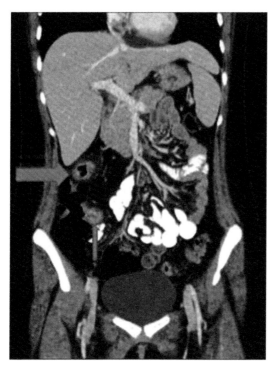

Fig. 4. Coronal view CT scan of another patient with Crohn's disease. The *thin arrow* points to the thickened and inflamed terminal ileum; the *thick arrow* points to the inflamed hepatic flexure colon.

The cumulative radiation dose of multiple CT scans over decades may increase cancer risk in patients with IBD. In one study, 371 patients with Crohn's disease were examined for radiation exposure from radiographic studies over 5 years.[4] The mean cumulative radiation exposure was 14 mSv, with a range of 0 to 303 mSv. Although most patients had a low radiation exposure, 27 patients (7%) had a

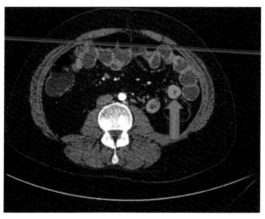

Fig. 5. Thickening of the small bowel as seen in Crohn's disease. The *arrow* points to the thickened small bowel loop.

cumulative exposure of more than 50 mSv (a cutoff suggesting a high risk of complications from radiation exposure). We advocate judicious use of studies using ionizing radiation, especially in children and young adults.

MRI

MRI and associated techniques, such as magnetic resonance enterography (MRE), are noninvasive, nonionizing imaging modalities used to evaluate gastrointestinal conditions, such as IBD. Current technology allows for fast-sequence, multiplanar, high-resolution imaging of soft tissues, such as the small and large bowel. In IBD, these images provide useful anatomic and functional information of the intestines and surrounding structures. At present, MRI technology is most useful for assessing small bowel disease and perineal disease including fistulas and sinus tracts.[5,6] This modality also allows clinicians to evaluate extraintestinal structures, such as the pelvic floor,[5] and help surgeons plan for operative interventions. The application of MRI technology to diagnosing IBD and informing treatment plans continues to grow and surgeons should be familiar with its advantages and disadvantages over other imaging modalities (**Box 1**).

Technique

MRI generates images by spatially localizing signal intensities from water molecules excited by oscillating magnetic fields. The theory was pioneered in the 1970s by Dr Paul Lauterbur at Stony Brook University and Dr Peter Mansfield at the University of Nottingham, England and won them the 2003 Nobel Prize in Physiology or Medicine. At appropriate resonance frequencies, excited hydrogen atoms emit radiofrequency signals that are captured by receiving coils. The rate at which these atoms return to equilibrium states helps determine differences between tissue types. Image contrast is controlled by varying the time between signal detection and magnetization to produce T1 (spin-lattice) and T2 (spin-spin) images. T1-weighted imaging is useful for assessing fatty tissue, liver lesions, and morphologic information. T2-weighted imaging better assesses edema and inflammation. Contrast agents, usually chelates of gadolinium, are administered intravenously to improve imaging quality. MRI contrast agents have far fewer nephrotoxic effects than intravenous CT contrast agents.[7]

Patients are placed either prone or supine on a sliding table that advances into a magnetic bore of varying strength, typically rated 1.5 T in medical applications with commercial ranges of 0.2 to 7 T. Because of the strong magnetic field, all patients are prescreened for MRI-unsafe devices and objects, either attached or implanted including metallic material. Ear plugs or audio systems are often used to minimize the loud noise level generated from the oscillating magnetic coils. Because multiple imaging sequences are obtained, the entire examination can last from 20 to 60 minutes.

Box 1 MRI	
Advantages	**Disadvantages**
Differentiates active inflammation from fibrosis	Cost
Nonionizing radiation, noninvasive	Time-consuming
Excellent soft tissue resolution	Less available than CT
Provides structural and functional anatomy	Need experienced radiologists
Provides information on extraintestinal pathology	—
MRI contrast less toxic than CT intravenous contrast	—

Postprocessing workstations receive the image sets and construct multiplanar views for radiographic interpretation. Several sequences including T2-weighted, gadolinium-enhanced T1-weighted, and fast-imaging with steady-state precession provide the most diagnostic information relevant to IBD, such as active inflammation.

MRE is an MRI with the addition of bowel-distending luminal contrast. MRE is similar to CTE in its intent to detect luminal and submucosal pathology but completely avoids the use of ionizing radiation. Unlike MR enterolysis where contrast agents are introduced via a nasojejunal tube, patients undergoing MRE drink a large volume (1–1.5 L) of a water-based oral contrast agent that promotes bowel distention. To maintain distention and provide the clearest lumen-to-bowel wall contrast, osmotic viscous agents, such as mannitol, are also administered to decrease water absorption. These oral mixtures are administered 20 to 30 minutes before imaging. MRE then requires an additional 30 to 45 minutes of table time. Although it takes longer to perform than CTE, MRE produces high-quality images with comparable results with other types of enterographies.

Indication for Use

Current evidence supports the use of MRI as an imaging modality in evaluating patients with Crohn's disease. Its chief strength is the ability to discern active inflammation from fibrosis in abnormal and thickened bowel.[8] Active inflammation appears bright on T2 single-shot fast spin echo sequences because of increased water within inflamed bowel walls and has a layered pattern of enhancement on T1 sequencing because of gadolinium specificity for active disease.[9] Distinguishing between the two pathophysiologic processes has direct therapeutic implications. Fibrotic bowel, for example, reflects permanent physical changes and is likely irreversible with additional medical therapy. Surgery with resection is favored. On the contrary, active inflammation in a segment of bowel suggests that permanent, physical changes have not occurred and more aggressive medical therapy may be effective (**Fig. 6**). In this situation, surgery is not the recommended first-line intervention. Imaging modalities, such as SBFT and even CT scans, cannot readily distinguish between these detailed characteristics of the bowel wall. MRI therefore has special ability in the evaluation of small bowel Crohn's disease because it can significantly alter treatment plans from medical to surgical or vice versa.

The advantages of MRI over conventional methods, such as SBFT, were reported in a recent prospective study comparing MRI with SBFT in 30 adult patients with recurrent Crohn's disease.[10] Although SBFTs demonstrated strictures and enteric fistulas, MRI identified active inflammation within those strictures based on transmural changes, vascular effects, and lymph node enlargement. MRI also identified extraintestinal abnormalities, such as gallstones and liver lesions. Based on these radiographic findings, the authors concluded that SBFT is a reasonable diagnostic tool to use in Crohn's disease, but if available, MRI should be the preferred imaging choice in assessing recurrent Crohn's disease. Whether the overall treatment plan and outcomes of these patients were affected by these additional MRI findings was not examined.

MRE and CTE have comparable diagnostic yields in assessing small bowel disease in Crohn's disease.[11] Both require luminal distention with oral contrast agents and can similarly identify disease localization, wall thickening, bowel wall enhancement, enteroenteric fistulas, and mesenteric lymphadenopathy.[12] Although CTE may provide higher-resolution image quality, MRE is an acceptable alternative as a diagnostic tool and most importantly does not use ionizing radiation. Because many patients with IBD are young, their lifetime risk of radiation from repeat imaging, such as CT

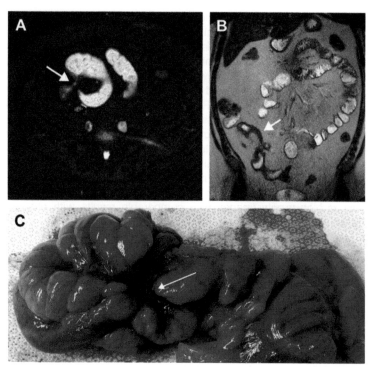

Fig. 6. MRI of abdomen (T2-weighted) of patient with Crohn's disease with enteroenteric fistulas and obstructing fibrosis (*arrows*) of the distal ileum in (*A*) axial (T2) and (*B*) coronal (T2) planes. Minimal active inflammation was observed and the patient underwent surgical resection of the distal ileum and cecum, which confirmed dense fibrosis and interloop fistulas (*C*).

scans, is substantial and unrealized.[13] In children with known IBD, MRI is now recommended as first-line imaging versus CT, which should be reserved only in emergency situations or when MRI is contraindicated.[14,15]

MRI is superior to other imaging modalities including CT in detecting perineal fistulas and sinus tracts with reported sensitivities of more than 80%.[16–18] Additional studies have shown that MRI is more accurate than an experienced surgeon's assessment of fistulas in the operating room and can detect tracts that would otherwise go undetected.[19,20] Although routine MRI scanning for anorectal fistulas is likely not necessary, in difficult Crohn's cases MRI can delineate complex and high fistulas (**Fig. 7**). MRI is less effective for mapping short, superficial fistula tracts. The preoperative assessment of fistula anatomy can guide surgeons during surgical interventions by better visualizing the relationships of the fistula to the internal sphincter muscle and pelvic floor. In equivocal cases, MRI can even exclude the presence of a fistula. These diagnostic data better inform treatment decisions in IBD cases, such as Crohn's disease, and many would argue that for perineal disease, MRI of the pelvis has become the imaging gold standard.

The role of MRI in diagnosing and treating chronic ulcerative colitis (CUC) is less clear. Early studies suggested that MRI was comparable with endoscopy in distinguishing CUC from Crohn's and in assessing disease severity when compared with tissue biopsies.[6] These findings are contradicted by more recent studies in children

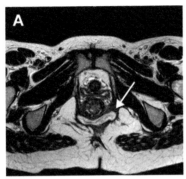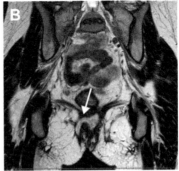

Fig. 7. MRI of pelvis (T2-weighted) showing in (*A*) axial and (*B*) coronal views a complex Crohn fistula with transsphincteric components and posterior bilateral extension in the intersphincteric plane (*arrows*).

demonstrating that MRI could not distinguish between Crohn's and CUC unless the terminal ileum was involved.[21] Comparisons of MRI with colonoscopy suggest that MRI can detect more fistulas arising from the colon than endoscopic evaluation, but these cases were likely related to Crohn's disease involving the colon instead of CUC.[22] Until more studies establish the clinical benefit of MRI over endoscopy in the evaluation of the colon, there is at present a limited role of MRI in evaluating CUC.

Limitations

MRI is significantly more expensive than plain radiograph, ultrasound (US), and CT. The costs arise from the at least $1 million average price for a 1.5-T MRI scanner, lifetime equipment maintenance, facility charges, and professional charges for radiologists. Cost-effectiveness research comparing MRI with other modalities is sparse, but available studies have suggested that the high cost may be justifiable in the long-term for certain situations, such as patients who are at high-risk for intravenous contrast agents[23] or in young patients who have more life-years to be exposed to radiation.[13] For the young IBD population, repeat imaging is common and MRI may therefore be cost-effective when balanced against the costs of complications from excess radiation exposure.

MRI technology is far less available than imaging modalities, such as CT scans. In 2010, the Centers for Disease Control and Prevention estimated that the United States had 26.5 MRI units versus 34.3 CT units per million population.[24] Smith-Bindman and colleagues[25] analyzed electronic records from six large integrated US health systems and found that MRI use increased from 17 to 65 MRIs per 1000 enrollees from 1996 to 2010. Concurrently, CT scans increased from 52 to 149 CTs per 1000 enrollees, more than twice the rate of MRI use. Widespread adoption of MRI is increasing but limited by available MRI units and experienced radiologists who can interpret results, such as MREs. As a result, CT technology, such as CTEs, is more commonly used in the evaluation of IBD.

Future Direction

MRI will be increasingly used in the diagnosis and management of IBD especially in Crohn's disease. Although its role in CUC remains to be determined, MRI has demonstrated clear benefit in assessing perineal disease for fistulas and sinus tracts. Its diagnostic use in assessing Crohn's small bowel disease is also becoming increasingly evident when compared with other imaging modalities. For young patients who will undergo repeat imaging, MRI likely has long-term benefit with its avoidance of ionizing radiation. As MRI continues to progress in availability and technique, future studies will need to more firmly establish its cost-effectiveness on diagnosis, treatment, and outcomes compared with the other available imaging modalities for IBD.

ULTRASOUND

US for IBD requires high-frequency (5–17 MHz) linear array probes for the US machine. High-frequency linear-array probes provide increased spatial resolution of the intestinal wall, which is essential for the assessment of wall diameter and wall layer discrimination. Compounding technology allows image reconstruction using signal responses from different frequencies or from viewing in different directions that results in an increase in contrast resolution and border definition of bowel wall architecture. Color or power Doppler imaging and contrast-enhanced US provide detailed information on mural and extraintestinal vascularity, which reflects inflammatory disease activity.[26]

For US diagnosis of IBD, one must understand of the anatomic location of Crohn's disease and ulcerative colitis. US does not provide a continuous and complete examination of the small and large bowel. The ileocecal region and the sigmoid colon can be identified in all patients. The left and right colon is adequately evaluated in most patients. The colonic flexures (especially the left flexure) are more difficult to visualize because of their cranial position and ligamentous fixation to the diaphragm. The transverse colon is identified in most patients, but complete examination is not easy to achieve because of its variable anatomy. The rectum and anal region cannot be visualized accurately by the transabdominal route because of their pelvic location. Transperineal US is useful in the evaluation of the perianal region and the distal rectum.[26,27]

US is used for small bowel imaging of IBD more frequently in Europe and at some centers in the United States. The sensitivity and specificity vary depending on operator experience, but are reported to be between 75% and 88%, and 93% and 97%, respectively.[28–30] Sonographic features suggesting small bowel involvement with Crohn's disease include bowel wall thickening and stiffness, and changes in the bowel wall stratification, but intestinal gas frequently obscures the bowel wall. Mucosal abnormalities are not detectable by US. The clinical role of US in ulcerative colitis is less well established as compared with Crohn's disease.

Future Directions

Small intestine contrast US is a new technique in which a nonabsorbable contrast solution (eg, polyethylene glycol 3350) is given orally before abdominal US. As with all US tests, small intestine contrast US sensitivity and specificity highly depends on the experience of the operator and is not commonly performed at this time.[31]

CAPSULE ENDOSCOPY

Wireless capsule endoscopy (CE) is an advanced imaging technique that is being increasingly used in the evaluation of IBD. Developed originally to evaluate small bowel for sources of occult bleeding with Food and Drug Administration approval in 2001, CE is emerging as an alternative method to evaluate the small bowel in IBD, particularly in Crohn's disease. Among patients with Crohn's disease, more than 30% have small bowel involvement only and 40% have both small bowel and colon involvement.[32] In many situations, the diagnosis of IBD, such as Crohn's disease, may be unclear. When traditional diagnostic attempts, such as endoscopy or SBFT, fail or are equivocal, CE may be considered an alternative modality to aid with the diagnosis and evaluation of the small bowel.

Technique

CE is a painless and radiation-free technique that requires no patient sedation. Additional benefits of CE include its ease-of-administration in the outpatient setting and patient satisfaction. Patients swallow an approximately 11 × 26 mm pill that contains a video camera, LED lights, a radio transmitter, and battery (**Fig. 8**). The pill transits through the small bowel in approximately 4 hours and colon in 24 to 48 hours before being excreted. Video images up to six frames per second are wirelessly transmitted to a portable device and downloaded to a computer. Equipment costs including the capsule ($500) are estimated to total $20,000 to $33,000.[33] In most cases, an experienced gastroenterologist reviews the series of images, which takes 30 minutes to 2 hours.[34] The first capsule developed was called the PillCam SB (Given, Yoqnem, Israel), which has now been updated to the third-generation PillCam SB3 with wider viewing angles and automatic light control. In 2007, Olympus (Lake Success, NY) developed a competing capsule (EndoCapsule), which may have longer battery life but comparable diagnostic yield compared with the PillCam.[35] A third pill approved by the Food and Drug Administration in 2013 called the (MiroCam, Seoul, Korea) uses a novel mode of transmission called electric field propagation to transmit images. Comparisons with EndoCapsule demonstrated similar diagnostic yields in 50 patients but the concordance between the two models was only 68%.[36] These studies illustrate a technical limitation in that pills often tumble through the small bowel and transmit an incomplete picture of the luminal surface.

History

One of the first reports of CE being used specifically in patients with IBD was in 2003.[37] Fireman and colleagues[37] used CE to evaluate 17 patients with normal colonoscopies and small bowel radiographs but clinical suspicion for Crohn's disease. Twelve (71%) patients were found to have mucosal changes, such as erosions, ulcers, and strictures, which were visually consistent with Crohn's. Other case studies have further demonstrated that CE can visually confirm small bowel lesions in 43% to 65% of

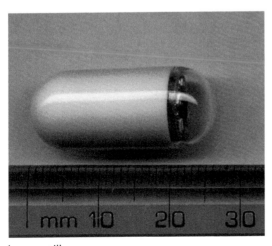

Fig. 8. Capsule endoscopy pill.

patients with completely negative colonoscopies and small bowel radiographs.[38–40] These early studies suggested that CE was sensitive in detecting mucosal abnormalities and might be useful in aiding diagnosis for equivocal cases in Crohn's disease.

Comparison of CE with other imaging modalities, such as small bowel enterography, SBFT,[41] and CTE,[42] consistently shows that CE can detect small bowel abnormalities that are missed by conventional tests (**Box 2**). In these cases, the detected mucosal lesions are often small and located in the proximal ileum or jejunum, areas that are poorly accessible with endoscopic techniques. These studies indicate that CE is a more sensitive test in detecting mucosal lesions compared with small bowel enterography, SBFT, and CTE. CE provided only visual documentation, however, and it remained unproven whether these abnormalities represented pathologic Crohn's disease because no biopsies were available for confirmation. Further research is needed to investigate whether the higher detection of mucosal abnormalities changes overall prognosis and therapeutic plans in IBD.

Indication for Use

Although CE has a clear role in the management of occult gastrointestinal bleeding,[43] there is no established role of this new technology in the present management of IBD. CE is at most a useful alternative method to evaluate the bowel in IBD when other conventional methods fail or are equivocal. Current best-practice recommendations are based on small, heterogeneous studies. A recent meta-analysis[44] that included 223 patients from 11 studies concluded that CE significantly increased diagnostic yields by 25% to 40% over barium studies and CT imaging. It is important to recognize that these higher diagnostic yields simply meant that a greater number of positive findings were detected. There was no gold standard diagnosis to confirm the clinical relevance of these findings. These challenges limit many of the studies on comparative effectiveness of CE in IBD.

Additional evidence needs to be accumulated before CE becomes first-line imaging in IBD. In 2008, Solem and colleagues[45] directly compared CE with CTE, ileocolonoscopy, and SBFT in 41 patients with suspected or known Crohn's disease. Each patient underwent all four tests in 4 consecutive days, which minimized the preparation required for each study. CE had the highest sensitivity (83%) but was not statistically significant when compared with the other three modalities. Calculated specificity was the lowest for CE (53%). Several patients (17%) had partial small bowel obstructive findings, but none experienced capsule retention. The authors were cautious in their recommendations for CE based on these findings and suggested that CE should not be used as a first-line diagnostic test in IBD. These findings are consistent with opinions that CE is more sensitive than conventional imaging modalities but specificity and positive predictive values are not fully established.[46]

Box 2 **Wireless capsule endoscopy**	
Advantages	**Disadvantages**
Sensitive to identifying mucosal abnormalities	Specificity and positive predictive values not known
Useful test when other imaging modalities negative	Cost
Easy to administer	Requires experienced gastroenterologist to review
Nonionizing radiation	Capsule retention
No sedation required	Nontherapeutic, no biopsies possible

Limitations

Capsule retention is the most feared complication from CE. In one of the largest reported series of more than 900 patients evaluated for obscure bleeding, capsule retention occurred in 0.75% patients that required surgical intervention.[47] Capsule retention rates are higher in the IBD population, particularly among Crohn's disease with its associated strictures, and have been reported in the 1.4% to 6.7% range.[39,40,48] Generally, if there is concern for capsule retention, a plain abdominal radiograph at 14 days after capsule ingestion visualizes the pill. Known obstructions and stricturing disease are a relative contraindication for undergoing CE. As a result of these concerns for capsule retention, a "patency" capsule (M2A, Given Imaging) was developed with an impermeable but absorbable membrane of lactose/barium. The M2A patency capsule membrane dissolves in 40 to 100 hours[49] but studies have shown persistent complication rates of 3% to 13%, probably because the dissolution times are too long.[33] A newer version of the patency capsule, the Agile (Given Imaging), has been recently developed with earlier onset of membrane dissolution (<30 hours) after ingestion. The Agile patency capsule has been tested and found to be safe in small studies.[50]

Besides higher costs, additional limitation for CE includes its nontherapeutic capabilities. In its current technology, CE is purely diagnostic and can only take static images of the luminal intestinal wall. Positive findings, such as mucosal erythema or ulcerations, need to be correlated to clinical suspicion and no biopsies or tattooing are possible. If a test were positive, then additional, invasive testing may need to be performed.

Future Direction

At present, CE is an alternative imaging modality and adds to the armament of radiographic tools for clinicians to use in IBD. Several clinical questions remain to be answered with CE. These include better defining the role of CE in IBD therapy and its use in determining severity of disease, medical response to therapy, and clinical usefulness in managing indeterminate colitis and CUC.[51] Future studies need to investigate the comparative effectiveness of CE with other imaging modalities and account for patient preferences during diagnostic work-up with comparable tools.

REFERENCES

1. Cutinha AH, De Nazareth AG, Alla VM, et al. Clues to colitis: tracking the prints. West J Emerg Med 2010;11(1):112–3.
2. Gore RM, Balthazar EJ, Ghahremani GG, et al. CT features of ulcerative colitis and Crohn's disease. AJR Am J Roentgenol 1996;167(1):3–15.
3. Siddiki HA, Fidler JL, Fletcher JG, et al. Prospective comparison of state-of-the-art MR enterography and CT enterography in small-bowel Crohn's disease. AJR Am J Roentgenol 2009;193(1):113–21.
4. Kroeker KI, Lam S, Birchall I, et al. Patients with IBD are exposed to high levels of ionizing radiation through CT scan diagnostic imaging: a five-year study. J Clin Gastroenterol 2011;45(1):34–9.
5. Koelbel G, Schmiedl U, Majer MC, et al. Diagnosis of fistulae and sinus tracts in patients with Crohn's disease: value of MR imaging. AJR Am J Roentgenol 1989; 152(5):999–1003.
6. Shoenut JP, Semelka RC, Magro CM, et al. Comparison of magnetic resonance imaging and endoscopy in distinguishing the type and severity of inflammatory bowel disease. J Clin Gastroenterol 1994;19(1):31–5.

7. Prince MR, Arnoldus C, Frisoli JK. Nephrotoxicity of high-dose gadolinium compared with iodinated contrast. J Magn Reson Imaging 1996;6(1):162–6.
8. Masselli G, Brizi GM, Parrella A, et al. Crohn's disease: magnetic resonance enteroclysis. Abdom Imaging 2004;29(3):326–34.
9. Koh DM, Miao Y, Chinn RJ, et al. MR imaging evaluation of the activity of Crohn's disease. AJR Am J Roentgenol 2001;177(6):1325–32.
10. Bernstein CN, Greenberg H, Boult I, et al. A prospective comparison study of MRI versus small bowel follow-through in recurrent Crohn's disease. Am J Gastroenterol 2005;100(11):2493–502.
11. Jensen MD, Ormstrup T, Vagn-Hansen C, et al. Interobserver and intermodality agreement for detection of small bowel Crohn's disease with MR enterography and CT enterography. Inflamm Bowel Dis 2011;17(5):1081–8.
12. Fiorino G, Bonifacio C, Peyrin-Biroulet L, et al. Prospective comparison of computed tomography enterography and magnetic resonance enterography for assessment of disease activity and complications in ileocolonic Crohn's disease. Inflamm Bowel Dis 2011;17(5):1073–80.
13. Brenner DJ, Hall EJ. Computed tomography: an increasing source of radiation exposure. N Engl J Med 2007;357(22):2277–84.
14. Athanasakos A, Mazioti A, Economopoulos N, et al. Inflammatory bowel disease-the role of cross-sectional imaging techniques in the investigation of the small bowel. Insights Imaging 2015;6(1):73–83.
15. Sanka S, Gomez A, Set P, et al. Use of small bowel MRI enteroclysis in the management of paediatric IBD. J Crohn's Colitis 2012;6(5):550–6.
16. Haggett PJ, Moore NR, Shearman JD, et al. Pelvic and perineal complications of Crohn's disease: assessment using magnetic resonance imaging. Gut 1995;36(3):407–10.
17. Ziech M, Felt-Bersma R, Stoker J. Imaging of perianal fistulas. Clin Gastroenterol Hepatol 2009;7(10):1037–45.
18. Chapple KS, Spencer JA, Windsor AC, et al. Prognostic value of magnetic resonance imaging in the management of fistula-in-ano. Dis Colon Rectum 2000;43(4):511–6.
19. Mullen R, Deveraj S, Suttie SA, et al. MR imaging of fistula in ano: indications and contribution to surgical assessment. Acta Chir Belg 2011;111(6):393–7.
20. Halligan S, Buchanan G. MR imaging of fistula-in-ano. Eur J Radiol 2003;47(2):98–107.
21. Ziech ML, Hummel TZ, Smets AM, et al. Accuracy of abdominal ultrasound and MRI for detection of Crohn's disease and ulcerative colitis in children. Pediatr Radiol 2014;44(11):1370–8.
22. Jiang X, Asbach P, Hamm B, et al. MR imaging of distal ileal and colorectal chronic inflammatory bowel disease: diagnostic accuracy of 1.5 T and 3 T MRI compared to colonoscopy. Int J Colorectal Dis 2014;29(12):1541–50.
23. Lessler DS, Sullivan SD, Stergachis A. Cost-effectiveness of unenhanced MR imaging vs contrast-enhanced CT of the abdomen or pelvis. AJR Am J Roentgenol 1994;163(1):5–9.
24. (OECD), O.f.E.C.-o.a.D., 2007 Computed tomography (CT) and magnetic resonance imaging (MRI) census. Benchmark report: IMV, Limited, Medical Information Division, 2007.
25. Smith-Bindman R, Miglioretti DL, Johnson E, et al. Use of diagnostic imaging studies and associated radiation exposure for patients enrolled in large integrated health care systems, 1996-2010. JAMA 2012;307(22):2400–9.
26. Strobel D, Goertz RS, Bernatik T. Diagnostics in inflammatory bowel disease: ultrasound. World J Gastroenterol 2011;17(27):3192–7.

27. Maconi G, Ardizzone S, Greco S, et al. Transperineal ultrasound in the detection of perianal and rectovaginal fistulae in Crohn's disease. Am J Gastroenterol 2007; 102(10):2214–9.

28. Hiorns MP. Imaging of inflammatory bowel disease. How? Pediatr Radiol 2008; 38(Suppl 3):S512–7.

29. Horsthuis K, Stokkers PC, Stoker J. Detection of inflammatory bowel disease: diagnostic performance of cross-sectional imaging modalities. Abdom Imaging 2008;33(4):407–16.

30. Fraquelli M, Colli A, Casazza G, et al. Role of US in detection of Crohn's disease: meta-analysis. Radiology 2005;236(1):95–101.

31. De Franco A, Di Veronica A, Armuzzi A, et al. Ileal Crohn's disease: mural microvascularity quantified with contrast-enhanced US correlates with disease activity. Radiology 2012;262(2):680–8.

32. Munkholm P. Crohn's disease–occurrence, course and prognosis. An epidemiologic cohort-study. Dan Med Bull 1997;44(3):287–302.

33. Swaminath A, Legnani P, Kornbluth A. Video capsule endoscopy in inflammatory bowel disease: past, present, and future redux. Inflamm Bowel Dis 2010;16(7): 1254–62.

34. Hara AK. Capsule endoscopy: the end of the barium small bowel examination? Abdom Imaging 2005;30(2):179–83.

35. Hartmann D, Eickhoff A, Damian U, et al. Diagnosis of small-bowel pathology using paired capsule endoscopy with two different devices: a randomized study. Endoscopy 2007;39(12):1041–5.

36. Dolak W, Kulnigg-Dabsch S, Evstatiev R, et al. A randomized head-to-head study of small-bowel imaging comparing MiroCam and EndoCapsule. Endoscopy 2012;44(11):1012–20.

37. Fireman Z, Mahajna E, Broide E, et al. Diagnosing small bowel Crohn's disease with wireless capsule endoscopy. Gut 2003;52(3):390–2.

38. Ge ZZ, Hu YB, Xiao SD. Capsule endoscopy in diagnosis of small bowel Crohn's disease. World J Gastroenterol 2004;10(9):1349–52.

39. Herrerias JM, Caunedo A, Rodríguez-Téllez M, et al. Capsule endoscopy in patients with suspected Crohn's disease and negative endoscopy. Endoscopy 2003;35(7):564–8.

40. Mow WS, Lo SK, Targan SR, et al. Initial experience with wireless capsule enteroscopy in the diagnosis and management of inflammatory bowel disease. Clin Gastroenterol Hepatol 2004;2(1):31–40.

41. Liangpunsakul S, Maglinte DD, Rex DK. Comparison of wireless capsule endoscopy and conventional radiologic methods in the diagnosis of small bowel disease. Gastrointest Endosc Clin N Am 2004;14(1):43–50.

42. Voderholzer WA, Beinhoelzl J, Rogalla P, et al. Small bowel involvement in Crohn's disease: a prospective comparison of wireless capsule endoscopy and computed tomography enteroclysis. Gut 2005;54(3):369–73.

43. Raju GS, Gerson L, Das A, et al. American Gastroenterological Association (AGA) Institute medical position statement on obscure gastrointestinal bleeding. Gastroenterology 2007;133(5):1694–6.

44. Triester SL, Leighton JA, Leontiadis GI, et al. A meta-analysis of the yield of capsule endoscopy compared to other diagnostic modalities in patients with non-stricturing small bowel Crohn's disease. Am J Gastroenterol 2006;101(5):954–64.

45. Solem CA, Loftus EV Jr, Fletcher JG, et al. Small-bowel imaging in Crohn's disease: a prospective, blinded, 4-way comparison trial. Gastrointest Endosc 2008;68(2):255–66.

46. Legnani P, Kornbluth A. Video capsule endoscopy in inflammatory bowel disease 2005. Curr Opin Gastroenterol 2005;21(4):438–42.
47. Barkin JS, Friedman S. Wireless capsule endoscopy requiring surgical intervention: the world's experience. Am J Gastroenterol 2002;97(9):S298.
48. Buchman AL, Miller FH, Wallin A, et al. Videocapsule endoscopy versus barium contrast studies for the diagnosis of Crohn's disease recurrence involving the small intestine. Am J Gastroenterol 2004;99(11):2171–7.
49. Delvaux M, Ben Soussan E, Laurent V, et al. Clinical evaluation of the use of the M2A patency capsule system before a capsule endoscopy procedure, in patients with known or suspected intestinal stenosis. Endoscopy 2005;37(9):801–7.
50. Herrerias JM, Leighton JA, Costamagna G, et al. Agile patency system eliminates risk of capsule retention in patients with known intestinal strictures who undergo capsule endoscopy. Gastrointest Endosc 2008;67(6):902–9.
51. Redondo-Cerezo E. Role of wireless capsule endoscopy in inflammatory bowel disease. World J Gastrointest Endosc 2010;2(5):179–85.

Medical Therapy for Inflammatory Bowel Disease

Panayiotis Grevenitis, MD, Arul Thomas, MD, Nilesh Lodhia, MD*

KEYWORDS

- Inflammatory bowel disease • Crohn's disease • Ulcerative colitis • Fistula
- Fulminant colitis • Perioperative management

KEY POINTS

- The goal of medical treatment in inflammatory bowel disease (IBD) is to suppress inflammation and induce mucosal healing.
- There are multiple different classes of medications that are effective in IBD, many of which can be used concomitantly.
- The perioperative medical management of IBD can be challenging, and physicians must weigh the possible increased risk of surgical complications versus the potential for recurrent disease without appropriate therapy.

INTRODUCTION

Surgeons often care for patients with inflammatory bowel disease (IBD) who are receiving therapies that can include 5-aminosalicylic acid (5-ASA) compounds, steroids, immunomodulators, and biologics. The goal of these agents is to suppress intestinal inflammation, ultimately improving the quality of life in patients afflicted with IBD. Conventional IBD treatment paradigms have followed a stepwise treatment approach, with intensified therapies used only when symptoms are not resolved with an earlier treatment (**Fig. 1**). However, more recent data suggest that initiation of higher-tiered disease modification therapies early in the course of disease can modify disease progression and thus alter the natural history of IBD.

Initial IBD treatment is aimed at inducing remission, whereas subsequent therapies are chosen to maintain remission. Traditionally, an acceptable therapeutic endpoint was the resolution of symptoms, defined as clinical remission. However, as a result

The authors have nothing to disclose.
Division of Gastroenterology & Hepatology, Medical University of South Carolina, 114 Doughty Street, Suite 249, MSC 702, Charleston, SC 29425-2900, USA
* Corresponding author.
E-mail address: lodhia@musc.edu

Surg Clin N Am 95 (2015) 1159–1182
http://dx.doi.org/10.1016/j.suc.2015.08.004
0039-6109/15/$ – see front matter © 2015 Elsevier Inc. All rights reserved.

surgical.theclinics.com

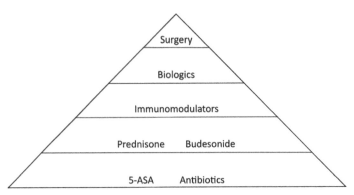

Fig. 1. A simplified approach to stepwise treatment of IBD.

of recent advances in therapy, clinicians can now strive to achieve more stringent end-points, such as endoscopic and histologic remission. Although there is variability regarding the precise endoscopic and histologic criteria required to achieve mucosal healing, the concept of mucosal healing refers to the normalization of gut mucosa. Numerous studies have demonstrated that mucosal healing can reduce relapse rates as well as the need for corticosteroids, hospitalizations, and surgeries.[1–6] In addition, chronic colonic inflammation is a risk factor for colorectal cancer in patients with IBD.[7,8] Therefore, mucosal healing may also potentially decrease the risk for colorectal malignancy.

Many different classes of agents can be used, individually or in combination, to achieve mucosal healing. Treatment must be individualized based on the aggressive nature of a patient's disease, their treatment goals, and their tolerability of various medications. Recent data have illustrated a synergistic effect of combination therapy with biologics and immunomodulators,[9–12] which is used frequently for patients with more aggressive disease. Patients on advanced therapies require special care, counseling, and consideration with regards to not only efficacy of the drugs but also adverse effects as well as the perioperative and peripartum use of these medications.

INFLAMMATORY BOWEL DISEASE MEDICATIONS
5-Aminosalicyclic Acid Compounds

5-ASA compounds are a class of medication used for the induction and maintenance of remission in patients with IBD. They have been the traditional first-line therapy in the treatment of mild to moderate ulcerative colitis (UC); efficacy in Crohn's disease (CD) remains controversial.

Action and metabolism

Sulfasalazine, oral mesalamine (Pentasa, Asacol HD, Delzicol, Lialda, and Apriso), rectal mesalamine (Rowasa and Canasa), olsalazine, and balsalazide are drugs that deliver 5-ASA to various parts of the gut (**Table 1**). Sulfasalazine, the first drug developed in this class, is a prodrug composed of 5-ASA and sulfapyridine that was originally proposed as a treatment for rheumatoid arthritis. It was soon discovered to be effective in the treatment of IBD. Isolation of the active 5-ASA compound was undertaken because most adverse effects patients experienced were secondary to the sulfapyridine moiety. As a result, multiple other formulations have been developed for use in IBD, many of which target different areas of the gastrointestinal tract. The precise mechanism responsible for the clinical efficacy of the 5-ASA compounds is unknown,

Table 1
5-Aminosalicyclic acid compounds

Generic Name	Trade Name	Formulation	Sites of Delivery
Mesalamine	Rowasa	Enema suspension	Rectum to splenic flexure
	Canasa	Suppository	Rectum
	Pentasa	Ethylcellulose-coated granules	Duodenum, jejunum, ileum, colon
	Asacol HD	Eudragit-S-coated tablets (dissolves at pH ≥ 7)	Terminal ileum, colon
	Delzicol	Eudragit-S-coated tablets (dissolves at pH ≥ 7)	Terminal ileum, colon
	Apriso	Enteric coating around polymer matrix (dissolves at pH ≥ 6)	Terminal ileum, colon
	Lialda	Enteric coating around polymer matrix (dissolves at pH ≥ 7)	Terminal ileum, colon
Olsalazine	Dipentum	5-ASA dimer linked by azo bond	Colon
Sulfasalazine	Azulfidine	5-ASA dimer linked to sulfapyridine by azo bond	Colon
Balsalazide	Colazal	5-ASA dimer linked to inert carrier by azo bond	Colon
	Giazo	5-ASA dimer linked to inert carrier by azo bond	Colon

although they are thought to act topically. One proposed mechanism is the inhibition of cytokine synthesis by upregulating peroxisome proliferator activated receptor-γ and its target genes, which in turn suppresses the activation of Nuclear factor-kappa beta (NFkB) and toll-like receptors. It is also thought to inhibit the biologic functions of proinflammatory cytokines interleukin (IL)-1, tumor necrosis factor-α (TNF-α), IL-2, IL-8, and NFkB.[13–15] 5-ASA compounds have also been shown to inhibit both cyclo-oxygenase and lipoxygenase enzymes in arachidonic acid metabolism, thereby preventing formation of proinflammatory prostaglandins and leukotrienes.[16–20] Other proposed mechanisms of action include antioxidant activity, immunosuppressive activity, and impairment of white cell adhesion and function.[21–26]

Efficacy

A large, systemic review of 11 randomized controlled trials (RCTs) revealed 5-ASA compounds to be effective at both inducing and maintaining remission in mildly to moderately active UC, especially when doses of 2.0 g/d or greater were used.[27] In contrast, the role of 5-ASA compounds in the induction or maintenance of remission CD remains uncertain, as the preponderance of data does not show benefit.[28]

Safety

Adverse reactions and toxicity are common with sulfasalazine, with about 20% to 25% of patients discontinuing the drug secondary to side effects. Most common dose-related adverse reactions include headache, epigastric pain, nausea and vomiting, and rash. Rare idiosyncratic reactions include hepatitis, fever, autoimmune hemolysis, aplastic anemia, agranulocytosis, and pancreatitis. These reactions should result in immediate discontinuation of the drug. Patients on sulfasalazine should be supplemented with folic acid because it can cause a deficiency resulting in megaloblastic anemia. It is also known to cause reversible oligospermia, but is safe in pregnancy and breast-feeding.[29,30] Mesalamine, olsalazine, and balsalazide are generally better tolerated that sulfasalazine. Headache, nausea, and abdominal pain are the most common side effects. The 5-ASA compounds can also rarely cause a paradoxic worsening of colitis, which would warrant drug discontinuation. In addition, olsalazine can induce a secretory diarrhea that can be controlled with gradual dose titration or administration with food.[31] Serious adverse events, such as hepatitis, pancreatitis, or interstitial nephritis, can also occur.[32,33] Like sulfasalazine, mesalamine, olsalazine, and balsalazide are safe in pregnancy and breast-feeding.

IMMUNOMODULATOR THERAPY

Thiopurines and methotrexate are commonly used immunomodulator therapies. Cyclosporine has a role in fulminant colitis.

Thiopurines

Action and metabolism
The thiopurine analogues azathioprine and 6-mercaptopurine (6-MP) gained widespread acceptance as established treatments for IBD in the early 1980s. These medications work through multiple mechanisms to control the dysregulated immune response in IBD. The thiopurine metabolite 6-thioguanine is a purine antagonist and therefore interferes with DNA and RNA synthesis. The reduction in DNA and RNA synthesis inhibits the proliferation of T and B lymphocytes.

Azathioprine is converted to 6-MP by a nonenzymatic reaction occurring within erythrocytes. There is significant genetic variation in thiopurine S-methyltransferase (TPMT) enzymatic activity and determining enzyme activity before initiation can help guide dosing (**Fig. 2**). TPMT testing, however, does not preclude the need for

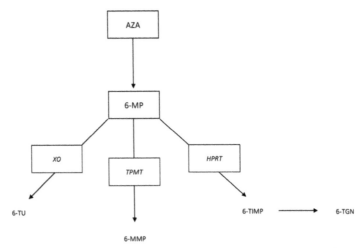

Fig. 2. A simplified approach to azathioprine (AZA) metabolism. TPMT breaks down 6-MP into the hepatotoxic metabolite 6-methylmercaptopurine (6-MMP). Besides TPMT metabolism, there are 2 other major pathways from 6-MP that should be considered. One is driven by the hypoxanthine phosphoribosyl transferase (HPRT) enzyme, leading to 6-thioguanine nucleotide (6-TGN), the metabolite responsible for the therapeutic benefit in inflammatory bowel disease and myelosuppression. The other pathway is driven by xanthine oxidase (XO), leading to production of 6-thiouric acid (6-TU), an inactive metabolite. 6-TIMP, 6-thioinosine monophosphate.

monitoring for hepatotoxicity or leukopenia. Although enzyme testing is expensive, it has been shown to reduce long-term costs from inappropriate dosing.[34,35]

Efficacy

Azathioprine and 6-MP promote clinical remission and steroid sparing in patients with IBD.[36] A recent *Cochrane Database Systemic Review* showed an odds ratio (OR) of 2.43 (95% confidence interval [CI], 1.62–3.64) for response in patients with CD who were treated with azathioprine or 6-MP compared with placebo. The steroid-sparing effect was also significant, with an OR of 3.69 (95% CI, 2.12–6.42).[37] Earlier data estimated that one-half to two-thirds of patients will respond to thiopurine treatment. Thiopurines have a delayed onset of action, requiring at least 3 to 4 months for a clinical benefit.[36]

Side effects

The side-effect profiles of azathioprine and 6-MP are significant, and 9.3% of patients develop adverse effects serious enough to stop therapy.[36] Allergic reactions include fever, rash, arthralgias, and pancreatitis; these are dose independent and resolve with discontinuation of the drug. Acute pancreatitis can be seen in 3% to 7% of patients, typically during the first month of treatment. Chronic pancreatitis attributable to azathioprine or 6-MP has not been reported.[38,39] Switching between azathioprine and 6-MP may help obviate side effects. However, patients who develop acute pancreatitis while taking either agent should be considered intolerant to both medications.

Myelosuppression is an important and potentially lethal complication of thiopurine therapy, and the white cell line is most commonly affected. Although typically associated with low TPMT enzyme activity, myelosuppression can also occur with normal enzymatic activity. Hepatotoxicity can be seen in up to 2% of patients and is typically caused by increased synthesis of 6-methylmercaptopurine.[40] Both myelosuppression and hepatotoxicity are dose-dependent responses, and management consists of dose reduction and possibly drug cessation.

For many patients and physicians, the most alarming adverse effect associated with thiopurine therapy is the potential risk of malignancy; the strongest associations have been linked with lymphoma and nonmelanoma skin cancer. A recent analysis of almost 20,000 French patients suggested that the risk of lymphoma in patients with IBD who were receiving thiopurines increased from 0.26 to 0.9 per 1000 patient-years, with a multivariate hazard ratio of 5.28 (95% CI, 2.01–13.9).[41] Furthermore, there have been 36 case reports of hepatosplenic T-cell lymphoma associated with thiopurine use, which most commonly occurs in young men and is usually fatal. Twenty of these cases were associated with the concomitant use of biologic therapy, and 16 involved thiopurine use alone.[42] A study of patients taking thiopurines for greater than 1 year showed a relative risk of 4.27 (95% CI, 3.08–5.92) for the development of nonmelanoma skin cancer. This risk further increased in those taking dual therapy with thiopurines and anti-TNF biologics.[43] Patients should ensure regular use of sunscreen during sun exposure and have annual skin examinations by their primary care provider or dermatologist.

Methotrexate

Action

Methotrexate was pioneered for the treatment of rheumatoid arthritis in the 1950s. It should be considered an alternative to thiopurines. Methotrexate has numerous anti-inflammatory effects, including blocking production of IL-1, IL-2, IL-6, and IL-8.[44]

Efficacy

RCTs have shown the efficacy of methotrexate in the induction and maintenance of remission in CD.[45–47] Based solely on existing data, methotrexate cannot be considered a major treatment of UC. For active UC, a single RCT including 67 patients showed similar remission rates after 4 months between the oral methotrexate group and the placebo group.[48] However, this study was limited in size and its use of oral methotrexate. In clinical practice, methotrexate is frequently successful in treating UC. A large RCT is currently ongoing to determine the efficacy of high-dose subcutaneous methotrexate in patients with UC. A clinical response can be expected within 8 weeks of starting therapy.[45]

Side effects

Although usually well-tolerated, the side-effect profile of methotrexate includes nausea, stomatitis, diarrhea, hair loss, leukopenia, interstitial pneumonitis, and hepatic fibrosis. Nausea is the most common side effect and usually improves with time. It is frequently managed supportively with ondansetron. Furthermore, daily folic acid can reduce nausea as well as stomatitis. Although the risk of hepatic fibrosis is low in patients with IBD, cirrhosis is the most worrisome adverse effect of methotrexate. The risk of cirrhosis is directly related both to the cumulative exposure to methotrexate and to the presence of other risk factors for liver disease. Therefore, patients with a history of excessive alcohol use and nonalcoholic fatty liver risk factors (eg, diabetes, obesity, hyperlipidemia) should avoid methotrexate. Elevated aminotransferase levels do not always correlate with the presence of hepatic fibrosis, and a liver biopsy should be considered if there is reasonable clinical suspicion for hepatic fibrosis, particularly if the cumulative dose has exceeded 1.5 g.[49] Methotrexate has high abortifacient and teratogenic effects, and patients should be counseled appropriately.

In general, potentially hepatotoxic and myelosuppressive medications should be avoided with methotrexate. Furthermore, the concurrent use of nonsteroidal anti-inflammatory drugs can increase methotrexate concentrations, thus increasing the risk of methotrexate toxicity.

Cyclosporine

Actions and characteristics

The development of cyclosporine greatly improved the success of solid organ transplantation. Cyclosporine selectively inhibits calcineurin, thus downregulating the transcription of many inflammatory cytokines (most notably IL-2) and reducing the proliferation of lymphocytes. The dramatic success of cyclosporine in organ transplantation has led investigators to explore its use in the treatment of immune-related disease. Over the last 2 decades, cyclosporine has been used in UC for the treatment of severe or fulminant colitis refractory to corticosteroids.

Efficacy

Cyclosporine was first shown to be an effective rescue or salvage therapy in corticosteroid-refractory UC in 1994 when a small, randomized placebo controlled trial showed that 9 of 11 patients treated with cyclosporine 4 mg/kg responded well enough to avoid colectomy, compared with 0 of 9 patients in the placebo arm. A comparison of 4 mg/kg versus 2 mg/kg continuous infusion showed that there was no difference in the response rate (approximately 85%) in each group.[50] Overall, studies have shown short-term response rates ranging from 64% to 100% and colectomy-free survival rates of 14% to 55% within 3 to 7 years.[51] A systematic review and meta-analysis in 2013 showed that cyclosporine and infliximab were comparable in

3-month and 12-month colectomy rates, adverse drug reactions, and postoperative complications in patients with fulminant colitis.[52]

In contrast to UC, the data do not support its efficacy in CD. Three large controlled trials illustrated that low-dose (5 mg/kg/d) oral cyclosporine is ineffective for both induction and maintenance of remission in CD.[53–55] Although there are no controlled trials with intravenous cyclosporine in CD, these trials are unlikely to be performed in the era of biologic therapy.

Safety
The side effects of cyclosporine can be significant. Trough levels between 150 and 250 ng/mL are recommended. Patients' renal function, magnesium levels, and cholesterol should be assessed before starting therapy. Patients should be carefully monitored for cyclosporine-induced hypertension, tremor, seizures, renal insufficiency, hypercholesterolemia, hypomagnesemia, and opportunistic infections.[56]

BIOLOGIC THERAPY
Tumor Necrosis Factor Antagonists

Actions and characteristics
Infliximab, adalimumab, golimumab, and certolizumab pegol are biologic agents that target TNF activity, decreasing mucosal inflammation through multiple mechanisms. Infliximab is a chimeric immunoglobulin (Ig) G1 antibody that binds to TNF, and in the late 1990s, it was the first biologic approved for use in IBD. It is administered intravenously. Adalimumab and golimumab are humanized IgG1 antibodies that bind to TNF and are administered subcutaneously. Certolizumab pegol is a pegylated Fab fragment an anti-TNF monoclonal antibody and also is given as a subcutaneous injection.

Efficacy
Sixty percent of patients will clinically respond to anti-TNF treatment within 2 to 6 weeks of initiation.[57] Multiple trials have shown that induction dosing with regular maintenance dosing, compared with intermittent dosing based on symptoms, ensures the highest efficacy and prevents loss of response. Nonetheless, response declines in 30% to 50% of initial responders while on maintenance therapy within 1 to 3 years. Loss of response can be attributed to the formation of antibodies, altered pharmacokinetics, or changes in the dominant mechanism of inflammation.[57] Antibody and metabolite testing of anti-TNF agents can better characterize loss of response and guide further management. When patients decompensate clinically without evidence of active inflammation on endoscopy, other processes such as a stricture, enteric infection (eg, *Clostridium difficile*), and concomitant irritable bowel syndrome should be considered. Anti-TNF treatment also has been found to be efficacious in the long-term treatment of fistulas associated with CD.[58–60]

Side effects
Reactions at the sites of subcutaneous injection (adalimumab, certolizumab, and golimumab) and intravenous infusion (infliximab) can occur during biologic therapy. Patients who have developed anti-infliximab antibodies are most prone to infusion reactions and can present with a syndrome of chest pain, dyspnea, rash, and hypotension.[58,61] A delayed hypersensitivity reaction, occurring within a few days to 2 weeks after infusion, can also occur. Symptoms include severe polyarthralgia, myalgia, facial edema, urticaria, and rash.[62] General management includes supportive care and a short course of oral steroids. Infections are a dreaded complication of anti-TNF therapy, and the use of concomitant immunosuppressants can increase infection risk.

There is an overall 2% to 4% risk of serious infection in the major trials of the anti-TNF agents.[62–64] Fungal, atypical, and mycobacterial (eg, reactivation of tuberculosis) infections should be considered in the workup of these patients. A chest radiograph along with hepatitis B and tuberculosis testing are mandatory before beginning treatment. Data on whether biologic therapy poses an increased risk for lymphoma are conflicting, but the preponderance of the data suggests that the increased risk for lymphoma from IBD therapy is principally attributable to thiopurines.[65,66] The formation of antinuclear antibodies and anti-double-stranded DNA can also occur with the use of anti-TNF biologic therapy over the long term.[11] Although drug-induced lupus is a possible side effect, the mere presence of antibodies is not pathogenic. Central and peripheral demyelination and polyneuropathy are uncommon neurologic side effects of anti-TNF biologic therapy.[67]

Anti-adhesion Molecules

Actions, characteristics, and efficacy

Natalizumab is a humanized monoclonal antibody that antagonizes both the α-4 β-1 and the α-4-β-7 integrins, blocking leukocyte adhesion and migration into areas of inflammation in both the central nervous system and the gastrointestinal tract. Data have shown efficacy for moderate to severe CD.[68,69] Natalizumab is US Food and Drug Administration–approved for inducing and maintaining clinical remission in adult patients with moderate to severe CD after failure of anti-TNF inhibitors.

Vedolizumab is also a humanized monoclonal antibody that targets only the α-4 β-7 integrin, which is limited to the gastrointestinal and nasopharyngeal mucosa.[70] It was found to be effective in both induction and remission therapy for UC and CD.[70–74] It also demonstrated efficacy for inducing clinical remission and mucosal healing. Vedolizumab is approved for the treatment of adult patients with moderate to severe IBD after failure of one or more standard therapies (corticosteroids, immunomodulators, or TNF antagonist). Given its impressive efficacy in UC, it is also being used as first-line therapy for maintenance of remission in patients with moderate to severe UC.

Side effects

Concerns over progressive multifocal leukoencephalopathy (PML) due to John Cunningham (JC) virus reactivation have prevented routine use of natalizumab as a therapy for IBD. Although the α-4 β-7 integrin subunit is relatively gut-specific, the α-4 β-1 subunit is present in numerous tissues, including the central nervous system. As a result, natalizumab affects leukocyte trafficking into the central nervous system, thereby increasing the risk of PML. This risk, along with hepatotoxicity, has reserved use of this biologic for only specific cases. Antibody testing for JC virus before initiating therapy, as well as during therapy, is recommended.[75]

In contrast, vedolizumab has been well tolerated in patients with either UC or CD, with no cases of PML in more 3000 patients.[76] As one could surmise based on the mechanism, the incidence of gastrointestinal and nasopharyngeal infections was higher with vedolizumab than with placebo.[74]

Overall, biologic therapies have few absolute drug-drug interactions. However, the risks and benefits of concomitant immunosuppressant use should be carefully considered.

CORTICOSTEROIDS
Actions and Characteristics

Corticosteroids, like many of the other drugs used in the treatment of IBD, were first developed to treat rheumatoid arthritis. Corticosteroids work by inhibiting almost every aspect of the immune response. They inhibit expression of adhesion molecules and trafficking of inflammatory cells of all target tissues, including the intestines. They also induce apoptosis of activated lymphocytes and decrease expression of inflammatory cytokines.[77–81] As early as 1954, an RCT demonstrated efficacy of cortisone in UC. Because of this, systemic corticosteroids continue to remain widely used for the induction of remission and treatment of acute exacerbations of UC and CD. However, their long-term use has been limited by their adverse effects. The side-effect profile associated with systemic corticosteroids prompted the development of 2 oral preparations of budesonide: the controlled ileal-release preparation (Entocort), and multimatrix system colonic delivery form known as budesonide multi-matrix system (MMX) (Uceris). Budesonide has an extensive first-pass hepatic metabolism, and therefore, a lower systemic bioavailability compared with prednisone.[82] Given their targeted delivery, budesonide and budesonide MMX may be able to achieve many of the beneficial effects of systemic corticosteroids with a lower adverse event profile.[83–85]

Efficacy

A large systematic review of 5 RCTs involving 445 patients found that both oral systemic corticosteroids and budesonide were effective at inducing remission in active UC with a number needed to treat of 3. In the corticosteroid arm, 46% of patients achieved remission, compared with 21% with placebo.[86] For the induction of remission in active CD, an analysis of 2 RCTs showed the efficacy of oral corticosteroids, with remission rates of 60% compared with 31% with placebo.[87,88] In a systematic review comparing traditional corticosteroids to budesonide in the treatment of active CD, budesonide was not quite as effective as standard corticosteroids at inducing remission, but had a better adverse event profile.[86] Despite efficacy in the induction of remission, there are no data to support the use of either traditional or second-generation corticosteroids for the maintenance of remission in IBD.

Safety

The side effects of corticosteroids have been well described. Short-term adverse effects include immunosuppression, glaucoma, fluid retention, hypertension, hyperglycemia, weight gain, and psychiatric illness.[89–92] Long-term consequences can also include decreased bone mineral density, cataracts, adrenal insufficiency, impaired wound healing, and diabetes mellitus.[93] Patients who have had long-term exposure to corticosteroids should be screened with a dual-energy radiograph absorptiometry scan. Second-generation corticosteroids, such as budesonide and budesonide MMX, have less systemic bioavailability than systemic steroids and are generally well-tolerated with minimal corticosteroid-related clinical effects.[94–96] However, caution should be exercised in patients with cirrhosis, where systemic bioavailability is increased by 2.5-fold,[97] as well as those on prolonged courses of budesonide.[98]

FISTULIZING CROHN'S DISEASE

The transmural inflammatory nature of CD predisposes to the formation of fistulae, a complication indicating a more aggressive and refractory disease phenotype.[99] Neither oral nor topical 5-ASA compounds have any utility in the treatment of fistulizing CD. Antibiotics (most commonly ciprofloxacin and metronidazole) have commonly been used in the treatment of enterocutaneous and perianal fistulae and are often effective at improving symptoms.[100,101] However, there are no placebo-controlled studies of oral antibiotics to demonstrate fistula closure. In addition, discontinuation of antibiotics leads to a high rate of recurrence.[102] A randomized placebo-controlled trial of topical metronidazole did not show a significant improvement in fistula closure, but did improve perianal discharge and pain.[103]

The data also suggest that azathioprine and 6-MP are effective in perianal fistula closure. This effectiveness has only been examined as a secondary endpoint,[38] and the advent of biologic therapy has resulted in a scarcity of clinical trials examining the efficacy of thiopurine therapy for fistulizing CD.[104] There are minimal data evaluating the efficacy of methotrexate for fistulizing CD.

TNF antagonists are the mainstay of medical therapy in fistulizing CD. The first RCT to demonstrate their efficacy randomized 94 CD patients with either abdominal or perianal fistulas to 3 months of treatment with placebo, 5 mg/kg, or 10 mg/kg of infliximab with standard dosing intervals. Reduction of draining fistulae by at least 50% was seen in 26% in the placebo group, compared with 68% and 56% in the infliximab 5 mg/kg and 10 mg/kg groups ($P = .002$ and $P = .02$). Complete closure of all fistulas was seen in 55% in the 5 mg/kg and 38% in the 10 mg/kg infliximab groups, compared with only 13% in the placebo group.[105] Follow-up studies confirmed the greater than 50% efficacy noted in this landmark trial.[106,107] Efficacy of adalimumab for perianal fistula closure, even in patients that are refractory to infliximab, has also been demonstrated.[59,108–110] Although limited data suggest a possible benefit for fistula closure with vedolizumab and natalizumab,[74,111] there is not enough evidence to recommend integrin inhibitors for fistulizing CD.

In summary, fistulizing CD is an aggressive phenotype, and medical therapy should involve a TNF inhibitor with strong consideration of concomitant treatment with a thiopurine. Metronidazole and ciprofloxacin can provide temporary benefit until combination therapy takes full effect.

FULMINANT COLITIS

Fulminant colitis secondary to IBD is a clinical scenario in which the surgeon should be intimately involved. It is more commonly described in UC, but can occur in CD as well. Despite the complexities and challenges that these patients present, the approach is simple: aggressive medical management, and early surgery in nonresponders.[112]

The cornerstone of initial therapy is intravenous corticosteroids with a dose equivalent to 60 mg methylprednisolone daily (which can be given either as a continuous infusion or in separate doses). Studies investigating higher doses have failed to show additional benefit with an increased risk of adverse effects.[113] The time period that one could be considered a nonresponder to corticosteroids is debated among experts, but generally ranges between 5 and 10 days.[112,114,115] Between 30% and 40% of patients with fulminant colitis do not respond to intravenous corticosteroids. For this group of patients, the decision to intensify medical treatment or proceed with surgery should be a joint discussion between the patient, gastroenterologist, and surgeon.[112]

For those patients who do not respond to corticosteroids, rescue therapy with infliximab or cyclosporine should at least be considered before surgery. The one open-label RCT directly comparing infliximab (5 mg/kg on days 0, 14, 42) and cyclosporine (2 mg/kg/d for 1 week, followed by oral medication until day 98) showed them to be similar in efficacy and adverse event profile. Despite some success, treatment failure (defined by the absence of a clinical response at day 7, a relapse between day 7 and day 98, absence of steroid-free remission at day 98, severe adverse event leading to treatment interruption, colectomy, or death) occurred in 54% and 60% of patients on infliximab and cyclosporine, respectively.[116] A systemic review and meta-analysis comparing cyclosporine and infliximab for the treatment of fulminant colitis showed a comparable 3-month colectomy rate (OR = 0.86, 95% CI = 0.31–2.41, P = .775), 12-month colectomy rate (OR = 0.60, 95% CI = 0.19–1.89, P = .381), rate of adverse events (OR = 0.76, 95% CI = 0.34–1.70, P = .508), and postoperative complication rate (OR = 1.66, 95% CI = 0.26–10.50, P = .591).[52] A recent retrospective study, however, found the colectomy rates at 1, 2, and 3 years to be higher in the cyclosporine group. Predictive factors for cyclosporine failure included extensive disease, elevated C-reactive protein, and lack of azathioprine treatment.[117] One small series of 19 patients showed that initial failure of either infliximab or cyclosporine followed by treatment with the other drug resulted in approximately 70% of patients undergoing colectomy in 12 months.[118] Thus, it is generally advisable to proceed to colectomy after failure of either cyclosporine or infliximab.

Despite the inclusion of broad-spectrum antibiotics in many treatment protocols for fulminant colitis, controlled trials investigating oral vancomycin, intravenous metronidazole, and intravenous ciprofloxacin in the absence of proven infection have failed to show therapeutic benefit.[119–121] However, given the rising prevalence of C difficile in IBD patients,[122] and the variable sensitivity of available diagnostic modalities,[123] empiric treatment can be considered if clinical suspicion exists.

PERIOPERATIVE CONSIDERATIONS

Despite advances in medical management, surgical intervention is still necessary in many patients with IBD. The operative management of CD is generally reserved for patients who have an obstructing fibrotic stricture, perforation, cancer, or fistulae or active luminal inflammation refractory to medical management. Indications for surgery in UC include fulminant colitis, dysplasia, neoplasia, medically intractable disease, and patient preference. The perioperative medical management of IBD has become especially challenging as the paradigm of treatment of IBD has shifted to more advanced immunosuppressive therapies.

Patients who are malnourished, are greater than 60 years of age, require emergent surgery, or have penetrating disease have increased perioperative morbidity.[124] The nature of the surgical procedure is also an important factor in perioperative morbidity. For example, total proctocolectomy (TPC) with J pouch is more likely to result in postoperative infection when compared with TPC with ileostomy. Laparoscopic surgery has consistently been associated with decreased postoperative length of stay and complication rate when compared with open procedures.[125]

Consideration should also be given to whether UC or CD is the underlying disease process. In UC, the most common surgery, TPC with ileal pouch-anal anastomosis (IPAA), is theoretically curative, which tends to simplify postoperative medical therapy. Conversely, when CD patients progress to surgery, decisions regarding perioperative and postoperative medical therapies pose more of a challenge. Most patients with CD who progress to surgery will require continued immunosuppressive therapy postoperatively. Perioperative management of immunosuppressive therapy needs to be individualized. Physicians must weigh the possible increased risk of surgical complications versus the potential for recurrent disease without appropriate therapy.

Immunomodulators

The data for perioperative use of azathioprine and 6-MP are sparse and unfortunately conflicting in regards to postoperative infectious complications. A retrospective cohort study of 159 patients with IBD undergoing elective bowel surgery evaluated the risk of postoperative infections in 3 groups of patients: corticosteroids alone, thiopurines (with or without corticosteroids), and neither thiopurines nor corticosteroids. Although the preoperative use of corticosteroids was associated with increased risk of postoperative infections (OR 3.69, 95% CI 1.24–10.97), the use of thiopurines was not (OR 1.68, 95% CI 0.65–4.27).[126] Conversely, prospective data from 343 consecutive patients with CD who underwent abdominal operations at a single tertiary referral center showed that thiopurine therapy was associated with an increase in intra-abdominal septic complications.[127]

Both azathioprine and 6-MP have some renal elimination, which harbors the potential for toxic metabolite accumulation in patients with decreased glomerular filtration. In rare circumstances, this could lead to severe myelotoxicity.[128] The authors recommend discontinuing thiopurines a day before surgery with resumption no sooner than 3 days after surgery.[124] The limited data investigating perioperative infectious complications on methotrexate are focused on orthopedic surgery in the rheumatoid arthritis population, not patients with IBD. Moreover, these data are conflicting, are of poor quality, and do not sufficiently address the risks of myelosuppression, pneumonitis, hepatotoxicity, and nephrotoxicity during the perioperative period. Therefore, the authors recommend that in patients with a history severe septic complication, it may be reasonable to discontinue methotrexate 1 week before surgery and resume it no sooner than 1 week after surgery.[124]

Cyclosporine is most typically used in patients with corticosteroid-refractory UC as a rescue therapy before colectomy. The most worrisome adverse effects of cyclosporine in the perioperative setting are nephrotoxicity and opportunistic infections. Mortalities secondary to opportunistic infections as high as 3.5% have been reported,[129] and prophylaxis of *Pneumocystis jiroveci* with trimethoprim-sulfamethoxazole should be considered.[124] Multiple small case series exploring the use of preoperative cyclosporine in UC have not shown an increase in adverse events during and after surgery.[130–132] Unfortunately, current clinical data are insufficient for further recommendations regarding cyclosporine in the perioperative period in CD; however, patients being treated should be closely monitored for deterioration in renal function and opportunistic infections.[124]

Biologics

Infliximab is the most widely studied biologic therapy for IBD. Although there is some conflicting evidence, the vast majority of data suggest that infliximab (and by extension the other TNF-α inhibitors adalimumab, certolizumab pegol, and golimumab) does not seem to increase peri-postoperative complications in IBD.

One study evaluated 45 patients who were randomized to infliximab or placebo after a failed trial of corticosteroids for severe or fulminant UC. Seven of the patients in the infliximab group and 14 in the placebo group required a colectomy within 3 months. There was no increase in the postoperative complication rate in the infliximab arm. In fact, 3 patients in the placebo group (compared with none of the infliximab-treated patients) required operation for septic complications.[133]

Although infliximab has decreased the rates of surgeries in patients with UC,[106] many were concerned that it merely delayed (but did not prevent) surgical intervention. Postponing surgery in this manner would lead to performing surgeries in patients who are more chronically ill, therefore increasing the risk of emergent procedures with associated greater morbidity and mortality.[134,135] To answer this question, Bordeianou and colleagues[136] retrospectively compared outcomes in 44 patients on infliximab with medically refractory UC undergoing a TPC or subtotal colectomy with 127 patients with a similar disease severity without exposure to biologic therapy. Infliximab exposure did not seem to affect the rate of emergent surgery (4.5% vs 4.4%, P = .98), rate of subtotal colectomy (19.2% vs 18.0%, P = .99), or rate of ileoanal J-pouch reconstruction (53.8% vs 62%, P = .98). Intraoperative findings such as perforation, toxic megacolon, and active disease were similar in both groups. Furthermore, short-term postoperative complications, defined as within 30 days of loop ileostomy closure in TPC and IPAA, have been shown to be comparable in perioperative infliximab and non-infliximab-treated patients.[137] Thus, the preoperative use of infliximab does not seem to increase surgical morbidity or mortality in UC.

Most of the data in CD show a similar safety profile. A cohort study compared 40 patients with CD on infliximab before intestinal resection (more than 75% within 12 weeks) to 39 biologic-naïve patients adjusted for age, gender, and surgical procedure. Early (10 days) and late (3 months) major or minor complications were identified. The incidence of early minor (15.0% vs 12.8%) and major (12.5% vs 7.7%) and late minor (2.5% vs 5.1%) and major (17.5% vs 12.8%) complications and the mean hospital stay after surgery (10.3 ± 4.0 days vs 9.9 ± 5.5 days) were similar in both groups.[138]

However, some studies indicate that biologic therapy during the perioperative period can increase the rate of perioperative complications. A large retrospective study showed that patients with CD who received infliximab within 12 weeks of ileocolonic resection had increased rates of postoperative sepsis, intra-abdominal abscess, and 30-day hospital readmissions. However, the presence of a diverting stoma in patients with infliximab seemed to decrease the risk of these complications.[139] Similarly, much of the data that seem to indicate a higher complication rate with infliximab when performing a TPC with IPAA in UC suggest that this risk may be mitigated with a 2- or 3-stage surgery.[134,140,141] Although it is likely that much of the data suggesting an increase in perioperative complications with infliximab reflect the higher burden of comorbidities in patients on biologic therapies,[124,142] the data are limited by the lack of RCTs.

Based on the available data, the authors generally recommend continuing anti-TNF therapy during the perioperative period. Although data are not available for natalizumab and vedolizumab in the perioperative period, the authors generally recommend continuing anti-integrin therapy. However, as with all immunosuppressive therapy in the perioperative period, decisions regarding the continuation of biologic therapy should be based on a comprehensive discussion between the patient, gastroenterologist, and surgeon.

POSTOPERATIVE RECURRENCE OF CROHN'S DISEASE

Greater than 75% of patients diagnosed with CD will eventually require surgical intervention.[143] Unfortunately, recurrence is very common. After ileal or ileocolonic resection, there is a 20% to 30% symptomatic recurrence rate in the first year after surgery, with a 10% increase each subsequent year. Most patients will eventually suffer recurrence, and a reoperation rate of 50% to 60% is generally reported.[144] Most evidence-based assessments of postoperative CD to date have focused on symptom recurrence, which grossly underestimates the true rate of postoperative recurrence. Thus, the goal of endoscopic remission is of particular importance in postoperative CD.[145,146]

Rutgeerts and colleagues[147] illustrated the importance of endoscopic assessment when they followed a cohort of 89 patients after ileocolonic resection (**Table 2**). Endoscopic disease severity 1 year after surgery was a strong predictor of future clinical symptoms and reoperation. Patients with mild or inactive disease (i0, i1) rarely had symptoms at 1 year, and 80% of these patients continued to have mild or absent

Table 2
Rutgeert's grading system for postoperative Crohn's disease

Endoscopic Findings	Rutgeert's Score
Normal mucosa	i0
<5 Aphthous lesions	i1
≥5 Aphthous lesions with normal mucosa between the lesions, or skip areas of larger lesions, or lesions confined to the ileocolonic anastomosis	i2
Diffuse aphthous ileitis with diffusely inflamed mucosa	i3
Diffuse inflammation with ulcers that are already larger, nodules, and/or narrowing	i4

From Rutgeerts P, Geboes K, Vantrappen G, et al. Predictability of the postoperative course of Crohn's disease. Gastroenterology 1990;99(4):956–63; with permission.

endoscopic recurrence at 3 years. Thirty-three percent of patients in the intermediate group (i2) progressed to i4 lesions at 3 years. Patients with severe endoscopic disease (i3 or i4) were more likely to have clinical recurrence at 1 year; 92% of these patients had progressive, severe endoscopic disease at 3 years with a high likelihood for reoperation.

In addition to Rutgeert's grading system, there are well-established risk factors (**Table 3**) that predict disease recurrence.[145,148] Given the high likelihood of postsurgical recurrence in CD, appropriate medical treatment based on risk factors for disease recurrence should be started soon after surgery. Medical therapy should be intensified if endoscopic assessment shows moderate (i2) or severe (i3 or i4) disease. Aggressive postoperative treatment of CD may be able to avert or delay future surgeries. Therefore, individualized care with frequent endoscopic disease assessments is particularly important in the postoperative setting.

Both metronidazole and ornidazole have been shown to be effective in reducing the severity of endoscopic recurrence. A placebo-controlled trial compared patients who received metronidazole (20 mg/kg body weight) daily for 3 months after curative ileal resection and primary anastomosis to patients receiving placebo. At 12 weeks, 21 of 28 patients (75%) in the placebo group had recurrent lesions in the neoterminal ileum compared with 12 of 23 patients (52%) in the metronidazole group ($P = .09$). The incidence of severe endoscopic recurrence was significantly reduced by metronidazole (3 of 23; 13%) as compared with placebo (12 of 28; 43%; $P = .02$). Metronidazole therapy also reduced the clinical recurrence rates at 1 year (4% vs 25%). However,

Table 3
Predictors of recurrence

Strong Risk Factors	Inconclusive Risk Factors
Smoking[a]	Family history of IBD
Penetrating disease[a]	Anastomotic site of disease
History of prior resection[a]	Type of anastomosis
Short duration of disease (<10 y)	Gender
Small bowel and colon involvement	Disease extent (length of diseased intestine)
Progress to surgery despite immunomodulator and biologic therapy	Young age at disease onset

[a] Strongest risk factors.

reductions at 2 years (26% vs 43%) and 3 years (30% vs 50%) were not significant, suggesting that metronidazole may merely delay disease recurrence.[149] Ornidazole 1 g daily for 1 year after ileal or ileocolonic resection also reduced clinical and endoscopic recurrence compared with placebo at 1 year.[150] Unfortunately, adverse effects (neuropathy and gastrointestinal intolerance) preclude long-term use of both antibiotics. Nonetheless, nitroimidazole antibiotics should be considered after ileal or ileocolonic resection to reduce or delay recurrence.

A study of 81 patients undergoing ileal or ileocolonic resection with at least one risk factor for CD recurrence (age <30 years, active smoking, prior resection, penetrating disease) supports the benefit of thiopurines. In this study, all patients received 3 months of metronidazole 750 mg daily and either azathioprine or placebo for 12 months immediately after surgical resection. The primary endpoint was endoscopic recurrence at 3 and 12 months. After 3 months, moderate (≥i2) endoscopic recurrence was evident in 53% of patients receiving placebo, but only in 34% on azathioprine ($P = .11$). At 12 months, the rate of moderate (≥i2) endoscopic recurrence was significantly lower in the azathioprine group (44%) compared with placebo (69%; $P = .05$). Only 3% of patients receiving metronidazole/placebo had complete mucosal remission (i0) compared with 22% of those receiving metronidazole/azathioprine.[151] A recent study comparing azathioprine to mesalazine in patients who had undergone an ileocolonic anastomosis in the preceding 6 to 24 months and had developed moderate or severe (≥i2) endoscopic recurrence before initiation of the study showed a superior endoscopic response with azathioprine. The proportion of patients showing a 1 point or greater reduction in Rutgeert's score between baseline and month 12 was 63.3% and 34.4% in the azathioprine and mesalazine groups, respectively ($P = .023$).[152] There are no studies currently that assess methotrexate monotherapy as prophylaxis for postoperative recurrence.

The ability of TNF-α antagonist therapy to induce mucosal healing in IBD has led to trials evaluating their use in postoperative CD. An early RCT comparing infliximab (5 mg/kg) to placebo illustrates the efficacy of infliximab in the postoperative setting. The rate of endoscopic recurrence at 1 year was 9.1% in the infliximab group, compared with 84.6% with placebo ($P = .0006$).[153] The data for adalimumab for postoperative CD seem equally promising.[154,155] Unfortunately, there are no data available for the use of natalizumab or vedolizumab in the postoperative setting (although there are ongoing trials for vedolizumab).

In summary, there are currently no formal guidelines for the medical prophylaxis of postoperative CD recurrence. Despite the lack of current guidelines, the natural progression of CD after surgery is toward recurrence. Thus, medical management should be strongly considered in all postoperative patients. Patients with aggressive risk factors for recurrence should generally be treated with immunomodulator or biologic therapy soon after surgery. Endoscopic recurrence is predictive of long-term outcomes, and endoscopy should therefore be performed at frequent intervals starting 3 to 6 months after surgery. Medication adjustments should be individualized and based on endoscopic findings.

REFERENCES

1. Dave M, Loftus EV Jr. Mucosal healing in inflammatory bowel disease—a true paradigm of success? Gastroenterol Hepatol (N Y) 2012;8(1):29–38.
2. Papi C, Fasci-Spurio F, Rogai F, et al. Mucosal healing in inflammatory bowel disease: treatment efficacy and predictive factors. Dig Liver Dis 2013;45(12): 978–85.

3. Froslie KF, Jahnsen J, Moum BA, et al. Mucosal healing in inflammatory bowel disease: results from a Norwegian population-based cohort. Gastroenterology 2007;133(2):412–22.

4. Colombel JF, Rutgeerts PJ, Sandborn WJ, et al. Adalimumab induces deep remission in patients with Crohn's disease. Clin Gastroenterol Hepatol 2014; 12(3):414–22.e5.

5. Schnitzler F, Fidder H, Ferrante M, et al. Mucosal healing predicts long-term outcome of maintenance therapy with infliximab in Crohn's disease. Inflamm Bowel Dis 2009;15(9):1295–301.

6. Rutgeerts P, Van Assche G, Sandborn WJ, et al. Adalimumab induces and maintains mucosal healing in patients with Crohn's disease: data from the EXTEND trial. Gastroenterology 2012;142(5):1102–11.e2.

7. Herrinton LJ, Liu L, Levin TR, et al. Incidence and mortality of colorectal adenocarcinoma in persons with inflammatory bowel disease from 1998 to 2010. Gastroenterology 2012;143(2):382–9.

8. Ullman TA, Itzkowitz SH. Intestinal inflammation and cancer. Gastroenterology 2011;140(6):1807–16.

9. Fasci Spurio F, Aratari A, Margagnoni G, et al. Early treatment in Crohn's disease: do we have enough evidence to reverse the therapeutic pyramid? J Gastrointestin Liver Dis 2012;21(1):67–73.

10. Maser EA, Villela R, Silverberg MS, et al. Association of trough serum infliximab to clinical outcome after scheduled maintenance treatment for Crohn's disease. Clin Gastroenterol Hepatol 2006;4(10):1248–54.

11. Vermeire S, Noman M, Van Assche G, et al. Effectiveness of concomitant immunosuppressive therapy in suppressing the formation of antibodies to infliximab in Crohn's disease. Gut 2007;56(9):1226–31.

12. Colombel JF, Sandborn WJ, Reinisch W, et al. Infliximab, azathioprine, or combination therapy for Crohn's disease. N Engl J Med 2010;362(15):1383–95.

13. Rousseaux C, Lefebvre B, Dubuquoy L, et al. Intestinal antiinflammatory effect of 5-aminosalicylic acid is dependent on peroxisome proliferator-activated receptor-gamma. J Exp Med 2005;201(8):1205–15.

14. Shanahan F, Niederlehner A, Carramanzana N, et al. Sulfasalazine inhibits the binding of TNF alpha to its receptor. Immunopharmacology 1990;20(3):217–24.

15. Bantel H, Berg C, Vieth M, et al. Mesalazine inhibits activation of transcription factor NF-kappaB in inflamed mucosa of patients with ulcerative colitis. Am J Gastroenterol 2000;95(12):3452–7.

16. Sharon P, Ligumsky M, Rachmilewitz D, et al. Role of prostaglandins in ulcerative colitis. Enhanced production during active disease and inhibition by sulfasalazine. Gastroenterology 1978;75(4):638–40.

17. Hawkey CJ, Boughton-Smith NK, Whittle BJ. Modulation of human colonic arachidonic acid metabolism by sulfasalazine. Dig Dis Sci 1985;30(12):1161–5.

18. Ligumsky M, Karmeli F, Sharon P, et al. Enhanced thromboxane A2 and prostacyclin production by cultured rectal mucosa in ulcerative colitis and its inhibition by steroids and sulfasalazine. Gastroenterology 1981;81(3):444–9.

19. Miller DK, Gillard JW, Vickers PJ, et al. Identification and isolation of a membrane protein necessary for leukotriene production. Nature 1990;343(6255):278–81.

20. Stenson WF, Lobos E. Sulfasalazine inhibits the synthesis of chemotactic lipids by neutrophils. J Clin Invest 1982;69(2):494–7.

21. Ahnfelt-Ronne I, Nielsen OH, Christensen A, et al. Clinical evidence supporting the radical scavenger mechanism of 5-aminosalicylic acid. Gastroenterology 1990;98(5 Pt 1):1162–9.

22. Stevens C, Lipman M, Fabry S, et al. 5-Aminosalicylic acid abrogates T-cell proliferation by blocking interleukin-2 production in peripheral blood mononuclear cells. J Pharmacol Exp Ther 1995;272(1):399–406.
23. MacDermott RP, Schloemann SR, Bertovich MJ, et al. Inhibition of antibody secretion by 5-aminosalicylic acid. Gastroenterology 1989;96(2 Pt 1):442–8.
24. Rhodes JM, Bartholomew TC, Jewell DP. Inhibition of leucocyte motility by drugs used in ulcerative colitis. Gut 1981;22(8):642–7.
25. Neal TM, Winterbourn CC, Vissers MC. Inhibition of neutrophil degranulation and superoxide production by sulfasalazine. Comparison with 5-aminosalicylic acid, sulfapyridine and olsalazine. Biochem Pharmacol 1987;36(17):2765–8.
26. Rubinstein A, Das KM, Melamed J, et al. Comparative analysis of systemic immunological parameters in ulcerative colitis and idiopathic proctitis: effects of sulfasalazine in vivo and in vitro. Clin Exp Immunol 1978;33(2):217–24.
27. Ford AC, Achkar JP, Khan KJ, et al. Efficacy of 5-aminosalicylates in ulcerative colitis: systematic review and meta-analysis. Am J Gastroenterol 2011;106(4): 601–16.
28. Ford AC, Kane SV, Khan KJ, et al. Efficacy of 5-aminosalicylates in Crohn's disease: systematic review and meta-analysis. Am J Gastroenterol 2011;106(4): 617–29.
29. Box SA, Pullar T. Sulphasalazine in the treatment of rheumatoid arthritis. Br J Rheumatol 1997;36(3):382–6.
30. Azulfidine, EN-Tabs. In: Physicians Desk Reference. 52nd edition. Montvale (NJ): Medical Economics Company; 1998. p. 2239.
31. Stein RB, Hanauer SB. Comparative tolerability of treatments for inflammatory bowel disease. Drug Saf 2000;23(5):429–48.
32. Woltsche M, Woltsche-Kahr I, Roeger GM, et al. Sulfasalazine-induced extrinsic allergic alveolitis in a patient with psoriatic arthritis. Eur J Med Res 2001;6(11): 495–7.
33. Gisbert JP, Gonzalez-Lama Y, Mate J. 5-Aminosalicylates and renal function in inflammatory bowel disease: a systematic review. Inflamm Bowel Dis 2007; 13(5):629–38.
34. Dubinsky MC, Reyes E, Ofman J, et al. A cost-effectiveness analysis of alternative disease management strategies in patients with Crohn's disease treated with azathioprine or 6-mercaptopurine. Am J Gastroenterol 2005;100(10): 2239–47.
35. Priest VL, Begg EJ, Gardiner SJ, et al. Pharmacoeconomic analyses of azathioprine, methotrexate and prospective pharmacogenetic testing for the management of inflammatory bowel disease. Pharmacoeconomics 2006;24(8):767–81.
36. Pearson DC, May GR, Fick G, et al. Azathioprine for maintaining remission of Crohn's disease. Cochrane Database Syst Rev 2000;(2):CD000067.
37. Prefontaine E, Macdonald JK, Sutherland LR. Azathioprine or 6-mercaptopurine for induction of remission in Crohn's disease. Cochrane Database Syst Rev 2010;(6):CD000545.
38. Pearson DC, May GR, Fick GH, et al. Azathioprine and 6-mercaptopurine in Crohn disease. A meta-analysis. Ann Intern Med 1995;123(2):132–42.
39. Su C, Lichtenstein GR. Treatment of inflammatory bowel disease with azathioprine and 6-mercaptopurine. Gastroenterol Clin North Am 2004;33(2): 209–34, viii.
40. Bouhnik Y, Lemann M, Mary JY, et al. Long-term follow-up of patients with Crohn's disease treated with azathioprine or 6-mercaptopurine. Lancet 1996; 347(8996):215–9.

41. Beaugerie L, Brousse N, Bouvier AM, et al. Lymphoproliferative disorders in patients receiving thiopurines for inflammatory bowel disease: a prospective observational cohort study. Lancet 2009;374(9701):1617–25.

42. Kotlyar DS, Osterman MT, Diamond RH, et al. A systematic review of factors that contribute to hepatosplenic T-cell lymphoma in patients with inflammatory bowel disease. Clin Gastroenterol Hepatol 2011;9(1):36–41.e1.

43. Peyrin-Biroulet L, Khosrotehrani K, Carrat F, et al. Increased risk for nonmelanoma skin cancers in patients who receive thiopurines for inflammatory bowel disease. Gastroenterology 2011;141(5):1621–8.e1–5.

44. Cronstein BN, Naime D, Ostad E. The antiinflammatory mechanism of methotrexate. Increased adenosine release at inflamed sites diminishes leukocyte accumulation in an in vivo model of inflammation. J Clin Invest 1993;92(6):2675–82.

45. Feagan BG, Rochon J, Fedorak RN, et al. Methotrexate for the treatment of Crohn's disease. The North American Crohn's Study Group Investigators. N Engl J Med 1995;332(5):292–7.

46. Feagan BG, Fedorak RN, Irvine EJ, et al. A comparison of methotrexate with placebo for the maintenance of remission in Crohn's disease. North American Crohn's Study Group Investigators. N Engl J Med 2000;342(22):1627–32.

47. Arora S, Katkov W, Cooley J, et al. Methotrexate in Crohn's disease: results of a randomized, double-blind, placebo-controlled trial. Hepatogastroenterology 1999;46(27):1724–9.

48. Oren R, Moshkowitz M, Odes S, et al. Methotrexate in chronic active Crohn's disease: a double-blind, randomized, Israeli multicenter trial. Am J Gastroenterol 1997;92(12):2203–9.

49. Te HS, Schiano TD, Kuan SF, et al. Hepatic effects of long-term methotrexate use in the treatment of inflammatory bowel disease. Am J Gastroenterol 2000;95(11):3150–6.

50. Van Assche G, D'Haens G, Noman M, et al. Randomized, double-blind comparison of 4 mg/kg versus 2 mg/kg intravenous cyclosporine in severe ulcerative colitis. Gastroenterology 2003;125(4):1025–31.

51. Naganuma M, Fujii T, Watanabe M. The use of traditional and newer calcineurin inhibitors in inflammatory bowel disease. J Gastroenterol 2011;46(2):129–37.

52. Chang KH, Burke JP, Coffey JC. Infliximab versus cyclosporine as rescue therapy in acute severe steroid-refractory ulcerative colitis: a systematic review and meta-analysis. Int J Colorectal Dis 2013;28(3):287–93.

53. Jewell DP, Lennard-Jones JE. Oral cyclosporin for chronic active Crohn's disease: a multicenter controlled trial. Eur J Gastroenterol Hepatol 1994;6:499–505.

54. Feagan BG, McDonald JW, Rochon J, et al. Low-dose cyclosporine for the treatment of Crohn's disease. The Canadian Crohn's Relapse Prevention Trial Investigators. N Engl J Med 1994;330(26):1846–51.

55. Stange EF, Modigliani R, Pena AS, et al. European trial of cyclosporine in chronic active Crohn's disease: a 12-month study. The European Study Group. Gastroenterology 1995;109(3):774–82.

56. Sternthal MB, Murphy SJ, George J, et al. Adverse events associated with the use of cyclosporine in patients with inflammatory bowel disease. Am J Gastroenterol 2008;103(4):937–43.

57. Dassopoulos T, Sninsky CA. Optimizing immunomodulators and anti-TNF agents in the therapy of Crohn disease. Gastroenterol Clin North Am 2012;41(2):393–409, ix.

58. Sands BE, Anderson FH, Bernstein CN, et al. Infliximab maintenance therapy for fistulizing Crohn's disease. N Engl J Med 2004;350(9):876–85.

59. Colombel JF, Schwartz DA, Sandborn WJ, et al. Adalimumab for the treatment of fistulas in patients with Crohn's disease. Gut 2009;58(7):940–8.
60. Ng SC, Plamondon S, Gupta A, et al. Prospective evaluation of anti-tumor necrosis factor therapy guided by magnetic resonance imaging for Crohn's perineal fistulas. Am J Gastroenterol 2009;104(12):2973–86.
61. Sandborn WJ, Hanauer SB, Rutgeerts P, et al. Adalimumab for maintenance treatment of Crohn's disease: results of the CLASSIC II trial. Gut 2007;56(9): 1232–9.
62. Hanauer S, Rutgeerts P, Targan S, et al. Delayed hypersensitivity to infliximab (Remicade) re-infusion after 2–4 year interval without treatment. Gastroenterology 1999;116:A731.
63. Hanauer SB, Feagan BG, Lichtenstein GR, et al. Maintenance infliximab for Crohn's disease: the ACCENT I randomised trial. Lancet 2002;359(9317): 1541–9.
64. Sandborn WJ, Feagan BG, Stoinov S, et al. Certolizumab pegol for the treatment of Crohn's disease. N Engl J Med 2007;357(3):228–38.
65. Siegel CA, Marden SM, Persing SM, et al. Risk of lymphoma associated with combination anti-tumor necrosis factor and immunomodulator therapy for the treatment of Crohn's disease: a meta-analysis. Clin Gastroenterol Hepatol 2009;7(8):874–81.
66. Deepak P, Sifuentes H, Sherid M, et al. T-cell non-Hodgkin's lymphomas reported to the FDA AERS with tumor necrosis factor-alpha (TNF-alpha) inhibitors: results of the REFURBISH study. Am J Gastroenterol 2013;108(1):99–105.
67. Nozaki K, Silver RM, Stickler DE, et al. Neurological deficits during treatment with tumor necrosis factor-alpha antagonists. Am J Med Sci 2011;342(5): 352–5.
68. Sandborn WJ, Colombel JF, Enns R, et al. Natalizumab induction and maintenance therapy for Crohn's disease. N Engl J Med 2005;353(18):1912–25.
69. Targan SR, Feagan BG, Fedorak RN, et al. Natalizumab for the treatment of active Crohn's disease: results of the ENCORE Trial. Gastroenterology 2007; 132(5):1672–83.
70. Feagan BG, Greenberg GR, Wild G, et al. Treatment of ulcerative colitis with a humanized antibody to the alpha4beta7 integrin. N Engl J Med 2005;352(24): 2499–507.
71. Feagan BG, Greenberg GR, Wild G, et al. Treatment of active Crohn's disease with MLN0002, a humanized antibody to the alpha4beta7 integrin. Clin Gastroenterol Hepatol 2008;6(12):1370–7.
72. Feagan BG, Rutgeerts P, Sands BE, et al. Vedolizumab as induction and maintenance therapy for ulcerative colitis. N Engl J Med 2013;369(8):699–710.
73. Parikh A, Leach T, Wyant T, et al. Vedolizumab for the treatment of active ulcerative colitis: a randomized controlled phase 2 dose-ranging study. Inflamm Bowel Dis 2012;18(8):1470–9.
74. Sandborn WJ, Feagan BG, Rutgeerts P, et al. Vedolizumab as induction and maintenance therapy for Crohn's disease. N Engl J Med 2013;369(8):711–21.
75. Thomas A, Lodhia N. Advanced therapy for inflammatory bowel disease: a guide for the primary care physician. J Am Board Fam Med 2014;27(3):411–20.
76. Amiot A, Peyrin-Biroulet L. Current, new and future biological agents on the horizon for the treatment of inflammatory bowel diseases. Therap Adv Gastroenterol 2015;8(2):66–82.
77. Goulding NJ. The molecular complexity of glucocorticoid actions in inflammation—a four-ring circus. Curr Opin Pharmacol 2004;4(6):629–36.

78. Hayashi R, Wada H, Ito K, et al. Effects of glucocorticoids on gene transcription. Eur J Pharmacol 2004;500(1–3):51–62.
79. De Bosscher K, Vanden Berghe W, Haegeman G. The interplay between the glucocorticoid receptor and nuclear factor-kappaB or activator protein-1: molecular mechanisms for gene repression. Endocr Rev 2003;24:488–522.
80. Kagoshima M, Ito K, Cosio B, et al. Glucocorticoid suppression of nuclear factor-kappa B: a role for histone modifications. Biochem Soc Trans 2003; 31(Pt 1):60–5.
81. Buttgereit F, Saag KG, Cutolo M, et al. The molecular basis for the effectiveness, toxicity, and resistance to glucocorticoids: focus on the treatment of rheumatoid arthritis. Scand J Rheumatol 2005;34(1):14–21.
82. Lundin PD, Edsbacker S, Bergstrand M, et al. Pharmacokinetics of budesonide controlled ileal release capsules in children and adults with active Crohn's disease. Aliment Pharmacol Ther 2003;17(1):85–92.
83. Seow CH, Benchimol EI, Steinhart AH, et al. Budesonide for Crohn's disease. Expert Opin Drug Metab Toxicol 2009;5(8):971–9.
84. Klotz U, Schwab M. Topical delivery of therapeutic agents in the treatment of inflammatory bowel disease. Adv Drug Deliv Rev 2005;57(2):267–79.
85. De Cassan C, Fiorino G, Danese S. Second-generation corticosteroids for the treatment of Crohn's disease and ulcerative colitis: more effective and less side effects? Dig Dis 2012;30(4):368–75.
86. Ford AC, Bernstein CN, Khan KJ, et al. Glucocorticosteroid therapy in inflammatory bowel disease: systematic review and meta-analysis. Am J Gastroenterol 2011;106(4):590–9 [quiz: 600].
87. Summers RW, Switz DM, Sessions JT Jr, et al. National Cooperative Crohn's Disease Study: results of drug treatment. Gastroenterology 1979;77(4 Pt 2):847–69.
88. Malchow H, Ewe K, Brandes JW, et al. European Cooperative Crohn's Disease Study (ECCDS): results of drug treatment. Gastroenterology 1984;86(2):249–66.
89. Toruner M, Loftus EV Jr, Harmsen WS, et al. Risk factors for opportunistic infections in patients with inflammatory bowel disease. Gastroenterology 2008; 134(4):929–36.
90. Hanauer SB, Present DH. The state of the art in the management of inflammatory bowel disease. Rev Gastroenterol Disord 2003;3(2):81–92.
91. Marehbian J, Arrighi HM, Hass S, et al. Adverse events associated with common therapy regimens for moderate-to-severe Crohn's disease. Am J Gastroenterol 2009;104(10):2524–33.
92. Lichtenstein GR, Feagan BG, Cohen RD, et al. Serious infections and mortality in association with therapies for Crohn's disease: TREAT registry. Clin Gastroenterol Hepatol 2006;4(5):621–30.
93. Irving PM, Gearry RB, Sparrow MP, et al. Review article: appropriate use of corticosteroids in Crohn's disease. Aliment Pharmacol Ther 2007;26(3):313–29.
94. Lyckegaart E, HK, Bengtsson B. Compassionate use of budesonide capsules (Entocort EC) in patients with Crohn's disease. Gastroenterology 2002; 122(T-1665) [abstract: 500].
95. Sandborn WJ, Travis S, Moro L, et al. Once-daily budesonide MMX(R) extended-release tablets induce remission in patients with mild to moderate ulcerative colitis: results from the CORE I study. Gastroenterology 2012; 143(5):1218–26.e1–2.
96. Travis SP, Danese S, Kupcinskas L, et al. Once-daily budesonide MMX in active, mild-to-moderate ulcerative colitis: results from the randomised CORE II study. Gut 2014;63(3):433–41.

97. Edsbacker S, Andersson T. Pharmacokinetics of budesonide (Entocort EC) capsules for Crohn's disease. Clin Pharmacokinet 2004;43(12):803–21.
98. Greenberg GR, Feagan BG, Martin F, et al. Oral budesonide for active Crohn's disease. Canadian Inflammatory Bowel Disease Study Group. N Engl J Med 1994;331(13):836–41.
99. Beaugerie L, Seksik P, Nion-Larmurier I, et al. Predictors of Crohn's disease. Gastroenterology 2006;130(3):650–6.
100. Jakobovits J, Schuster MM. Metronidazole therapy for Crohn's disease and associated fistulae. Am J Gastroenterol 1984;79(7):533–40.
101. Bernstein LH, Frank MS, Brandt LJ, et al. Healing of perineal Crohn's disease with metronidazole. Gastroenterology 1980;79(3):599.
102. Brandt LJ, Bernstein LH, Boley SJ, et al. Metronidazole therapy for perineal Crohn's disease: a follow-up study. Gastroenterology 1982;83(2):383–7.
103. Maeda Y, Ng SC, Durdey P, et al. Randomized clinical trial of metronidazole ointment versus placebo in perianal Crohn's disease. Br J Surg 2010;97(9): 1340–7.
104. Wiese DM, Schwartz DA. Managing perianal Crohn's disease. Curr Gastroenterol Rep 2012;14(2):153–61.
105. Present DH, Rutgeerts P, Targan S, et al. Infliximab for the treatment of fistulas in patients with Crohn's disease. N Engl J Med 1999;340(18):1398–405.
106. Lichtenstein GR, Yan S, Bala M, et al. Infliximab maintenance treatment reduces hospitalizations, surgeries, and procedures in fistulizing Crohn's disease. Gastroenterology 2005;128(4):862–9.
107. Ng SC, Plamondon S, Gupta A, et al. Prospective assessment of the effect on quality of life of anti-tumour necrosis factor therapy for perineal Crohn's fistulas. Aliment Pharmacol Ther 2009;30(7):757–66.
108. Hanauer SB, Sandborn WJ, Rutgeerts P, et al. Human anti-tumor necrosis factor monoclonal antibody (adalimumab) in Crohn's disease: the CLASSIC-I trial. Gastroenterology 2006;130(2):323–33 [quiz: 591].
109. Jilani NZ, Akobeng AK. Adalimumab for maintenance of clinical response and remission in patients with Crohn's disease: the CHARM trial. Colombel JF, Sandborn WJ, Rutgeerts P, et al. Gastroenterology 2007;132:52–65. J Pediatr Gastroenterol Nutr 2008;46(2):226–7.
110. Lichtiger S, Binion DG, Wolf DC, et al. The CHOICE trial: adalimumab demonstrates safety, fistula healing, improved quality of life and increased work productivity in patients with Crohn's disease who failed prior infliximab therapy. Aliment Pharmacol Ther 2010;32(10):1228–39.
111. Chen CH, Kularatna G, Stone CD, et al. Clinical experience of natalizumab in Crohn's disease patients in a restricted distribution program. Ann Gastroenterol 2013;26(3):189–90.
112. Portela F, Lago P. Fulminant colitis. Best Pract Res Clin Gastroenterol 2013; 27(5):771–82.
113. Rosenberg W, Ireland A, Jewell DP. High-dose methylprednisolone in the treatment of active ulcerative colitis. J Clin Gastroenterol 1990;12(1):40–1.
114. Truelove SC, Jewell DP. Intensive intravenous regimen for severe attacks of ulcerative colitis. Lancet 1974;1(7866):1067–70.
115. Blomberg B, Jarnerot G. Clinical evaluation and management of acute severe colitis. Inflamm Bowel Dis 2000;6(3):214–27.
116. Laharie D, Bourreille A, Branche J, et al. Ciclosporin versus infliximab in patients with severe ulcerative colitis refractory to intravenous steroids: a parallel, open-label randomised controlled trial. Lancet 2012;380(9857):1909–15.

117. Mocciaro F, Renna S, Orlando A, et al. Cyclosporine or infliximab as rescue therapy in severe refractory ulcerative colitis: early and long-term data from a retrospective observational study. J Crohns Colitis 2012;6(6):681–6.

118. Maser EA, Deconda D, Lichtiger S, et al. Cyclosporine and infliximab as rescue therapy for each other in patients with steroid-refractory ulcerative colitis. Clin Gastroenterol Hepatol 2008;6(10):1112–6.

119. Dickinson RJ, O'Connor HJ, Pinder I, et al. Double blind controlled trial of oral vancomycin as adjunctive treatment in acute exacerbations of idiopathic colitis. Gut 1985;26(12):1380–4.

120. Chapman RW, Selby WS, Jewell DP. Controlled trial of intravenous metronidazole as an adjunct to corticosteroids in severe ulcerative colitis. Gut 1986;27(10):1210–2.

121. Mantzaris GJ, Petraki K, Archavlis E, et al. A prospective randomized controlled trial of intravenous ciprofloxacin as an adjunct to corticosteroids in acute, severe ulcerative colitis. Scand J Gastroenterol 2001;36(9):971–4.

122. Issa M, Ananthakrishnan AN, Binion DG. Clostridium difficile and inflammatory bowel disease. Inflamm Bowel Dis 2008;14(10):1432–42.

123. Deshpande A, Pasupuleti V, Rolston DD, et al. Diagnostic accuracy of real-time polymerase chain reaction in detection of Clostridium difficile in the stool samples of patients with suspected Clostridium difficile infection: a meta-analysis. Clin Infect Dis 2011;53(7):e81–90.

124. Kumar A, Auron M, Aneja A, et al. Inflammatory bowel disease: perioperative pharmacological considerations. Mayo Clin Proc 2011;86(8):748–57.

125. Ananthakrishnan AN, McGinley EL, Saeian K, et al. Laparoscopic resection for inflammatory bowel disease: outcomes from a nationwide sample. J Gastrointest Surg 2010;14(1):58–65.

126. Aberra FN, Lewis JD, Hass D, et al. Corticosteroids and immunomodulators: postoperative infectious complication risk in inflammatory bowel disease patients. Gastroenterology 2003;125(2):320–7.

127. Myrelid P, Olaison G, Sjodahl R, et al. Thiopurine therapy is associated with postoperative intra-abdominal septic complications in abdominal surgery for Crohn's disease. Dis Colon Rectum 2009;52(8):1387–94.

128. Connell WR, Kamm MA, Ritchie JK, et al. Bone marrow toxicity caused by azathioprine in inflammatory bowel disease: 27 years of experience. Gut 1993;34(8):1081–5.

129. Arts J, D'Haens G, Zeegers M, et al. Long-term outcome of treatment with intravenous cyclosporin in patients with severe ulcerative colitis. Inflamm Bowel Dis 2004;10(2):73–8.

130. Pinna-Pintor M, Arese P, Bona R, et al. Severe steroid-unresponsive ulcerative colitis: outcomes of restorative proctocolectomy in patients undergoing cyclosporin treatment. Dis Colon Rectum 2000;43(5):609–13 [discussion: 613–4].

131. Fleshner PR, Michelassi F, Rubin M, et al. Morbidity of subtotal colectomy in patients with severe ulcerative colitis unresponsive to cyclosporin. Dis Colon Rectum 1995;38(12):1241–5.

132. Hyde GM, Jewell DP, Kettlewell MG, et al. Cyclosporin for severe ulcerative colitis does not increase the rate of perioperative complications. Dis Colon Rectum 2001;44(10):1436–40.

133. Jarnerot G, Hertervig E, Friis-Liby I, et al. Infliximab as rescue therapy in severe to moderately severe ulcerative colitis: a randomized, placebo-controlled study. Gastroenterology 2005;128(7):1805–11.

134. Mor IJ, Vogel JD, da Luz Moreira A, et al. Infliximab in ulcerative colitis is associated with an increased risk of postoperative complications after

restorative proctocolectomy. Dis Colon Rectum 2008;51(8):1202–7 [discussion 1207–10].

135. Selvasekar CR, Cima RR, Larson DW, et al. Effect of infliximab on short-term complications in patients undergoing operation for chronic ulcerative colitis. J Am Coll Surg 2007;204(5):956–62 [discussion: 962–3].

136. Bordeianou L, Kunitake H, Shellito P, et al. Preoperative infliximab treatment in patients with ulcerative and indeterminate colitis does not increase rate of conversion to emergent and multistep abdominal surgery. Int J Colorectal Dis 2010; 25(3):401–4.

137. Gainsbury ML, Chu DI, Howard LA, et al. Preoperative infliximab is not associated with an increased risk of short-term postoperative complications after restorative proctocolectomy and ileal pouch-anal anastomosis. J Gastrointest Surg 2011;15(3):397–403.

138. Marchal L, D'Haens G, Van Assche G, et al. The risk of post-operative complications associated with infliximab therapy for Crohn's disease: a controlled cohort study. Aliment Pharmacol Ther 2004;19(7):749–54.

139. Appau KA, Fazio VW, Shen B, et al. Use of infliximab within 3 months of ileocolonic resection is associated with adverse postoperative outcomes in Crohn's patients. J Gastrointest Surg 2008;12(10):1738–44.

140. Gu J, Remzi FH, Shen B, et al. Operative strategy modifies risk of pouch-related outcomes in patients with ulcerative colitis on preoperative anti-tumor necrosis factor-alpha therapy. Dis Colon Rectum 2013;56(11):1243–52.

141. Hicks CW, Hodin RA, Bordeianou L. Possible overuse of 3-stage procedures for active ulcerative colitis. JAMA Surg 2013;148(7):658–64.

142. Narula N, Charleton D, Marshall JK. Meta-analysis: peri-operative anti-TNFalpha treatment and post-operative complications in patients with inflammatory bowel disease. Aliment Pharmacol Ther 2013;37(11):1057–64.

143. Achkar JP, Shen B. Medical management of postoperative complications of inflammatory bowel disease: pouchitis and Crohn's disease recurrence. Curr Gastroenterol Rep 2001;3(6):484–90.

144. Rutgeerts P. Protagonist: Crohn's disease recurrence can be prevented after ileal resection. Gut 2002;51(2):152–3.

145. Schwartz M, Regueiro M. Prevention and treatment of postoperative Crohn's disease recurrence: an update for a new decade. Curr Gastroenterol Rep 2011; 13(1):95–100.

146. Rutgeerts P, Feagan BG, Lichtenstein GR, et al. Comparison of scheduled and episodic treatment strategies of infliximab in Crohn's disease. Gastroenterology 2004;126(2):402–13.

147. Rutgeerts P, Geboes K, Vantrappen G, et al. Predictability of the postoperative course of Crohn disease. Gastroenterology 1990;99(4):956–63.

148. Cho SM, Cho SW, Regueiro M. Postoperative management of Crohn's disease. Med Clin North Am 2010;94(1):179–88.

149. Rutgeerts P, Hiele M, Geboes K, et al. Controlled trial of metronidazole treatment for prevention of Crohn's recurrence after ileal resection. Gastroenterology 1995; 108(6):1617–21.

150. Rutgeerts P, Van Assche G, Vermeire S, et al. Ornidazole for prophylaxis of postoperative Crohn's disease recurrence: a randomized, double-blind, placebo-controlled trial. Gastroenterology 2005;128(4):856–61.

151. D'Haens GR, Vermeire S, Van Assche G, et al. Therapy of metronidazole with azathioprine to prevent postoperative recurrence of Crohn's disease: a controlled randomized trial. Gastroenterology 2008;135(4):1123–9.

152. Reinisch W, Angelberger S, Petritsch W, et al. Azathioprine versus mesalazine for prevention of postoperative clinical recurrence in patients with Crohn's disease with endoscopic recurrence: efficacy and safety results of a randomised, double-blind, double-dummy, multicentre trial. Gut 2010;59(6):752–9.

153. Regueiro M, Schraut W, Baidoo L, et al. Infliximab prevents Crohn's disease recurrence after ileal resection. Gastroenterology 2009;136(2):441–50.e1 [quiz: 716].

154. Papamichael K, Archavlis E, Lariou C, et al. Adalimumab for the prevention and/or treatment of post-operative recurrence of Crohn's disease: a prospective, two-year, single center, pilot study. J Crohns Colitis 2012;6(9):924–31.

155. Kotze PG, Yamamoto T, Danese S, et al. Direct retrospective comparison of adalimumab and infliximab in preventing early postoperative endoscopic recurrence after ileocaecal resection for Crohn's disease: results from the MULTIPER database. J Crohns Colitis 2015;9(7):541–7.

Crohn's Disease of the Foregut

Kurt G. Davis, MD

KEYWORDS

- Crohn's disease • Esophagus • Gastric • Foregut

KEY POINTS

- Crohn's disease of the foregut is underrecognized.
- The most common location of Crohn's disease in the proximal intestine is in the gastric antrum.
- Surgical management of esophageal Crohn's disease is reserved for complications such as strictures or fistulas.
- The most common indication for surgical management of gastroduodenal Crohn's disease is obstruction.
- The surgical options are gastric bypass or strictureplasty with or without concomitant vagotomy.

INTRODUCTION

In 1932, New York physicians Crohn, Ginzburg, and Oppenheimer published the seminal work describing the small bowel inflammatory process that would carry the eponymous name of its first author.[1] At that time, the disease was believed to be limited to the terminal portion of the small intestine. The authors and others quickly realized that the disease could be more extensively distributed, however. Two years after this initial publication, Crohn asserted that the disease "could involve other segments than the terminal ileum"[2] and he thereby favored the term regional ileitis. That same year, also in New York, the first operation for Crohn's disease involving the foregut likely occurred when Eggers performed an esophagectomy with plastic tube reconstruction for a young man with a benign esophageal stricture.[3]

Although the understanding of Crohn's disease has grown greatly since its first description, the experience with foregut disease remains sparse. It is now well-recognized that Crohn's disease can affect any part of the intestinal tract from the mouth to the anus. The recognition and documentation of foregut Crohn's disease remains underappreciated, however. The exact incidence of proximal intestinal Crohn's is difficult to define and the preponderance of the literature centers around

Colon and Rectal Surgery, Department of Surgery, William Beaumont Army Medical Center, 4756 Loma de Plata Drive, El Paso, TX 79934, USA
E-mail address: kurtdavis88@gmail.com

Surg Clin N Am 95 (2015) 1183–1193
http://dx.doi.org/10.1016/j.suc.2015.07.004
0039-6109/15/$ – see front matter Published by Elsevier Inc.

surgical.theclinics.com

case reports and small case series. Estimates of foregut Crohn's disease range between 1% and 13% in patients with documented ileocolic disease.[4] The diagnosis is often made only in patients who have significant symptoms from their upper intestinal disease. Patients that have documented proximal Crohn's disease typically have evidence of the disease in their distal small intestine or colon.[4,5] However, finding the evidence of proximal Crohn's disease often depends on how diligently it is sought.

In 1975, an extensive experience involving more than 8000 cases of regional enteritis was presented. There were no patients demonstrating any involvement of the proximal intestinal tract.[6] Korelitz and associates[7] performed one of the first series specifically looking for evidence of Crohn's disease in the proximal intestine. This evaluation of 45 patients with Crohn's disease distally was performed and histologic lesions were found in almost one-half of the patients, and 24% were diagnostic for Crohn's. An even larger evaluation involving 225 patients suffering from Crohn's disease of the lower gastrointestinal tract was also performed. The authors performed an upper endoscopic examination and found 49% of patients demonstrated evidence of gastric Crohn's disease, whereas 34% had evidence of disease in the duodenum.[8] In another study, Alcantara and colleagues[9] found that 56% of Crohn's disease patients demonstrated upper endoscopic abnormalities. Again, the most frequently affected site was the gastric antrum, followed by the duodenum. In the largest study to date, Oberhuber and coworkers[10] performed a retrospective study of 792 patients with known distal disease. Crohn's disease was identified histologically in the antrum and body in 40% of patients and was found in the duodenum or duodenal bulb in 13% of patients.[10] Clearly, the incidence of foregut Crohn's disease is greater than previously documented and finding it requires only seeking it in patients already diagnosed with the disease distally.

Granulomas, considered to be pathognomonic for the diagnosis of Crohn's disease, are frequently unseen. Despite a diagnosis of Crohn's in the distal bowel, granulomas are seen in only 20% to 30% of grossly abnormal tissue biopsies.[8,9,11] Although they are more commonly found in grossly abnormal lesions, they can be detected in more than 10% of grossly normal tissue as well.[9]

Despite being more common than previously recognized, symptomatic proximal disease is indeed rare. Even patients with concomitant disease tend to seek medical care for their lower intestinal symptoms.[12] It remains imperative that physicians who treat patients with Crohn's disease remain vigilant for the possibility of foregut Crohn's and query for any upper intestinal complaints and perform an upper intestinal investigation if the clinical scenario presents itself.

ESOPHAGEAL CROHN'S DISEASE

First described by Franklin and Taylor in 1950,[13] Crohn's disease of the esophagus is the least common location for the disease in the intestinal tract. A 1983 review of the English-language literature to that point revealed reports of only 20 patients with Crohn's disease of the esophagus.[14] Several large reports have confirmed the scarcity of the condition. One study documents only 9 cases among 500 patients followed long term with Crohn's disease,[15] and a review of a 20-year experience at the Mayo Clinic showed only 20 patients (0.2%) identified as having esophageal involvement.[16] The majority of patients in these reports, however, came to medical attention owing to the severity of their condition. These patients were treated for the painful dysphagia, esophageal strictures, or fistulas associated with advanced, aggressive Crohn's disease. Indeed, 1 study group showed that more than 30% of the patients in their study had disease so severe that it required esophagectomy.[14]

This summary does not represent adequately all patients with esophageal involvement of Crohn's disease.

A higher incidence of esophageal disease has been noted in the pediatric population. One study documented a higher incidence in children with Crohn's disease who underwent upper endoscopy with biopsy.[17] A higher involvement was also documented when all children with Crohn's disease underwent upper endoscopy. Their findings demonstrated esophagitis or esophageal ulcers in 44% of their patients.[18] It is more likely that these findings stem from a more diligent search in the pediatric population than a higher prevalence, however. When adults with Crohn's disease underwent upper endoscopy, endoscopic lesions in the esophagus were observed in 15%.[8] The incidence of esophageal Crohn's disease clearly lags behind that found in the lower intestine but it is not as rare as once believed.

Signs and Symptoms

It must be emphasized that any patient with an existing diagnosis of Crohn's disease warrants the performance of an upper endoscopy with biopsy for even minor upper intestinal complaints. Most patients are asymptomatic, with only 33% of patients with documented esophageal disease having any esophageal complaints in 1 study.[19] When present, these symptoms can be difficult to differentiate from more common intestinal complaints such as gastritis or gastroesophageal reflux disease. Patients often complain of vague abdominal discomfort or heartburn. More advanced disease is heralded by dysphagia, nausea, vomiting, or odynophagia.[19,20] The radiographic or endoscopic findings of esophageal Crohn's disease mirror those of colonic disease. On endoscopic examination, inflammation or linear ulceration consistent with esophagitis is seen in 75% to 85% of patients.[15,16] More advanced disease shows aphthous ulcerations, mucosal nodularity or the typical cobblestone appearance in 30% to 40%. The histology typically shows inflammation, whereas granuloma formation is seldom identified.

The acute inflammatory process can progress to chronic fibrosis and stenosis and can lead to the development of an esophageal stricture.[21] Patients typically present with progressive dysphagia, odynophagia, or worsening reflux symptoms. Symptoms can progress to nausea and emesis with resultant weight loss. These patients are best evaluated with an esophagram in conjunction with upper endoscopy and biopsy, and the differentiation from malignancy can understandably be difficult. As with Crohn's disease found elsewhere in the gastrointestinal tract, fistula formation can occur. The most common location for a fistula is between the esophagus and the tracheobronchial tree, but can occur between any structure in the mediastinum or abdomen as well. Patients present similarly to and often have a coexisting esophageal stricture present. Epigastric or chest pain, dysphagia, weight loss, and odynophagia[22] are the most common complaints. A fistula can also present as recurrent pneumonia without concomitant esophageal complaints. Recurrent lower lobe pneumonia, pneumonitis, or abscess in patients with Crohn's disease should be considered signs of fistula formation and warrant evaluation of the esophagus with radiography and endoscopy.

Treatment

As with Crohn's disease in any anatomic location, medical management is the first line of therapy. Owing to the rarity of symptomatic presentation, and the fact that most cases presented the literature are severe, there is a dearth of literature regarding the medical management of esophageal Crohn's disease, and no randomized studies exist. The treatment that is defined is of variable efficacy. Successful medical therapy with symptom resolution has been reported with corticosteroids and acid suppression alone. Recurrent esophageal dilatations have been reported to control symptoms of esophageal stricture.[23] The largest published series consists of only 14 patients with Crohn's disease of the esophagus. All of the patients had concurrent evidence of Crohn's disease elsewhere and more than one-half experienced "complete healing" of their esophageal lesions when treated with corticosteroids after 2 to 4 weeks.[24] Several other treatment modalities have been reported in case reports. Topical steroid application with swallowed aerosolized budesonide has been reported as successful,[25] as has granulocyte/monocyte adsorption[26] and infliximab administration.[27] In an attempt to coalesce sparse data, the European consensus guidelines recommend that esophageal Crohn's disease is best managed with a proton pump inhibitor, systemic corticosteroids, and thiopurines or methotrexate.[28] The surgical management of these patients is limited typically to management of complications, such as persistent stricture of fistula formation.

Strictures

The treatment of intestinal strictures with endoscopic dilation is well documented. Although the occurrence of an esophageal stricture secondary to Crohn's disease is uncommon, numerous authors have reported an experience with the procedure.[23,29] These strictures often require multiple dilations and the recurrent stricture rate is high. The practitioner should always be cognizant of the fact that, although the surgical therapy required is typically an esophagectomy, there are reports of undiagnosed malignancy lurking within these strictures.[30]

Fistulas

The literature dealing with esophageal fistula from Crohn's disease involves case reports, with fewer than 20 described in the English literature.[31–33] These reports document fistula formation between the pleural cavity, bronchus, esophageal wall, as well as the stomach. Although there have been reports of successful fistula closure using liquid polymer sealant,[34] as well as using intravenous infliximab,[35] the majority of these require surgical repair. Esophagectomy with gastric pull-through and primary anastomosis offers definitive treatment of both the fistula and any resultant infectious complications and should be considered the standard for symptomatic fistula patients.

GASTRODUODENAL CROHN'S DISEASE

Gastroduodenal Crohn's disease is encountered more frequently than esophageal disease, but as with all foregut Crohn's disease the likelihood of finding it depends on how diligently it is sought. In the 1970s, Nugent and associates[36] published the largest series of patients to that time, documenting an incidence of gastroduodenal Crohn's of around 2%. At that time, slightly more than 150 total cases had been reported in the literature. These numbers remained consistent with later reports.[37] As with esophageal disease, a slightly greater incidence is documented in the pediatric population. Griffiths found an incidence of around 5%, but again only patients with suggestive symptoms were evaluated.[38]

These studies center on patients being evaluated for upper intestinal complaints. When all patients with lower intestinal Crohn's disease are subjected to esophagogastroduodenoscopy, much higher rates are encountered. In 1 such study, investigators found almost one-half of their patients with Crohn's demonstrated gastric lesions consistent with the disease whereas one-third had duodenal evidence of the disease.[8] In another evaluation, 10% of patients with distal Crohn's were found to harbor

Helicobacter pylori, but 32% of patients had evidence of *H pylori*–negative gastritis. The inflammation present closely resembled the inflammatory changes seen in Crohn's disease.[39] Clearly, as with esophageal Crohn's, the incidence of the disease depends on if whether is sought, because the majority of patients lack significant symptomology.

Signs and Symptoms

Although the majority of patients are asymptomatic, patients who do have symptoms of upper intestinal disease most commonly complain of upper abdominal pain. Nausea and emesis are the second most common complaints. Significant weight loss, and occasionally upper gastrointestinal bleeding or fever, have also been reported. Pancreatitis secondary to duodenal scarring has also been cited rarely.[40,41] In the pediatric population, the most common presenting symptom is weight loss, followed by epigastric pain and recurrent vomiting. Hematemesis and melena are noted to occur less commonly than in the adult population.[38] It should be emphasized, however, that even when upper intestinal disease is documented, the majority of patients remain more symptomatic from their lower intestinal disease.[42]

Endoscopic Findings

There should be a low threshold for performing upper endoscopy on any patient with Crohn's disease with any upper tract complaint. Endoscopy allows better visualization of mucosal defects for biopsy and allows monitoring of any therapeutic effect. Endoscopic biopsy is an invaluable tool for the diagnosis of gastroduodenal Crohn's disease. The mucosal lesions found at endoscopy are heterogeneous, but irregularly shaped ulcers and erosions are typical for gastroduodenal Crohn's disease.[37] The most common endoscopic findings in the upper intestine are similar to those encountered distally. These findings include mucosal nodularity or a cobblestone appearance of the mucosa. Aphthous or linear ulcerations, thickening or narrowing of the antrum, and duodenal strictures are also encountered.[43] Diffuse granularity, nodularity, and ulceration can be accompanied by the lack of distensibility of the involved area with insufflation.[36] Notching in the duodenal folds has been reported to be a strong indication for Crohn's disease.[44] Biopsies should be taken from endoscopically normal mucosa as well as grossly abnormal tissue.[45] Although the presence of the granulomas is conclusive for the diagnosis, these are identified in fewer than 33% of patients in most series. Confirmed Crohn's disease of the gastrointestinal tract or the presence of radiographic or endoscopic findings of diffuse inflammation involving the stomach or duodenum is consistent with a diagnosis of Crohn's disease, and more than 90% of patients have endoscopic abnormalities.[46]

Treatment

Even patients with symptomatic foregut disease will likely be amenable to medical management and are not likely to require surgical intervention for their foregut disease. For patients who do require surgical evaluation, most operative interventions are required for complications stemming from their disease. The most common indications for surgical therapy are in patients suffering from unrelenting duodenal obstruction secondary to strictures. Patients may also rarely come to surgery for fistulous disease or even less commonly for malignancy arising in the chronic inflammation.

Medical Management

There are no controlled, prospective studies evaluating the management of gastroduodenal Crohn's disease. Because the majority of patients already have documented, concomitant distal disease at the time of diagnosis, these patients are commonly already receiving medical management when the upper tract disease is diagnosed.[47,48] These patients do not need to have their medical management adjusted from those patients only with disease involving only the distal intestine.[38] Several experts recommend intense acid suppression with a proton pump inhibitor. Peptic ulcer disease and H pylori infection should be excluded and, if present, treated. Occasionally, this treatment alone is sufficient to allow healing of the gastroduodenal Crohn's disease.[49] Historically, the primary treatment recommendation was for systemic corticosteroids coupled with acid suppression.[49,50] In addition, there are reports of successful management with sucralfate, 6-mercaptopurine,[51] azathioprine, and H2 receptor antagonists used as adjunct therapy.[52] The role of infliximab remains to be defined. To reiterate, the European consensus guidelines recommend a proton pump inhibitor, systemic corticosteroids, and thiopurines or methotrexate for the management of upper intestinal Crohn's disease.[28]

Endoscopic Management

Strictures are the most common indication for intervention in patients with gastroduodenal Crohn's disease. Short pyloric or duodenal strictures are typically well-suited for endoscopic balloon dilation. Numerous reports of balloon dilation have been made, with a low risk of perforation of 1% to 2%, yet often repeated endoscopic dilation is required[53] to completely treat strictures. In 1 series, 5 patients with obstructive gastroduodenal Crohn's disease were treated with endoscopic balloon dilation. Each of the initial dilations was successful but 3 of the 5 patients had recurrent symptoms that required repeat dilations every 3 to 4 months. All 5 patients avoided surgery over a mean follow-up interval of 4 years with concomitant use of either a proton pump inhibitor or a histamine-2 receptor blocker.[54] In the largest study involving Crohn's strictures—the majority in the lower intestine—Singh and associates[55] performed 29 dilations with a mean follow-up period of 18 months. Technical success was achieved in 28 of 29 stricture dilations. The recurrence rate was noted to be lower when steroid injections were performed concurrently with the dilation. Three perforations, all in the colon, occurred for a complication rate of 10%, and there were no mortalities.[55]

Surgical Management

The most common indication for surgical intervention in patients with gastroduodenal disease is also duodenal obstruction. The most common symptoms of duodenal obstruction are nausea and emesis, occasionally coupled with refractory ulcer-type abdominal pain. Additional indications for surgery include massive or persistent upper gastrointestinal hemorrhage, and less commonly fistula formation or the development of malignancy in the setting of the chronic inflammation.

Duodenal Obstruction

Surgical options for managing gastroduodenal Crohn's disease include bypass surgery, typically with either gastrojejunostomy or gastroduodenostomy reconstruction. These procedures can be performed either with or without a concurrent vagotomy. The other commonly used surgical procedure is a stricturoplasty, performed similarly to that performed elsewhere in the intestine. Most patients either remain asymptomatic or are adequately managed medically and the requirement to perform these procedures is rare. As a result, there are no randomized trials comparing results and the literature stems primarily from case series based on single-institution experiences.

In 1983, 1 assessment of the long-term follow-up of patients treated surgically was performed. Ross and coworkers[56] evaluated 10 patients with Crohn's disease who had been managed surgically at the Cleveland Clinic and had a follow-up of on average 14 years. Eight of the patients had a gastrojejunostomy performed, 3 with concomitant vagotomy. They found that 7 of the patients required reoperation for recurrent duodenal Crohn's disease. The indications for subsequent operations were marginal ulceration, recurrent obstruction, or duodenal fistula. Their conclusions were that vagotomy should be part of the operative management of these patients.[57] The following year, Murray and associates[58] published the Lahey clinic experience of 25 patients who required an operation for duodenal Crohn's disease. Duodenal obstruction was the indication for operation in 22 of these patients, and duodenoenteric fistula was the cause for the other 3. After a median follow-up of 12 years, one-third of the patients required reoperation for duodenal disease. Marginal ulceration and recurrent gastroduodenal obstruction again were the primary reasons for reoperation. The addition of vagotomy was not noted to protect against subsequent marginal ulceration, yet the absence of appreciable morbidity associated with vagotomy and the high incidence of marginal ulcers reported with gastroenterostomy led the authors to recommend vagotomy at the primary operation for duodenal Crohn's disease.[58]

The largest series was reported by Nugent and Roy,[46] who documented 33 patients who required surgery. Again, the most common indication for surgery was for gastroduodenal obstruction. Reoperation was required in only 8 patients; however, 7 of these patients also had a vagotomy performed. Based on their findings that vagotomy did not mitigate the presence of marginal ulceration or the need for reoperation, these authors thought that their results did not support the routine use of vagotomy when a bypass procedure is performed.[46] Poggioli and colleagues[59] added their results of 8 surgical patients spanning a 15-year period. Three patients had surgery for a duodenal fistula, and 5 had evidence of duodenal obstruction. Of the patients with obstruction, 3 were treated with strictureplasty and 2 with duodenojejunostomy.[59] One of the stricturoplasty patients required revision and was treated with a subsequent gastroduodenal resection.

Worsey and associates[60] updated the Cleveland Clinic experience after adopting strictureplasty as the primary procedure. They documented a total cohort of 34 patients requiring surgery. The authors performed intestinal bypass in 21 patients, whereas strictureplasty was favored in 13. Vagotomy was performed concurrently with 16 of 21 bypasses and 7 of 13 strictureplasty procedures. Although follow-up was shorter, strictureplasty was felt to be a safe and effective operation for duodenal Crohn's disease and no additional benefit could be seen with the addition of vagotomy.[60] Yamamoto and coworkers[61] added their strictureplasty experience with an additional 13 patients spanning a 20-year period. Ten patients underwent strictureplasty as the primary procedure, and in 3 strictureplasty was performed as a revision. Symptoms of obstruction persisted in 4 patients after strictureplasty with 1 requiring revision to a gastrojejunostomy. Six patients developed recurrent stricture, and 5 required repeat strictureplasty and the other patient underwent duodenojejunostomy. Overall 9 of 13 patients required additional surgery after the strictureplasty.[61]

Shapiro and associates[62] have documented the most recent experience with the surgical management of gastroduodenal Crohn's disease. Thirty patients required surgical intervention over a 10-year period. Four patients underwent operation for fistulas, and 26 underwent surgery for obstructive symptoms. The operations performed were 11 open bypasses, 13 laparoscopic bypasses, and 2 strictureplasty procedures. Only 1 vagotomy was done. Patients resumed oral diet and were discharged sooner after laparoscopic bypass, compared with the open procedure. Two patients experienced disease recurrence, requiring revision 1 in each of the open and laparoscopic groups. Despite not using vagotomy frequently, the authors did not notice an increased incidence of gastroduodenal ulcers in their patients.[62,63]

It is apparent that there are insufficient data to definitively favor 1 operative technique over another. Strictureplasty is a viable treatment option for this patient population, but does seem to have a higher recurrence rate than intestinal bypass. Intestinal bypass can be safely performed laparoscopically with a more rapid return of diet and a faster discharge from the hospital. Owing to a lack of clear benefit, the routine use of vagotomy in a patient population that is already prone to disabling diarrhea should be questioned.

Fistulas

The surgical management of duodenal fistulas from Crohn's disease does not share the operative dilemmas that those of duodenal obstruction carry. Although there are reports of isolated fistulous disease arising in the stomach with no evidence of disease elsewhere,[64] fistula formation typically originates in the colon or small intestine in areas of active Crohn's disease and forms a fistulous connection to the stomach or duodenum. The fistula most commonly involves an ileocolic anastomosis that is positioned adjacent to the duodenum.[65,66] Surgical management consists of resection of the source of the fistula with primary closure of the duodenum.[59] If a large duodenal defect exists, then a duodenojejunostomy is recommended, provided there is no evidence of jejunal Crohn's disease.[66] Prevention should be stressed, and any ileocolonic anastomosis should be positioned away from the stomach or duodenum or protected with omentum in an attempt to prevent fistulization.

Malignancy

Malignant degeneration is possible in upper tract Crohn's disease, as it is in inflammatory bowel disease elsewhere. There are reports of malignant degeneration and malignancy may not be clearly identified preoperatively.[67,68] Resection may be the most prudent course for disease that fails other management.

SUMMARY

Proximal intestinal Crohn's disease is likely more common than previously recognized, and the incidence of diagnosis depends on the diligence with which it is sought. The majority of patients with proximal Crohn's disease has concurrent disease distally or will likely develop it in the future. Patients that have demonstrated colonic or ileocolic disease that complain of upper abdominal complaints such as pain, gastric reflux, or dysphagia should be evaluated with an upper endoscopy and biopsy. The most common surgical indication for gastroduodenal disease is for obstructive symptoms. These patents are adequately served with strictureplasty, but have a higher recurrence rate than with intestinal bypass procedures that can safely be performed laparoscopically. There is no definitive benefit to adding vagotomy in these patients. Fistulas most commonly originate in the colon or distal small intestine and are best prevented or treated with resection and duodenal or gastric closure.

REFERENCES

1. Crohn BB, Ginzburg L, Oppenheimer GD. Regional ileitis. A pathologic and clinical entity. JAMA 1932;99:1323–9.
2. Crohn BB. The broadening concept of regional ileitis. Am J Dig Dis Nutr 1934;1:97–9.
3. Eggers C. Plastic reconstruction of the esophagus. Ann Surg 1938;107(1):50–4.
4. Wagtmans MJ, van Hogezand RA, Griffioen G, et al. Crohn's disease of the upper gastrointestinal tract. Neth J Med 1997;50(2):S2–7.

5. Levine MS. Crohn's disease of the upper gastrointestinal tract. Radiol Clin North Am 1987;25:79–91.
6. Marshak RH. Granulomatous disease of the intestinal tract (Crohn's disease). Radiology 1975;114(1):3–22.
7. Korelitz BI, Waye JD, Kreuning J, et al. Crohn's disease in endoscopic biopsies of the gastric antrum and duodenum. Am J Gastroenterol 1981;76(2):103–9.
8. Schmitz-Moormann P, Malchow H, Pittner PM. Endoscopic and bioptic study of the upper gastrointestinal tract in Crohn's disease patients. Pathol Res Pract 1985;179(3):377–87.
9. Alcantara M, Rodriguez R, Potenciano JL, et al. Endoscopic and bioptic findings in the upper gastrointestinal tract in patients with Crohn's disease. Endoscopy 1993;25(4):282–6.
10. Oberhuber G, Hirsch M, Stolte M. High incidence of upper gastrointestinal tract involvement in Crohn's disease. Virchows Arch 1998;432(1):49–52.
11. Abdullah BA, Gupta SK, Croffie JM, et al. The role of esophagogastroduodenoscopy in the initial evaluation of childhood inflammatory bowel disease: a 7-year study. J Pediatr Gastroenterol Nutr 2002;35:636–40.
12. Wagtmans MJ, Verspaget HW, Lamers CB, et al. Clinical aspects of Crohn's disease of the upper gastrointestinal tract: a comparison with distal Crohn's disease. Am J Gastroenterol 1997;92:1467–71.
13. Franklin RH, Taylor S. Nonspecific granulomatous (regional) esophagus. J Thorac Surg 1950;19:292–7.
14. Davidson JT, Sawyers JL. Crohn's disease of the esophagus. Am Surg 1983; 49(3):168–72.
15. Geboes K, Janssens J, Rutgeerts P, et al. Crohn's disease of the esophagus. J Clin Gastroenterol 1986;8:31–7.
16. Decker GA, Loftus EV, Pasha TM, et al. Crohn's disease of the esophagus: clinical features and outcomes. Inflamm Bowel Dis 2001;7(2):113–9.
17. Mashako MN, Cezard JP, Navarro J, et al. Crohn's disease lesions in the upper gastrointestinal tract: Correlation between clinical, radiological. Endoscopic, and histological features in adolescents and children. J Pediatr Gastroenterol Nutr 1989;8:442–6.
18. Ruuska T, Vaajalahti P, Arajarvi P, et al. Prospective evaluation of upper gastrointestinal mucosal lesions in children with ulcerative colitis and Crohn's disease. J Pediatr Gastroenterol Nutr 1994;19:181–6.
19. Ramaswamy K, Jacobson K, Jevon G, et al. Esophageal Crohn disease in children: a clinical spectrum. J Pediatr Gastroenterol Nutr 2003;36:454–8.
20. Rudolph I, Goldstein F, DiMarino AJ Jr. Crohn's disease of the esophagus: three cases and a literature review. Can J Gastroenterol 2001;15:117–22.
21. Pantanowitz L, Nasser I, Gelrud A, et al. Crohn's disease of the esophagus. Ear Nose Throat J 2004;83(6):420–3.
22. Wang W, Ni Y, Ke C, et al. Isolated Crohn's disease of the esophagus with esophago-medistinal fistula formation. World J Surg Oncol 2012;10:208.
23. Rahhal RM, Banerjee S, Jensen CS. Pediatric Crohn disease presenting as an esophageal stricture. J Pediatr Gastroenterol Nutr 2007;45(1):125–9.
24. D'Haens G, Rutgeerts P, Geboes K, et al. The natural history of esophageal Crohn's disease: three patterns of evolution. Gastrointest Endosc 1994;40:296–300.
25. Zezos P, Kouklakis G, Oikonomou A, et al. Esophageal Crohn's disease treated topically with swallowed aerosolized budesonide. Case Rep Med 2010;2010.
26. Fefferman DS, Shah SA, Alsahlil M, et al. Successful treatment of refractory esophageal Crohn's disease with infliximab. Dig Dis Sci 2001;46:1733–5.

27. Moribata K, Kato J, Iimura S, et al. Mucosal healing of esophageal involvement of Crohn's disease with granulocyte/monocyte adsorption. J Clin Apher 2011;26(4): 225–7.
28. Dignass A, van Assche G, Lindsay JO, et al. The second European evidence-based consensus on the diagnosis and management of Crohn's disease: current management. J Crohns Colitis 2010;4(1):28–62.
29. Naranjo-Rodriguez A, Solorzano-Peck G, Lopez-Rubio F, et al. Isolated oesopha-geal involvement of Crohn's disease. Eur J Gastroenterol Hepatol 2003;15(10): 1123–6.
30. Mahdi SI, Elhassan AM, Ahmed ME. Crohn's disease masquerading carcinoma of the esophagus. Saudi Med J 2007;28(8):1287–8.
31. Rholl JC, Yavorski RT, Cheney CP, et al. Esophagogastric fistula: a complication of Crohn's disease–case report and review of the literature. Am J Gastroenterol 1998;93:1381–3.
32. Cynn WS, Chon H, Gureghian PA, et al. Crohn's disease of the esophagus. Am J Roentgenol Radium Ther Nucl Med 1975;125(2):359–64.
33. Clarke BW, Cassara JE, Morgan DR. Crohn's disease of the esophagus with esophago-bronchial fistula formation: a case report and review of the literature. Gastrointest Endosc 2010;71(1):207–9.
34. Rieder F, Hamer O, Gelbmann C, et al. Crohn's disease of the esophagus: treat-ment of an esophagobronchial fistula with the novel liquid embolic polymer "onyx". Z Gastroenterol 2006;44:599–602.
35. Ho IK, Guarino DP, Pertsovskiy Y, et al. Infliximab treatment of an esophagobron-chial fistula in a patient with extensive Crohn's disease of the esophagus. J Clin Gastroenterol 2002;34:488–9.
36. Nugent FW, Richmond M, Park SK. Crohn's disease of the duodenum. Gut 1977; 18:115–20.
37. Rutgeerts P, Onette E, Vantrappen G, et al. Crohn's disease of the stomach and duodenum: a clinical study with emphasis on the value of endoscopy and endo-scopic biopsies. Endoscopy 1980;12:288–94.
38. Griffiths AM, Alemayehu E, Sherman P. Clinical features of gastroduodenal Crohn's disease in adolescents. J Pediatr Gastroenterol Nutr 1989;8(2):166–71.
39. Halme L, Karkkainen P, Rautelin H, et al. High frequency of helicobacter negative gastritis in patients with Crohn's disease. Gut 1996;38:379–83.
40. Altman HS, Phillips G, Bank S, et al. Pancreatitis associated with duodenal Crohn's disease. Am J Gastroenterol 1983;78(3):174–7.
41. Spiess SE, Braun M, Vogelzang RL, et al. Crohn's disease of the duodenum complicated by pancreatitis and common bile duct obstruction. Am J Gastroen-terol 1992;87:1033–6.
42. Lossing A, Langer B, Jeejeebhoy KN. Gastroduodenal Crohn's disease: diag-nosis and selection of treatment. Can J Surg 1983;26(4):358–60.
43. Danzi JT, Farmer RG, Sullivan BH, et al. Endoscopic features of gastroduodenal Crohn's disease. Gastroenterology 1976;70(1):9–13.
44. Van Hogezand RA, Witte AM, Veenendaal RA, et al. Proximal Crohn's disease: review of the clinicopathologic features and therapy. Inflamm Bowel Dis 2001;7:328–37.
45. Gad A. The diagnosis of gastroduodenal Crohn's disease by endoscopic biopsy. Scand J Gastroenterol Suppl 1989;167:23–8.
46. Nugent FW, Roy MA. Duodenal Crohn's disease: an analysis of 89 cases. Am J Gastroenterol 1989;84(3):249–54.
47. Wagtmans MJ, van Hogezand RA, Griffioen G, et al. Crohn's disease of the upper gastrointestinal tract. Neth J Med 1997;50:S2–7.

48. Isaacs KL. Upper gastrointestinal tract endoscopy in inflammatory bowel disease. Gastrointest Endosc Clin N Am 2002;12:451–62.
49. Valori RM, Cockel R. Omeprazole for duodenal ulceration in Crohn's disease. BMJ 1990;300:438–9.
50. Miehsler W, Puspok A, Oberhuber T, et al. Impact of different therapeutic regimens on the outcome of patients with Crohn's disease of the upper gastrointestinal tract. Inflamm Bowel Dis 2001;7:99–105.
51. Korelitz BI, Adler DJ, Mendelsohn RA, et al. Long-term experience with 6-mercaptopurine in the treatment of Crohn's disease. Am J Gastroenterol 1993;88:1198–205.
52. Oberhuber G, Puspok A, Oesterreicher C, et al. Focally enhanced gastritis: a frequent type of gastritis in patients with Crohn's disease. Gastroenterology 1997;112:698–706.
53. Murthy UK. Repeated hydrostatic balloon dilation in obstructive gastroduodenal Crohn's disease. Gastrointest Endosc 1991;37:484–5.
54. Matsui T, Hatakeyama S, Ikeda K, et al. Longterm outcome of endoscopic balloon dilation in obstructive gastroduodenal Crohn's disease. Endoscopy 1997;29:640–5.
55. Singh VV, Draganov P, Valentine J. Efficacy and safety of endoscopic balloon dilation of symptomatic upper and lower gastrointestinal Crohn's disease strictures. J Clin Gastroenterol 2005;39(4):284–90.
56. Farmer RG, Hawk WA, Turnbull RB Jr. Crohn's disease of the duodenum (transmural duodenitis): clinical manifestations. Report of 11 cases. Am J Dig Dis 1972;17(3):191–8.
57. Ross TM, Fazio VW, Farmer RG. Long-term results of surgical treatment for Crohn's disease of the duodenum. Ann Surg 1983;197:399–406.
58. Murray JJ, Schoetz DJ, Nugent FW, et al. Surgical management of Crohn's disease involving the duodenum. Am J Surg 1984;147(1):58–65.
59. Poggioli G, Stocchi L, Laureti S, et al. Duodenal involvement of Crohn's disease: three different clinicopathologic patterns. Dis Colon Rectum 1997;40:179–83.
60. Worsey MJ, Hull T, Ryland L. Strictureplasty is an effective option in the operative management of duodenal Crohn's disease. Dis Colon Rectum 1999;42(5):596–600.
61. Yamamoto T, Bain IM, Connolly AB, et al. Outcome of Strictureplasty for duodenal Crohn's disease. Br J Surg 1999;86:259–62.
62. Shapiro M, Greenstein AJ, Byrn J. Surgical management and outcomes of patients with duodenal Crohn's disease. J Am Coll Surg 2008;207(1):36–42.
63. Pichney LS, Fantry GT, Graham SM. Gastrocolic and duodenocolic fistulas in Crohn's disease. J Clin Gastroenterol 1992;15:205–11.
64. Gary ER, Tremaine WJ, Banks PM, et al. Isolated Crohn's disease of the stomach. Mayo Clin Proc 1989;64:776–9.
65. Wilk PJ, Fazio V, Turnbull RB Jr. The dilemma of Crohn's disease: ileoduodenal fistula complicating Crohn's disease. Dis Colon Rectum 1977;20:387–92.
66. Yamamoto T, Bain IM, Connolly AB, et al. Gastrodu- duodenal fistulas in Crohn's disease: clinical features and management. Dis Colon Rectum 1998;41:1287–92.
67. Meiselman MS, Ghahremani GG, Kaufman MW. Crohn's disease of the duodenum complicated by adenocarcinoma. Gastrointest Radiol 1987;12:333–6.
68. Slezak P, Rubio C, Blomqvist L, et al. Duodenal adenocarcinoma in Crohn's disease of the small bowel: a case report. Gastrointest Radiol 1991;16:15–7.

Crohn's Disease of the Colon, Rectum, and Anus

William J. Harb, MD

KEYWORDS

- Crohn's Disease • Perianal Crohn's Disease • Colonic Crohn's Disease
- Crohn fistula • Ileostomy

KEY POINTS

- Intra-abdominal abscesses associated with colonic Crohn's Disease (CD) that are addressed before definitive surgery may be associated with fewer stomas.
- Segmental colectomy for colonic CD is a viable option for patients with limited disease.
- The definitive operation for the patient with colonic CD is total proctocolectomy with end ileostomy (TPC/I).
- Fecal diversion when done to decrease colonic inflammation, perianal inflammation, and sepsis may become permanent.

CD of the large intestine is one of the more challenging forms of the disease to treat.[1] CD of the small bowel and ileocolic disease are often treated surgically without the need for an ostomy, whereas the decision tree for surgical treatment of CD of the colon, rectum, and anus frequently has an ostomy at an early branching point. Also, because an ostomy has such a life-changing impact, CD of the large intestine can require difficult decisions. Delays in treatment because of the fear of an ostomy can also lead to more complicated procedures. This review focuses on the less-common complications of CD of the colon, rectum, and anus as well as the surgical treatment options.

PRESENTATIONS OF CROHN'S DISEASE
Intra-Abdominal Abscess

Intra-abdominal abscesses can complicate the treatment of patients with CD and add additional steps in management. These steps can include percutaneous drainage, surgical drainage, and/or fecal diversion. Ideally, preoperative drainage of an abscess would obviate surgery in the acute setting, make future surgery technically easier for the surgeon and patient, and decrease the likelihood of the need for an ostomy.

The author has no conflicts of interest.
The Colorectal Center, 2011 Church Street, Suite 703, Nashville, TN 37203, USA
E-mail address: BillH@TheColorectalCenter.com

Surg Clin N Am 95 (2015) 1195–1210
http://dx.doi.org/10.1016/j.suc.2015.07.005
0039-6109/15/$ – see front matter © 2015 Elsevier Inc. All rights reserved.

da Luz and colleagues[2] retrospectively reviewed the Cleveland Clinic, Ohio, experience with abdominal and pelvic abscesses in patients with CD from 1997 to 2007 and evaluated the efficacy of percutaneous drainage of abscesses in 94 patients. Patients with postoperative and perirectal abscesses were excluded from this review. Of this group of patients, 82% had ileocolic CD and 16% had colonic CD. An abscess was the initial presentation of CD in only 5 patients; 31 of 48 patients (65%) had what was considered a successful delay in surgery (median delay of surgery of 43 days). Factors associated with failure of percutaneous drainage were steroid use, colonic disease phenotype, and multiloculated abscesses. However, the size of the abscess was not associated with success or failure. As should be the goal with preoperative percutaneous drainage of intra-abdominal abscesses, initial percutaneous drainage did reduce the incidence of stoma creation when compared with initial surgical intervention (23% vs 58%, $P = .01$).

The nonsurgical viewpoint of intra-abdominal abscesses was summarized by an article from Massachusetts General Hospital.[3] Gutierrez and colleagues[3] reviewed 66 patients who were treated for intra-abdominal abscesses from 1991 to 2001. Of these, 37 patients had percutaneous drainage and 29 patients had surgical drainage of abscesses. The evaluation focused on the time to resolution of abscesses, which was not different between percutaneous and surgical drainage. The investigators also evaluated the need for surgery after percutaneous drainage and found that one-third of patients required surgery within 1 year. The investigators did not comment on whether or not patients treated with percutaneous drainage had a lower incidence of stoma creation.

Abdominal Wall Abscesses

In contrast to intra-abdominal abscesses, abdominal wall abscesses are less common. Abscesses of the abdominal wall typically indicate an underlying fistula. Neufeld and colleagues[4] identified 13 patients over a 10-year period who were diagnosed with abdominal wall abscesses resulting from CD. Mean patient age was 32.8 years. In 2 patients, the abscess was the initial presentation of CD; 6 patients were found to have colonic CD, and 5 patients had ileocecal CD. All 13 patients ultimately had definitive surgery with resection of the source of the fistula. As the fistula is the source of the abscess, it must be addressed. The investigators noted that draining the abdominal wall abscess without addressing the fistula led to a 100% failure rate, and this is in contrast to percutaneous drainage of intra-abdominal abscesses that are not associated with fistulae. It was concluded that the presence of an abdominal wall abscess indicates complicated CD and that preoperative drainage can prepare the patient for definitive surgery.[4]

Unfortunately, much of the literature describing abdominal wall abscesses does not differentiate intra-abdominal abscesses from retroperitoneal (psoas) abscesses. A psoas abscess is most commonly the result of a mesenteric abscess extending through the mesentery into the retroperitoneal space overlying the psoas muscle.[4] The formerly (now rare) classic presentation of an iliopsoas abscess is septic arthritis of the hip.[5] While this was previously most commonly seen with spondylitis resulting from tuberculosis, CD is now a much more common cause.[4]

Toxic Megacolon

Toxic megacolon is uncommon in both ulcerative colitis (UC) and CD, occurring in only 1% to 5% of patients with CD. This condition may occur as an exacerbation of inflammatory bowel disease (IBD), but it is the initial manifestation of IBD in more than 60% of patients.[6] Multiple factors have been shown to precipitate toxic megacolon, including antidiarrheal agents, belladonna alkaloids, and opiates.[7] The criteria for toxic megacolon are not only dilation of the colon but also systemic symptoms of toxicity. Jalan and colleagues[8] proposed criteria for the diagnosis of toxic megacolon in 1969. These criteria, which are still commonly used, include a colonic diameter of 6 cm or greater and 3 of the following:

1. Temperature greater than 38 °C
2. Heart rate greater than 120 beats per minute
3. Anemia
4. White blood cell count greater than $10.5 \times 10^9/L$.

The criteria also require that one of the following conditions be present:

1. Hypotension
2. Altered mental status
3. Dehydration
4. Electrolyte abnormalities[9]

Treatment of toxic megacolon includes broad-spectrum antibiotics as well as corticosteroids. Early surgical consultation is recommended.[8] If improvement does not occur within 24 to 72 hours, surgery is recommended; TAC with end ileostomy is the procedure of choice.[7] Early surgical intervention may prevent colonic perforation. Colonic perforation that occurs with toxic megacolon is associated with a mortality rate of 20%, when compared with a 4% mortality associated with toxic megacolon without perforation.[10] Unlike other cases of megacolon such as colonic pseudo-obstruction (Ogilvie syndrome), colonoscopy is generally contraindicated in cases of toxic megacolon. *Clostridium difficile* colitis, as well as colitis resulting from cytomegalovirus infection should be excluded.[10,11]

Bleeding

Massive gastrointestinal (GI) tract bleeding may occur in the setting of CD and can be particularly difficult to treat. Typical diagnostic procedures that are used in patients with lower GI tract bleeding without IBD are often also used in patients with bleeding resulting from CD. These procedures include colonoscopy and angiography. Kostka and Lukas[12] identified 6 of 156 patients with CD over an 18-year span who had massive GI tract bleeding; 3 patients had a previous diagnosis of CD, whereas 3 patients presented with bleeding as the initial symptom of CD. These 6 patients had a total of 11 episodes of bleeding. The site of bleeding was identified preoperatively by angiography in 2 patients and by colonoscopy in 2 patients. The most common procedure required was an ileocecal resection (3 patients). Of the 6 patients, 4 ultimately underwent surgery, which led the investigators to conclude that a conservative approach may be tried as first-line therapy, but surgery is inevitable.

Robert and colleagues[13] reviewed the Mount Sinai, New York, experience with massive GI tract bleeding resulting from CD. At a center with an extensive experience with IBD, over a 26-year period (1960–1986), only 21 of 1526 patients developed severe GI tract bleeding. The group of 11 men and 10 women had a median age of 27 years. A total of 12 surgical procedures were done including 6 subtotal colectomies, 4 ileocolonic resections, 1 sigmoid colectomy, and 1 right hemicolectomy. Interestingly, 9 of the 10 patients with ileocolonic CD also had colonic involvement. The frequency of bleeding was much higher among patients with colonic involvement (17/929; 1.9%) when compared with patients with small bowel disease (4/597; 0.7%) (*P*<.001). Recurrent bleeding was quite unusual.[13] Although the differences were not statistically significant, they commented that surgery at the time of the initial bleeding seemed to lead to a lower mortality and a lower chance of recurrent bleeding.

Several investigators have stated that ileocecal CD was the most common form of CD that caused bleeding, whereas Belaiche and colleagues[14] found the opposite. These investigators retrospectively identified 34 cases of CD with GI tract bleeding. The site of bleeding was attributed to the colon in 85% of cases when compared with isolated small bowel disease in only 15% ($P<.0001$). An ulcer was identified to be the cause of the bleeding in 95% of patients, and this ulcer was most commonly in the descending colon.

However, not all investigators think that surgical resection is the only treatment option. A recent retrospective review from Thailand identified 7 patients who were not considered fit for surgery (3 were poor surgical candidates, and 6 were thought to be at high risk of short bowel syndrome). Of the 7 patients, 5 presented with bleeding as their first presentation of CD. These patients did not undergo angiographic embolization because of the risk of short bowel syndrome. These patients were treated with infliximab (5 mg/kg). Bleeding stopped within 24 hours in 6 of 7 patients, and 1 patient had an episode of rebleeding, which stopped 10 days after the initial infusion of infliximab. The median number of doses of infliximab was 2.[15]

Obstruction Because of Stricture

Strictures do occur in the large bowel in patients with CD, but the frequency is less than that in the small bowel. Colonic strictures are more common in patients with UC than in those with CD, occurring in approximately 5% to 17% of patients with UC and 5% of patients with CD.[16] Although many would think that colonic strictures are more likely to be malignant in patients with CD than in those with UC, the converse has actually been shown. Gumaste and colleagues[17] from Mount Sinai Hospital in New York found 29% incidence of malignancy in patients with UC who had colonic strictures, when compared with a 6.8% incidence of malignancy in those with Crohn strictures.[18]

Strictures may be classified as either inflammatory or fibrostenotic lesions. Differentiating between the 2 is important for determining appropriate treatment.[19] The type of stricture may be differentiated based on imaging studies. Characteristics such as edema, bowel wall thickness, and vascularization help make this differentiation. The typical location of obstruction and strictures in CD is ileocecal.

It should be recalled that any stricture found in the colon or rectum should be biopsied because these should be considered malignant until proven otherwise. The role of strictureplasty in patients with colonic strictures has yet to be defined, but many consider it contraindicated.[16]

OPERATIONS AND TECHNIQUES FOR CROHN'S DISEASE OF THE COLON AND RECTUM

Multiple different surgical operations exist for the patient with CD of the colon and rectum. Several pieces of information should be taken into consideration when deciding which operation is most ideally suited for the individual patient. The amount of colon involved with the colitis should be considered, as well as whether or not the rectum is involved. A digital examination of the anus and distal rectum should be done because perianal CD may contraindicate a sphincter-saving operation and cause the surgeon to recommend an operation with an ostomy. In addition, the function of the anus should be considered, and any underlying fecal incontinence may lead to a change in procedure.

Segmental Resection

A common dilemma for the surgeon faced with a patient with colonic CD and rectal sparing is whether the patient should have a segmental resection or a TAC. Martel and colleagues[20] reviewed their experience with segmental colectomy for colonic CD. A total of 84 patients underwent segmental colectomy, 32% patients required an ostomy, and 36 patients underwent reoperation. The mean time to reoperation was 4.5 years. The investigators concluded that there was no higher risk of surgical recurrence in patients undergoing segmental colectomy when compared with those undergoing TAC/IRA.

Fichera and colleagues[21] reviewed their outcomes of patients with Crohn colitis undergoing surgery. Over an 18-year period, 179 patients with colonic CD had surgery, and 54 patients (30%) had a segmental colectomy done. Patients who had a segmental colectomy done had a statistically significantly higher risk of surgical recurrence than those who underwent TAC/IRA or TPC/I. Significantly, after 1 year, 30 patients who had segmental colectomy (61%) were still taking steroids or immunomodulators; 17 patients required a permanent stoma (34.7%). There was a statistically significant higher chance of the need for a stoma in patients with distal disease when compared with those with proximal disease. The investigators concluded that patients with involvement of multiple colonic segments, especially if the disease was distal (descending and rectosigmoid colon), had a much lower risk of recurrence if treated with TPC/I rather than segmental colectomy. However, they also noted that if patients have short-segment colonic CD (<20 cm), then segmental colectomy is a valuable alternative.[21]

Tekkis and colleagues[22] published a meta-analysis comparing TAC/IRA to segmental colectomy. Six studies from 1988 to 2002, which included 488 patients, were included. There was no difference in recurrence of CD between those undergoing TAC/IRA and those undergoing segmental colectomy. However, patients who had segmental colectomy did have recurrence of their disease a mean of 4.43 years earlier than patients undergoing TAC/IRA. It was concluded that segmental colectomy was an attractive option for select patients with colonic CD. However, in patients with colonic involvement of 2 or more segments, TAC/IRA was the preferred alternative.

Total Abdominal Colectomy with Ileorectal Anastomosis

An option for the patient with colonic CD without rectal disease (rectal sparing) or perianal disease is a TAC/IRA. The surgeon must ensure that not only the rectum but also the anus is free of inflammation. Although this will not be an option for all patients with CD of the colon and rectum, approximately 25% to 50% of patients will not have disease of both the rectum and anus and would therefore be candidates. The surgeon should exclude any other conditions, such as fecal incontinence, that would preclude an anastomosis.[23]

Fortunately, recurrence (or the new occurrence) of CD in the rectum or anus after TAC/IRA is uncommon. Longo and colleagues[23] reviewed 131 patients who underwent TAC/IRA. It should be noted that their statistical methods only included crude fractions and not a log rank test, such as Kaplan-Meier. Of the 118 patients with a functioning anastomosis, 30 patients required proctectomy and 16 patients required diversion with an ostomy. At a mean follow-up of 9.5 years, 72 patients retained a functional anastomosis. The mean bowel frequency was 4.7 per day.

O'Riordan and colleagues[24] also studied the long-term outcome of the IRA after TAC/IRA. Over a 28-year period, 81 patients underwent TAC/IRA for CD. The anastomotic leak rate was 7.4%. At 5 years, 87% of patients (95% confidence interval [CI], 75.5–93.3) had a functioning IRA, and at 10 years, 72.2% of patients had a functioning anastomosis (95% CI, 55.8–83.4). The investigators concluded that TAC/IRA is a good option for select patients but that the long-term risk of proctectomy is approximately 30%.

Restorative Proctocolectomy

While restorative proctocolectomy (proctocolectomy with ileal j-pouch-anal anastomosis [IPAA]) is considered by many to be the gold-standard operation for UC,[25] its use in patients with CD is controversial and much less common. In fact, many think that IPAA is contraindicated in patients with a preoperative diagnosis of CD.[26] The literature regarding IPAA is somewhat difficult to interpret because many patients with CD who undergo IPAA have a preoperative diagnosis of indeterminate colitis or UC and are only diagnosed with CD after surgery.[27] For those surgeons who do offer restorative proctocolectomy to patients with CD, preoperative requirements include the absence of both perianal and small bowel disease. Panis and colleagues[28] were some of the initial advocates for IPAA in the setting of CD because they began offering IPAA to patients with CD in 1985. Between 1985 and 1992, 31 patients with a preoperative diagnosis of CD underwent IPAA. Only 2 patients developed fistulae and 2 patients developed recurrent CD. No patients were lost to follow-up, and there was no statistically significant difference in stool frequency when their patients with CD were compared with 44 patients who had UC ($P = .68$).

Regimbeau and colleagues[29] have updated their experience with IPAA for CD. Although 26 patients had a preoperative diagnosis of CD, these results are still difficult to interpret because they are combined with the results of 15 patients who had CD diagnosed after IPAA was done. It is notable that 27% of the patients (11 of 41) had postoperative complications, including 7 patients who developed pouch-perineal fistulas. In addition, 38% of patients developed pouchitis and 3 patients (7% of the 41 patients) ultimately required pouch excision.[29]

The results of Regimbeau and colleagues[29] are in contrast to those of Sagar and colleagues[27] from the Mayo Clinic. These investigators reviewed 37 patients who underwent IPAA and were diagnosed postoperatively with CD. Of these 37 patients, 11 developed complex fistulas. Pouch failure occurred in 17 patients. The investigators concluded that IPAA done with a preoperative diagnosis of CD had a high failure rate (45%) but that long-term functional results were acceptable if the pouch was able to be preserved. Others have seen similar results to those of Sagar and colleagues.[27] Mylonakis and colleagues[30] identified 23 patients who had IPAA for CD. Of these patients, 48% had pouch excision after a mean follow-up of 10.2 years. Although IPAA for CD does have its advocates, CD remains an absolute contraindication to IPAA in the opinion of many surgeons.[21]

Total Abdominal Colectomy with Ileostomy Without Proctectomy

TAC with end ileostomy while leaving the rectum in situ (TAC/I) is an option for the patient with colonic CD in whom the pelvic dissection necessary for removal of the rectum is not thought to be wise. This option is an ideal one for a patient with an acute presentation of colonic CD requiring surgery (such as a patient with toxic megacolon or bleeding from a colonic source) or a patient with a more chronic disease presentation requiring surgery (ie, a patient on high doses of steroids).

Management of the Rectal Stump

When colectomy without proctectomy is done for an acute presentation of CD, there are different choices regarding how to deal with the rectal stump. One option is to merely close off the stump.[31] When this is done, drains should be placed in the pelvis; consideration should be given to placing a rectal tube for drainage as well. Some have noted that there is a chance of the stump blowing out when this option is chosen. In order to decrease the incidence of this event, some have placed the rectal stump in the subcutaneous tissue of the abdominal incision with the hopes that if this does occur, it will occur in the wound rather than intra-abdominally. This placement would hopefully avoid an intra-abdominal or pelvic abscess. Others have noted that it is difficult to make the rectal stump reach the abdominal wall, and they have placed abdominal/pelvic drains, as well as a rectal tube, to lessen the chance of this occurring.[32] Trickett and colleagues[33] reported the outcomes of 37 patients who had an emergency TAC. In 27 patients, the stump was left in an intraperitoneal position, and it was placed in a subcutaneous position in 10 patients. Two patients had leakage from an intraperitoneal stump, which did not require further surgery but did prolong their length of hospital stay; 3 patients had leakage from a subcutaneously placed stump, which resulted in a mucous fistula and a wound infection. However, the subcutaneous placement of the rectal stump and the resulting wound infection did not seem to prolong the length of the hospital stay. The incidence of pelvic sepsis seems to be related to the length of the remaining rectum. The highest incidence seems to be with a short intrapelvic stump (33%), followed by an intraperitoneal stump (6%–12%), with a subcutaneously placed stump having the lowest risk of pelvic sepsis (3%–4%).[33] While one advantage of a longer stump is a lower incidence of pelvic sepsis, another advantage is that any future pelvic surgery is technically easier because it should be easier to dissect a longer stump. For example, in some situations, one may not be able to differentiate between CD and UC before surgery and a restorative proctocolectomy may be planned at some point in the future for the patient with UC.

Secondary Proctectomy

When the rectum is not removed at the time of the initial operation, secondary proctectomy may be required at a later time for Crohn proctitis or diversion proctitis. Common symptoms of diversion proctitis that develop after colectomy with an ostomy, such as mucous per anus and rectal bleeding, may become symptomatic enough to require treatment. Although Crohn proctitis does not usually require treatment after colectomy with an ostomy, diversion proctitis that develops may require treatment in a minority of patients.[34] If such treatment (commonly topical therapy) fails, secondary proctectomy may be required.

Cattan and colleagues[35] retrospectively reviewed 144 patients who underwent TAC for CD over a 17-year period. Of these, 118 patients had an IRA (the majority were not done at the time of the initial surgery, but were done a median of 3 months after surgery). Most patients who did not have an IRA done, had proctitis (the minority had perianal disease only or both proctitis and perianal disease). Thirteen patients underwent a secondary proctectomy, which was most commonly done for intractable proctitis (10 patients).

Geoghegan and colleagues[36] have also reviewed the need for secondary proctectomy in patients with CD who underwent TAC. A total of 44 patients had surgery for colonic CD. Secondary proctectomy was done in 5 of 12 patients who had surgery for acute colitis, but only in 1 patient who had an elective colectomy. None of their patients developed cancer in the retained rectal stump.

Rieger and colleagues[37] reviewed 38 patients who had TAC for CD between 1968 and 1994. Fourteen patients ultimately underwent secondary proctectomy (9 of these 14 patients had secondary proctectomy after TAC/I and 5 required proctectomy after TAC/IRA). The reader would be wise to recall that the experiences of both Rieger and colleagues[37] and Geoghegan and colleagues[36] was reported before the era of biological therapy for IBD, hence the requirement for secondary proctectomy is most likely lower now after the initiation of this therapy.

Additional reasons for proctectomy after TAC/I are the development of cancer or the inability to exclude cancer, as well as persistently symptomatic perianal CD. The development of cancer in the retained rectum after TAC/I is rare.[38]

Total Proctocolectomy with Ileostomy

The definitive operation for CD involving the colon and rectum is the removal of the entire colon and rectum with a permanent ileostomy. This operation has the advantage of removing the diseased intestine in one operation without a frequent need for secondary operations. Therefore, diseases and complications related to the rectum and rectal stump are not a concern. Recurrence of CD in patients undergoing TPC/I is much less than that in patients undergoing operations in which an anastomosis is done (such as segmental colectomy or TAC/IRA). Yamamoto and colleagues[39] reviewed their experience with TPC/I in 103 patients who had surgery between 1958 and 1997. The 5-, 10-, and 15-year recurrence rates were 13%, 17%, and 25%, respectively, after a median follow-up of 18.6 years. The investigators concluded that TPC/I carried a low long-term recurrence rate but that young males were at an increased risk of recurrence. Fichera and colleagues[21] reviewed 179 patients who had surgery for colonic CD. A total of 75 patients had TPC/I, and only 4 of these patients developed recurrent disease. The investigators noted that patients undergoing TPC/I were less likely to be taking medications 1 year after surgery than patients who had either segmental colectomy or TAC/IRA. They concluded that TPC/I was associated with low morbidity, longer time to recurrence, and a lower overall risk of recurrence.

Abdominoperineal Resection for Distal Crohn's Disease

For the patient with CD of the rectum or perineal CD, when the proximal colon is normal, an option is removal of the rectum and anus only with an intersphincteric proctectomy. de Buck van Overstraeten and colleagues[40] reviewed 10 patients who underwent abdominoperineal resection (APR) for CD. The proximal colon was found to be normal at colonoscopy. The investigators identified recurrent disease in 9 of 10 patients at a median of 9.5 months. Even with medical treatment, completion colectomy was done in 5 of these 9 patients. It was concluded that even with a normal-appearing proximal colon, TPC/I was a more appropriate procedure than APR in patients with Crohn proctitis and perineal disease because of the severe and early recurrence of CD.

MANAGEMENT OF SPECIFIC COMPLICATIONS AFTER SURGERY FOR CROHN'S DISEASE
Perineal Wound after Proctectomy

The perineal wound that is created after proctectomy for CD does not always heal primarily, and delayed healing after proctectomy has been a common difficulty. This fact is especially true in the patient who has perineal CD.[41] In some patients, this can be averted. The patient with an anorectal abscess should have this drained before definitive proctectomy. In addition, some patients with severe perianal CD with abscesses and fistulae may benefit from fecal diversion before definitive proctectomy. This procedure may increase the chance of primary healing and decrease the incidence of the nonhealed perineal wound. Yamamoto and colleagues[39] retrospectively reviewed 145 patients who underwent proctocolectomy for CD from 1970 to 1997; 33 patients (23%) developed a persistent perineal sinus after TPC/I. Multivariate analysis showed age, rectal involvement of CD, and fecal contamination at the time of surgery as risk factors for persistent perineal sinus. The investigators also noted that an extrasphincteric dissection was an additional risk factor for a persistent perineal sinus.

High Ileostomy Output after Total Proctocolectomy with End Ileostomy

High ileostomy output, known also as ileostomy diarrhea, can be quite disabling for some patients with CD who have had TPC/I. Some patients seem prone to this complication, such as those who have had a previous cholecystectomy (bile-acid-induced diarrhea) or the patient who has had a prior ileal resection for CD. In addition, dehydration is common when output is greater than 2 L/d (normal ileostomy output is 800–1000 mL/d).[42] Other common complaints in the patient with dehydration from high stoma output include decreased urine output and concentrated-appearing urine.[42]

Treatment should begin with the restriction of hypotonic fluids. The luminal concentration of sodium must be increased in order to cause sodium to be reabsorbed. Sodium absorption in the jejunum is coupled with glucose absorption; therefore, oral intake of a glucose-saline solution will lead to increased sodium reabsorption and a concomitant decrease in ileostomy output.[42]

Initial medical therapy should begin with antimotility agents, such as loperamide. Loperamide has the advantages of being an over-the-counter product and being nonaddictive. Other medical treatment options for patients with continued high ileostomy output include codeine phosphate, Lomotil (diphenoxylate hydrochloride and atropine sulfate), and tincture of opium. The use of the long-acting somatostatin analog octreotide has been reported in patients with high stoma output.[43]

While treatment of ileostomy diarrhea is usually successful with loperamide, other more novel treatment regimens have been studied. One novel treatment option for ileostomy diarrhea is the use of budesonide. Ecker and colleagues[44] studied 23 patients with CD and high ileostomy output (defined as >1000 mL/d). No other antiinflammatory agents were allowed. The patients were treated with budesonide 3 mg orally thrice daily for 4 weeks. Preoperative evaluation revealed no evidence of active inflammation. Budesonide was withdrawn, and there was a statistically significant increase in ileostomy output of 295 g/d; 20 of 22 patients had an increase in ileostomy output. Budesonide was reintroduced, and ileostomy output decreased by 323.7 g/d. Twenty patients had a decrease in ileostomy output. The investigators concluded that the antidiarrheal effect of budesonide is independent of its antiinflammatory effect.[44]

Perianal Crohn's Disease

Although CD was first described as a unique entity in 1932,[45] perianal disease was first described in 1959.[46] Perianal Crohn's Disease (PCD) is more commonly found in patients with CD involving both the colon and rectum.[47] Hellers and colleagues[48] found that 92% of patients with CD involving the colon and rectum had perianal disease, whereas only 41% of patients with CD with rectal sparing had perianal involvement. PCD is much less common in patients with small bowel or ileocolic CD, as Hellers and colleagues[48] found that patients with isolated ileal disease had an incidence of perianal disease of 12%, whereas 15% of patients with ileocolic CD had perianal disease.

Anorectal findings in PCD include not only anal fistulae but also anal tags, anal fissures, hemorrhoids, perianal abscesses, and strictures. Michelassi and colleagues[49] reported on 224 patients with anorectal complications of CD; 66 patients had a combination of anorectal findings. Other common findings included anal fistulae (51 patients) and anorectal abscesses (36 patients). Forty patients had anal stenosis.[49]

Besides anatomic findings, PCD can also be classified by the activity and impact on quality of life. A scoring system for gauging the activity of PCD has been developed.[50] The Perianal Disease Activity Index takes into account fistula activity, restriction of activities, and the severity of perianal disease. The score is based on a 5-point scale and has been validated. The status of the rectum is also an important consideration in selecting treatment options because active proctitis resulting from CD will have a negative impact on perianal disease as well as decrease the number of possible treatment options for PCD.[51]

Treatment options for PCD depend on the type of findings. The anatomy of disease in CD is clearly different from that of a typical cryptoglandular disease, and therefore, the chance of healing after surgical treatment is also different. For patients with significant disease, fecal diversion in the form of an ostomy may be required.

Anal Fistulae

For patients with anal fistulae, several treatment options exist. Patients with simple (subcutaneous or intersphincteric) and singular anal fistulae may be treated with fistulotomy. However, in the patient with CD and multiple or complex anal fistulae, non–sphincter-preserving procedures such as fistulotomy should be used sparingly because of the risk of fecal incontinence.[51] Therefore, when a patient with PCD has multiple fistulae or fistulae that involve a significant amount of anal sphincter, consideration should be given to sphincter preservation. These patients are best treated with draining setons while control of their CD is obtained. As will be discussed, this may require medical therapy, and occasionally, fecal diversion. After this has been achieved, more definitive treatment of the fistulae can be initiated. This treatment may include anal fistula plugs, rectal advancement flaps, ligation of the intersphincteric fistula tract (LIFT procedure), or an anal fistulotomy.

Anal fistula plugs have also been used in patients with PCD. However, the use of such plugs has been studied much less extensively in patients with PCD than in those with cryptoglandular anal fistulae. In fact, several of the randomized trials studying anal fistula plugs have specifically excluded patients with CD.[52] A recent systematic review of the use of anal fistula plugs evaluated the efficacy in patients with fistulae related to CD.[53] Although the efficacy for anal fistula plugs was similar between patients with cryptoglandular anal fistulae and fistulae related to CD (55% vs 54%), the investigators concluded that the anal fistula plug had not been adequately studied in patients with CD.

Rectal mucosal advancement flaps have also been studied in PCD. A recent systematic review of endorectal advancement flap revealed that flaps done for cryptoglandular disease were much more successful than those done for CD (81% success rate vs 64% success rate). However, it should be noted that, in this review, many more patients were identified with cryptoglandular disease than with CD (1335 patients vs 91 patients).[54]

LIFT is a newer procedure, which has had early success in the treatment of patients with transsphincteric anal fistulae. Use of LIFT in patients with CD has been studied on a limited basis. Similar to other surgical options for patients with anal fistulae related to CD, success rates are lower. A recent prospective study of LIFT in 15 patients with CD revealed a 67% success rate at 12 months. The investigators concluded that patients with anal fistulae associated with CD could be treated with LIFT. No other studies of LIFT in patients with PCD are yet available.[55]

Anal Stenosis and Strictures

Anal stenosis and strictures are a common finding in patients with PCD and can be difficult to treat. Most strictures are thought to be the result of long-standing inflammation.[56] These strictures can be graded as either reversible (inflammatory) or irreversible (fibrostenotic). The location of strictures can be either anal or distal rectal. The location is important in determining the appropriate treatment. Brochard and colleagues[56] reviewed 102 patients with anorectal strictures in the setting of CD; 76% of strictures were inflammatory and 24% were fibrostenotic. It was observed that 34% patients developed an anal fistula. After a median follow-up of 2.8 years, 59% of the strictures had healed. As would be expected, inflammatory strictures were much more likely to heal. Factors associated with stricture healing were female sex, duration of CD less than 10 years, and presence of an anal fistula; 25% of patients required a stoma. The presence or absence of proctitis was not noted in their study, and it is unknown if this affected healing. The use of biological agents, particularly anti–tumor necrosis factor agents, contributed to the high healing rate of anorectal strictures.[56]

Fecal Diversion for Perianal Crohn's Disease

CD has a bimodal presentation with respect to age of onset. Therefore, it most commonly presents in both younger and older adults.[57] It has been shown that an earlier age at presentation is associated with a more severe phenotype. Also, it follows that more severe disease would require more extensive surgical treatment, including the possibility of a permanent ostomy. Understandably, the prospect of an ileostomy for the younger patient can provoke anxiety.[58]

The prospect of a temporary diverting ileostomy without intestinal resection has been discussed for some time for the patient with severe PCD. A loop ileostomy is the most common form of fecal diversion in this situation, and it can often be done laparoscopically.[59] It has been shown that medical therapy combined with fecal diversion can control the patient's sIBD.[60] One key issue that is important to discuss with the patient preoperatively is whether or not the ostomy is temporary because many of these ostomies may become permanent.

In 2007, Mueller and colleagues[61] reported a series of patients with perianal CD. From 1992 to 1995, 97 patients with CD (whose follow-up data were available) were treated. Of the 97 patients, 51 required temporary fecal diversion (again, most commonly by loop ileostomy). Of the 51 patients, 24 ultimately had stoma reversal (47%). The investigators concluded that the risk of permanent fecal diversion was high in patients with complicated perianal disease requiring colorectal resection, but in patients with perianal CD requiring small bowel resection or segmental colonic resection, there was no risk of a permanent stoma.[61]

Mennigen and colleagues[59] identified 33 patients between 2003 and 2012 who underwent what was intended to be a temporary ileostomy for CD; 22 of 29 patients (4 were excluded because of missing data) underwent fecal diversion for perianal CD. Stoma reversal was done in 19 of 25 patients for whom follow-up data was available. However, only 4 of 25 patients had stoma reversal without the need for further surgery. The investigators concluded that although most stomas were indeed temporary, most patients required surgery for the same reason for which they underwent the initial stoma; this was done at a median of 18.5 months after closure of the ileostomy. Of these 19 patients, 7 had a definitive stoma created.[59]

Biological therapy for treatment of IBD has had a significant impact, and treatment of IBD improved with the introduction of infliximab in 1998. Therefore, it would be expected that with improved treatment response rates, the patient with PCD could hope to have a lower risk of a permanent stoma. This fact has been investigated by Hong and colleagues.[62] The investigators identified 21 patients from 1990 to 2007 with perianal CD who underwent fecal diversion. The median age was 34 years. The median follow-up time was 22 months. At 22 months, 4 patients had undergone stoma closure, 11 had had proctocolectomy, and 6 patients still had a stoma. The investigators reviewed the effect of fecal diversion on the course of perianal CD in these patients. In 4 patients (19%), no effect was seen, and 6 patients had temporary improvement (29%). There was initial improvement with a later plateau in 7 patients (33%) and healing in 4 patients (19%). Of the 21 patients, 11 (52%) received infliximab. In this group, 4 patients underwent proctocolectomy and 2 had intestinal continuity restored. There was no statistically significant difference in stoma reversal between the infliximab and the noninfliximab group.

This view was echoed by Gu and colleagues[63] who reviewed 138 patients with PCD undergoing fecal diversion from 1994 to 2012 at the Cleveland Clinic, Ohio. Only 22% of patients had stoma closure. A total of 45 (33%) patients underwent proctectomy with a permanent stoma and 63 patients (45%) underwent proctectomy with permanent stoma formation after a mean follow-up of 5.7 years. No difference was identified in the outcome based on the type of medical treatment, including treatment with biological agents ($P = .25$).[63] However, when Coscia and colleagues[64] reviewed the course of 233 patients with anorectal CD who were treated between 1995 and 2010, they found that there was a decrease in the risk of permanent stoma from 60.8% in the prebiological therapy era to 19.2% in the biological therapy era. As there seems to be a difference of opinion regarding the impact of biological therapy on the risk of a permanent stoma, debate will most likely continue.

Several different clinical presentations of PCD can make it particularly difficult both to deal with and to treat. The first is the isolated finding of perianal disease without proximal intestinal (either small or large bowel) involvement; this only occurs in less than 5% of patients.[65] The physician who is confronted with unusual perianal disease should recall that CD does not always manifest with intestinal involvement, and this may create difficulty in diagnosis for the treating physician, especially because isolated perianal disease is relatively uncommon. Therefore, it is important for the treating clinician to be aware of isolated perianal CD.

Another presentation that can be difficult to deal with is the presentation of perianal disease in the patient who was previously diagnosed as having UC. While perianal disease is more common in patients with CD, any type of perianal disease, such as anal fissures, anal fistulae, anorectal abscesses, and hemorrhoids can occur in patients with UC. Zabana and colleagues[66] found that 5% of patients with UC had perianal disease. The investigators noted that the diagnosis was changed from UC to CD in one-third of their patients and found a higher requirement for steroids in patients with perianal disease. Therefore, it is uncommon for the patient with UC to have perianal disease. When confronted with the combination of perianal disease and UC, the diagnosis of UC should be questioned and the possibility of CD entertained.

SUMMARY

The management of patients with CD of the colon, rectum, and anus is complex and has changed since the introduction of biological agents. Timing of surgery, the optimal treatment of perianal CD, and the use and avoidance of a stoma are several of the difficult issues in the management of these patients. Segmental colectomy has a role in the management of patients with CD and rectal sparing. Patients with perianal CD should be evaluated for proximal intestinal involvement. Patients with severe perianal CD should have fecal diversion before proctectomy to prevent delayed perineal wound healing.

ACKNOWLEDGMENTS

The author would like to thank Marilyn Teolis for her assistance with researching this article.

REFERENCES

1. Zisman TL, Cohen RD. Pharmacoeconomics and quality of life of current and emerging biologic therapies for inflammatory bowel disease. Curr Treat Options Gastroenterol 2007;10(3):185–94.
2. da Luz MA, Stocchi L, Tan E, et al. Outcomes of Crohn's disease presenting with abdominopelvic abscess. Dis Colon Rectum 2009;52(5):906–12.
3. Gutierrez A, Lee H, Sands BE. Outcome of surgical versus percutaneous drainage of abdominal and pelvic abscesses in Crohn's disease. Am J Gastroenterol 2006;101(10):2283–9.
4. Neufeld D, Keidar A, Gutman M, et al. Abdominal wall abscesses in patients with Crohn's disease: clinical outcome. J Gastrointest Surg 2006;10(3):445–9.
5. Ogihara M, Masaki T, Watanabe T, et al. Psoas abscess complicating Crohn's disease: report of a case. Surg Today 2000;30(8):759–63.
6. Campieri M, Gionchetti P, Belluzzi A, et al. Efficacy of 5-aminosalicylic acid enemas versus hydrocortisone enemas in ulcerative colitis. Dig Dis Sci 1987; 32(12 Suppl):67S–70S.
7. Gordon PH, Nivatvongs S. Principles and practice of surgery for the Colon, rectum, and anus. London: Informa Healthcare USA, Inc; 2007.
8. Jalan KN, Sircus W, Card WI, et al. An experience of ulcerative colitis. I. Toxic dilation in 55 cases. Gastroenterology 1969;57(1):68–82.
9. Hefaiedh R, Cheikh M, Ennaifer R, et al. Toxic megacolon complicating a first course of Crohn's disease: about two cases. Clin Pract 2013;3(2):e24.
10. Heppell J, Farkouh E, Dube S, et al. Toxic megacolon. An analysis of 70 cases. Dis Colon Rectum 1986;29(12):789–92.
11. Greenstein AJ, Sachar DB, Gibas A, et al. Outcome of toxic dilatation in ulcerative and Crohn's colitis. J Clin Gastroenterol 1985;7(2):137–43.
12. Kostka R, Lukas M. Massive, life-threatening bleeding in Crohn's disease. Acta Chir Belg 2005;105(2):168–74.
13. Robert JR, Sachar DB, Greenstein AJ. Severe gastrointestinal hemorrhage in Crohn's disease. Ann Surg 1991;213(3):207–11.
14. Belaiche J, Louis E, D'Haens G, et al. Acute lower gastrointestinal bleeding in Crohn's disease: characteristics of a unique series of 34 patients. Belgian IBD Research Group. Am J Gastroenterol 1999;94(8):2177–81.
15. Aniwan S, Eakpongpaisit S, Imraporn B, et al. Infliximab stopped severe gastrointestinal bleeding in Crohn's disease. World J Gastroenterol 2012;18(21): 2730–4.
16. Coviello LC, Stein SL. Surgical management of nonpolypoid colorectal lesions and strictures in colonic inflammatory bowel disease. Gastrointest Endosc Clin N Am 2014;24(3):447–54.
17. Gumaste V, Sachar DB, Greenstein AJ. Benign and malignant colorectal strictures in ulcerative colitis. Gut 1992;33(7):938–41.
18. Yamazaki Y, Ribeiro MB, Sachar DB, et al. Malignant colorectal strictures in Crohn's disease. Am J Gastroenterol 1991;86(7):882–5.
19. Katsanos KH, Tsianos VE, Maliouki M, et al. Obstruction and pseudo-obstruction in inflammatory bowel disease. Ann Gastroenterol 2010;23(4):243–56.
20. Martel P, Betton PO, Gallot D, et al. Crohn's colitis: experience with segmental resections; results in a series of 84 patients. J Am Coll Surg 2002;194(4):448–53.
21. Fichera A, McCormack R, Rubin MA, et al. Long-term outcome of surgically treated Crohn's colitis: a prospective study. Dis Colon Rectum 2005;48(5): 963–9.

22. Tekkis PP, Purkayastha S, Lanitis S, et al. A comparison of segmental vs subtotal/total colectomy for colonic Crohn's disease: a meta-analysis. Colorectal Dis 2006; 8(2):82–90.

23. Longo WE, Oakley JR, Lavery IC, et al. Outcome of ileorectal anastomosis for Crohn's colitis. Dis Colon Rectum 1992;35(11):1066–71.

24. O'Riordan JM, O'Connor BI, Huang H, et al. Long-term outcome of colectomy and ileorectal anastomosis for Crohn's colitis. Dis Colon Rectum 2011;54(11):1347–54.

25. Scoglio D, Ahmed AU, Fichera A. Surgical treatment of ulcerative colitis: ileorectal vs ileal pouch-anal anastomosis. World J Gastroenterol 2014;20(37):13211–8.

26. Brown CJ, Maclean AR, Cohen Z, et al. Crohn's disease and indeterminate colitis and the ileal pouch-anal anastomosis: outcomes and patterns of failure. Dis Colon Rectum 2005;48(8):1542–9.

27. Sagar PM, Dozois RR, Wolff BG. Long-term results of ileal pouch-anal anastomosis in patients with Crohn's disease. Dis Colon Rectum 1996;39(8):893–8.

28. Panis Y, Poupard B, Nemeth J, et al. Ileal pouch/anal anastomosis for Crohn's disease. Lancet 1996;347(9005):854–7.

29. Regimbeau JM, Panis Y, Pocard M, et al. Long-term results of ileal pouch-anal anastomosis for colorectal Crohn's disease. Dis Colon Rectum 2001;44(6):769–78.

30. Mylonakis E, Allan RN, Keighley MR. How does pouch construction for a final diagnosis of Crohn's disease compare with ileoproctostomy for established Crohn's proctocolitis? Dis Colon Rectum 2001;44(8):1137–42.

31. Carter FM, McLeod RS, Cohen Z. Subtotal colectomy for ulcerative colitis: complications related to the rectal remnant. Dis Colon Rectum 1991;34(11):1005–9.

32. Ng RL, Davies AH, Grace RH, et al. Subcutaneous rectal stump closure after emergency subtotal colectomy. Br J Surg 1992;79(7):701–3.

33. Trickett JP, Tilney HS, Gudgeon AM, et al. Management of the rectal stump after emergency sub-total colectomy: which surgical option is associated with the lowest morbidity? Colorectal Dis 2005;7(5):519–22.

34. Strong SA, Koltun WA, Hyman NH, et al. Practice parameters for the surgical management of Crohn's disease. Dis Colon Rectum 2007;50(11):1735–46.

35. Cattan P, Bonhomme N, Panis Y, et al. Fate of the rectum in patients undergoing total colectomy for Crohn's disease. Br J Surg 2002;89(4):454–9.

36. Geoghegan JG, Carton E, O'Shea AM, et al. Crohn's colitis: the fate of the rectum. Int J Colorectal Dis 1998;13(5–6):256–9.

37. Rieger N, Collopy B, Fink R, et al. Total colectomy for Crohn's disease. Aust N Z J Surg 1999;69(1):28–30.

38. Cirincione E, Gorfine SR, Bauer JJ. Is Hartmann's procedure safe in Crohn's disease? Report of three cases. Dis Colon Rectum 2000;43(4):544–7.

39. Yamamoto T, Allan RN, Keighley MR. Audit of single-stage proctocolectomy for Crohn's disease: postoperative complications and recurrence. Dis Colon Rectum 2000;43(2):249–56.

40. de Buck van Overstraeten A, Wolthuis AM, Vermeire S, et al. Intersphincteric proctectomy with end-colostomy for anorectal Crohn's disease results in early and severe proximal colonic recurrence. J Crohns Colitis 2013;7(6):e227–31.

41. Genua JC, Vivas DA. Management of nonhealing perineal wounds. Clin Colon Rectal Surg 2007;20(4):322–8.

42. Tsao SK, Baker M, Nightingale JM. High-output stoma after small-bowel resections for Crohn's disease. Nat Clin Pract Gastroenterol Hepatol 2005;2(12):604–8.

43. Neef B, Horing E, von GU. Successful treatment of a life-threatening ileostomy diarrhea with the somatostatin analog octreotide. Dtsch Med Wochenschr 1994;119(24):869–74 [in German].

44. Ecker KW, Stallmach A, Loffler J, et al. Long-term treatment of high intestinal output syndrome with budesonide in patients with Crohn's disease and ileostomy. Dis Colon Rectum 2005;48(2):237–42.

45. Crohn BB, Ginzburg L, Oppenheimer GD. Regional ileitis: a pathologic and clinical entity. 1932. Mt Sinai J Med 2000;67(3):263–8.

46. Morson B, Lockhart-Mummery HE. Anal lesions in Crohn's disease. Lancet 1959; 2:1122–3.

47. Lewis RT, Bleier JI. Surgical treatment of anorectal Crohn's Disease. Clin Colon Rectal Surg 2013;26(2):90–9.

48. Hellers G, Bergstrand O, Ewerth S, et al. Occurrence and outcome after primary treatment of anal fistulae in Crohn's disease. Gut 1980;21(6):525–7.

49. Michelassi F, Melis M, Rubin M, et al. Surgical treatment of anorectal complications in Crohn's disease. Surgery 2000;128(4):597–603.

50. Irvine EJ. Usual therapy improves perianal Crohn's disease as measured by a new disease activity index. McMaster IBD Study Group. J Clin Gastroenterol 1995;20(1):27–32.

51. Sandborn WJ, Fazio VW, Feagan BG, et al. AGA technical review on perianal Crohn's disease. Gastroenterology 2003;125(5):1508–30.

52. Stamos MJ, Snyder M, Robb BW, et al. Prospective multicenter study of a synthetic bioabsorbable anal fistula plug to treat cryptoglandular transsphincteric anal fistulas. Dis Colon Rectum 2015;58(3):344–51.

53. O'Riordan JM, Datta I, Johnston C, et al. A systematic review of the anal fistula plug for patients with Crohn's and non-Crohn's related fistula-in-ano. Dis Colon Rectum 2012;55(3):351–8.

54. Soltani A, Kaiser AM. Endorectal advancement flap for cryptoglandular or Crohn's fistula-in-ano. Dis Colon Rectum 2010;53(4):486–95.

55. Gingold DS, Murrell ZA, Fleshner PR. A prospective evaluation of the ligation of the intersphincteric tract procedure for complex anal fistula in patients with Crohn's disease. Ann Surg 2014;260(6):1057–61.

56. Brochard C, Siproudhis L, Wallenhorst T, et al. Anorectal stricture in 102 patients with Crohn's disease: natural history in the era of biologics. Aliment Pharmacol Ther 2014;40(7):796–803.

57. Bayless TM, Tokayer AZ, Polito JM, et al. Crohn's disease: concordance for site and clinical type in affected family members–potential hereditary influences. Gastroenterology 1996;111(3):573–9.

58. Allison M, Lindsay J, Gould D, et al. Surgery in young adults with inflammatory bowel disease: a narrative account. Int J Nurs Stud 2013;50(11): 1566–75.

59. Mennigen R, Heptner B, Senninger N, et al. Temporary fecal diversion in the management of colorectal and perianal Crohn's disease. Gastroenterol Res Pract 2015;2015:286315.

60. Uzzan M, Stefanescu C, Maggiori L, et al. Case series: does a combination of anti-TNF antibodies and transient ileal fecal stream diversion in severe Crohn's colitis with perianal fistula prevent definitive stoma? Am J Gastroenterol 2013; 108(10):1666–8.

61. Mueller MH, Geis M, Glatzle J, et al. Risk of fecal diversion in complicated perianal Crohn's disease. J Gastrointest Surg 2007;11(4):529–37.

62. Hong MK, Craig LA, Bell S, et al. Faecal diversion in the management of perianal Crohn's disease. Colorectal Dis 2011;13(2):171–6.

63. Gu J, Valente MA, Remzi FH, et al. Factors affecting the fate of faecal diversion in patients with perianal Crohn's disease. Colorectal Dis 2015;17(1):66–72.

64. Coscia M, Gentilini L, Laureti S, et al. Risk of permanent stoma in extensive Crohn's colitis: the impact of biological drugs. Colorectal Dis 2013;15(9):1115–22.

65. Bell SJ, Williams AB, Wiesel P, et al. The clinical course of fistulating Crohn's disease. Aliment Pharmacol Ther 2003;17(9):1145–51.

66. Zabana Y, Van DM, Garcia-Planella E, et al. Perianal disease in patients with ulcerative colitis: a case-control study. J Crohns Colitis 2011;5(4):338–41.

Indications and Options for Surgery in Ulcerative Colitis

Jaime L. Bohl, MD*, Kathryn Sobba, MD

KEYWORDS

- Inflammatory bowel disease • Surgery • Ulcerative colitis • Total proctocolectomy
- Ileal pouch–anal anastomosis

KEY POINTS

- Current elective indications for surgical therapy in ulcerative colitis include cancer, risk for cancer (dysplasia), stricture, medical intractability, overwhelming side effects of medical treatment, and unresponsive extraintestinal manifestations.
- Patients with ulcerative colitis may require emergency surgery in the setting of acute severe colitis that fails to respond to rescue therapy, fulminant colitis, toxic megacolon, perforation, or stricture.
- Total abdominal colectomy is a surgical treatment option that allows patients who require emergency surgery to reestablish nutrition and withdraw immunosuppressive medication so that pelvic surgery and ileoanal pouch formation is performed when the patient is in good health.
- Anastomotic techniques included double-stapled anastomosis and hand-sewn techniques with mucosectomy. Outcomes for both techniques are acceptable and the clinical circumstances, such as dysplasia, need for oncologic margins, and pouch reach into the pelvis, should determine the technique used.

INTRODUCTION

Ulcerative colitis (UC) is a chronic inflammatory disease characterized by inflammation that is limited to the mucosa of the colon and rectum.[1] The disease starts at the rectum and extends proximally for varying lengths and in its greatest extent can reach the cecum.[2] Approximately 500,000 people in the United States carry a diagnosis of UC, with an incidence of around 12 per 100,000 per year.[3] Surgery to remove the colon and rectum is considered curative. Between 4% and 9% of

Disclosures: Neither author has a disclosure to make.
Department of Surgery, Wake Forest School of Medicine, Medical Center Boulevard, Winston Salem, NC 27157, USA
* Corresponding author.
E-mail address: jbohl@wakehealth.edu

patients with UC require proctocolectomy within the first year of diagnosis, and the risk of surgical treatment following that is 1% per year.[4–6] Patients with the following risk factors are more likely to develop complications requiring colectomy: disease that extends proximal to the splenic flexure, male gender, patients with corticosteroid resistance, and complications related to corticosteroid administration.[7] Ultimately, patients with UC may require surgery for presence of cancer, accumulating risk for cancer development, medical intractability, or development of a life-threatening complication such as toxic colitis, toxic megacolon, and hemorrhage. Surgical consultation can provide discussion of risks and benefits of surgery, type of surgery for which the individual patient is a candidate, and long-term outcomes of surgical treatment. This article discusses the indications and surgical options for patients with UC.

INDICATIONS FOR SURGERY IN PATIENTS WITH ULCERATIVE COLITIS
Cancer Risk

Colorectal cancer is one of the most common causes for mortality in patients with UC.[8] Cumulative risk for colorectal cancer in patients with ulcerative colitis is 2% after 10 years, 8% after 20 years, and 18% after 30 years of diagnosis.[8] Proctocolectomy is recommended in patients with ulcerative colitis who develop colon or rectal cancer, high-grade dysplasia, nonadenomalike dysplasia–associated lesion or mass, and adenoma associated with dysplasia at the base or surrounding areas of inflammation.[9–11] Proctocolectomy in patients with ulcerative colitis with low-grade dysplasia is controversial and should be recommended based on the individual patient's risk for carcinoma development versus surgical complication.[12] Stricture in the setting of ulcerative colitis should also prompt surgical therapy. Although only 25% of strictures that develop in the setting of UC are malignant,[13] biopsy to differentiate benign versus malignant stricture is unreliable.[14]

Intractability

The most common indication for elective surgical treatment of UC is intractable disease. Intractability is present when medical therapy fails to control disease symptoms or extraintestinal manifestations, when medication side effects produce poor quality of life or problems with patient compliance, or when effective long-term medication use results in accumulating or unacceptable risks.[12]

Emergency Situations

Acute severe UC, the most common indication for emergent surgery, has been defined by passage of more than 6 bloody stools per day with associated fever, tachycardia, hemoglobin level less than 75% of normal, and an increased sedimentation rate. Fulminant colitis occurs when patients have more than 10 bloody stools per day, anemia requiring transfusion, and colonic distention on abdominal radiographs.[15] Severe colitis that is refractory to intravenous steroid treatment may undergo medical salvage therapy with infliximab or cyclosporine. However, presence of impending perforation, multisystem organ dysfunction, or failure to respond to rescue medical therapy is an absolute indication for surgical therapy.[16] Toxic megacolon is defined as the presence of transverse colon dilatation greater than 6 cm, which can progress to pneumatosis and colonic perforation.[17] Because perforation is associated with a mortality between 27% and 57%,[18,19] patients should be taken for surgery if toxic megacolon persists or does not improve with medical treatment.

EMERGENT SURGICAL TECHNIQUES
Emergent Open Total Abdominal Colectomy with End Ileostomy

Open abdominal colectomy is the most common emergent procedure in patients with UC. This procedure can be performed quickly, thereby minimizing time under anesthesia. The risk of mortality and morbidity to the patient is half that of total proctocolectomy (TPC).[20] In addition, total colectomy allows for removal of the bulk of diseased colonic segment, patient symptoms to subside, steroid withdrawal, and nutritional improvement so further reconstruction can be performed when the patient is in optimal health.

Preoperative planning

All patients who undergo placement of a temporary or permanent ileostomy should have education regarding its function, complications, and effect on quality of life. Health care providers should show patients pictures of a stoma, explain the daily care of a stoma, and introduce the equipment necessary to pouch the stoma. Other patients who have recovered from surgeries in which a stoma was placed may volunteer to talk to patients on a peer basis to reduce fear. The patient's abdomen should be marked away from bony prominences and skin folds and in a position that the patient can visualize. The placement of a stoma should be assessed in the supine, sitting, and standing positions to visualize changes in the abdominal wall contour. Attention to these details preoperatively improves the function and care of a stoma postoperatively.

Prep and positioning

The patient is brought to the operating room and general anesthesia is induced. A Foley catheter is inserted and the patient is placed into lithotomy position. Lithotomy position allows the surgical assistant to move to a position between the patient's legs when mobilizing the splenic flexure and improve surgical visualization. The patient's abdomen is prepped and draped and preoperative antibiotics are administered.

Intra-abdominal access

A full midline laparotomy incision allows for visualization of the hepatic and splenic flexures for swift mobilization. Placement of self-retaining retractors such as a Bookwalter may be used to improve exposure. Alternatively, a large or extralarge rigid wound retractor can be placed, with rolled laparotomy pads used to assist with retraction and exposure.

Right colon mobilization

The right colon must be fully mobilized by incising the white line of Toldt from inferior to superior, thereby allowing rotation of the cecum, right colon, and mesocolon medially. As the right colon is rolled medially, the avascular, areolar plane between the right mesocolon and retroperitoneum is divided. In addition, the terminal ileum attachments to the retroperitoneum above the pelvic inlet and right common iliac vessels must be incised for ileal mobility (**Fig. 1**). Care must be taken to avoid injury to the gonadal vessels, ureter, and duodenum, which lay posterior to the areolar plane. The retroperitoneal location of these structures is preserved as the right colon is released and rolled medially. The gastrocolic ligament is incised by dissecting the omentum off the proximal transverse colon in a medial to right lateral fashion. In addition, the hepatocolic ligament is ligated (**Fig. 2**).

Pitfalls

Dissection in a plane lateral to the white line of Toldt and too far superior results in right kidney mobilization. Failure to retract the right colon medially while dissecting the areolar attachments may result in duodenal injury secondary to poor visualization.

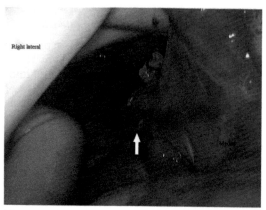

Fig. 1. The terminal ileum and its mesentery are lifted from the retroperitoneal attachments just above the iliac vessels and right ureter. *Arrow* marks right ureter.

However, excessive medial retraction of the right colon at the level of the duodenum can result in avulsion of a large venous collateral branch between the inferior pancreaticoduodenal vein and middle colic vein.

Omental preservation
The omentum is then dissected from the transverse colon by incising the avascular plane between them. The omentum with pale yellow fat is retracted superiorly as the transverse colon and deeper yellow epiploicae are retracted inferiorly. Entrance into the lesser sac can be confirmed by visualization of the posterior stomach superiorly and the transverse mesocolon and pancreas posteriorly. As the surgeon proceeds in the right to left direction, there is a double leaflet of the omentum, which should be dissected from the distal transverse colon for full mobilization. The surgeon should follow the superolateral movement of the colon into the left upper quadrant to avoid entry into the colonic lumen.

Left colon mobilization
The sigmoid colon is then identified and retracted medially in order to place the peritoneal reflection on stretch. Incision of the left line of Toldt from inferior to superior allows the

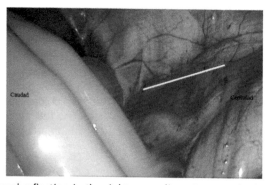

Fig. 2. The peritoneal reflection in the right paracolic gutter must be incised to rotate the right colon and its mesentery off the retroperitoneal attachments. The *white line* marks the plane required for incision.

surgeon to identify the loose areolar plane between the left mesocolon and retroperitoneum. Additional lateral attachments of the sigmoid colon may require incision to allow for full retraction in a right medial direction. As the left colon is retracted to the right side of the patient, the gonadal vessels and then more medially the ureter can be identified crossing over the iliac vessels (**Fig. 3**). Working in an inferior to superior direction the retroperitoneum is dissected from the mesocolon using a combination of blunt and sharp dissection. As the surgeon encounters the Gerota fascia more superiorly, this dissection becomes more difficult because the attachment between mesocolon and fascia is tougher (**Fig. 4**). The left colon is completely mobilized when the retroperitoneum has been released from the left mesocolon several centimeters short of the abdominal aorta.

Splenic flexure mobilization

Incision of the peritoneal reflection in the left paracolic gutter is carried cephalad past the splenic flexure. The peritoneal incision is carried cephalad past the splenic flexure of the colon. Careful medial retraction of the proximal left colon allows for further dissection of the left mesocolon off the Gerota fascia (**Fig. 5**). Cautery of the phrenocolic and splenocolic ligaments is performed. Eventually the surgeon should be able to encircle the splenic flexure by entering the plane from the previous omental dissection. The remaining attachments are then cauterized.

Pitfalls

The tendon of the iliopsoas muscle may be mistakenly identified as the ureter by the novice. This tendon is located superolateral to the ureter. Complete dissection of all fat from the iliopsoas muscle may signify that the retroperitoneal structures are retracted medially with the left mesocolon. Dissection in a plane more medial, between the left colon and retroperitoneum, should be identified. The surgeon should use the same areolar plane between the proximal left colon and Gerota fascia to avoid mobilizing the left kidney or bleeding from dissection within the pararenal fat. Tearing of the splenic capsule can occur from aggressive medial and inferior traction on the proximal left colon before ligament transection at the splenic flexure. If visualization of the plane from inferior to superior becomes difficult, the surgeon should approach the splenic flexure from the previous gastrocolic dissection used to remove the omentum from the transverse colon. In addition, failure to dissect the tough Gerota facial attachments to the proximal left mesocolon prevents full mobilization of the left colon and splenic flexure. These attachments are posterior to the colon and its mesentery, whereas splenic flexure attachments to the colon are lateral and superior.

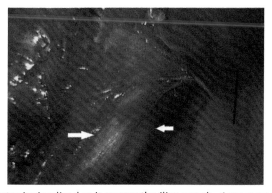

Fig. 3. The left ureter is visualized as it crosses the iliac vessels. *Arrows* mark left ureter as it crosses the iliac vessels.

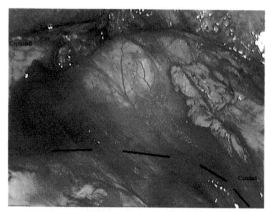

Fig. 4. The areolar attachments of the left colon mesentery must be incised to mobilize it from the Gerota fascia and the retroperitoneum. The *black dotted line* marks the line of left colon mesentery attachment to Gerota's fascia and the retroperitoneum.

Bowel transection
A linear stapler is fired across the terminal ileocecal junction and at the rectosigmoid junction.

Division of the vascular pedicles
Division of the mesocolon can now proceed in a right to left fashion. The surgeon can use an energy device or clamp-and-tie technique. A window above and below each of the vascular pedicles (ileocolic, right colic, middle colic, left colic, and inferior mesenteric vessels) can be made to ensure complete ligation of the pedicle.

Pitfalls
The surgeon should take care not to enter the areolar plane between the mesorectum and parietal fascia of the pelvis in order to preserve dissection planes for future surgical reconstruction. If necessary, the surgeon may leave a cuff of sigmoid colon on the distal staple line to avoid septic complications at the pelvic inlet. It is recommended to take the vascular pedicles midway between their origin and the mesenteric side of the

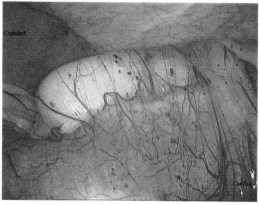

Fig. 5. Blunt dissection is used to visualize the splenocolic ligament for full splenic flexure mobilization.

colon. This method allows for control of the major vessels before branching into smaller vessels but preserves a proximal length that can be grasped and easily controlled in the event of bleeding. The 1 exception to this recommendation is the ileocolic vessel when future ileoanal pouch reconstruction is planned. Preservation of the entire ileocolic pedicle length is important for ileal collateral vessels that supply the future ileal pouch.

Ileostomy creation

The right lower quadrant of the abdominal wall is optimal for the new ileostomy. Start by making a small circumferential incision through the skin and dermis, which is amputated. The surgeon then dissects down through the subcutaneous tissues using a combination of cautery and blunt dissection. Retractors are then used to visualize the anterior rectus sheath, which is incised vertically. Heavy scissors are then placed vertically, opened, and rotated 90° to bluntly retract the rectus fibers and expose the posterior rectus sheath. Retractors are replaced to include the rectus fibers, and the posterior rectus fascia is incised vertically for several centimeters to allow inclusion of 2 fingers. The terminal ileum is delivered through this orifice without tension, while ensuring that the mesentery does not become twisted through the ileostomy orifice.

Pitfalls

The terminal ileum should sit at the abdominal wall without tension. Failure to mobilize the terminal ileal mesentery from the retroperitoneum limits the mobility of the ileostomy. Inability to lift the terminal ileum through the abdominal wall orifice may be secondary to a bulky small bowel mesentery. This technique requires opening of the fascia and skin orifice to accommodate further ileal mobilization.

Procedure completion

The abdomen is irrigated and inspected to ensure hemostasis in all quadrants. The midline incision is closed. The ileostomy is matured in a Brooke fashion by amputating the distal staple line and folding the ileum over itself for 1 to 2 cm before suturing the distal ileal to the deep dermis.

Additional Considerations

Fate of preserved rectum

A total abdominal colectomy with end ileostomy and Hartmann pouch of the rectal stump is the preferred procedure for patients with UC who are acutely ill. Before reconstructive surgery, a pathologic assessment of resected tissue can confirm or change the initial diagnosis. In addition, this procedure allows patients to assess the impact of an ileostomy on their lives. This assessment allows patients to be more informed about choices for future elective surgery. If present, rectal symptoms before proctectomy can be controlled with mesalamine enemas. However, because of ongoing low-grade symptoms from the rectal pouch and the risk for rectal cancer, proctectomy should be performed whether the patient desires ileal anal anastomosis or not.[21]

Laparoscopic versus open approach

Although the technical aspects of laparoscopic colectomy, proctectomy, and ileal anal pouch creation are beyond the scope of this article, some surgeons have shown that a minimally invasive approach in patients with fulminant UC is a reasonable operative strategy. Such an approach by experienced surgeons has a low complication rate, low conversion rate, and increased ability to pursue a laparoscopic completion proctectomy with ileal pouch–anal anastomosis (IPAA) in the future.[22–24]

Poor rectal tissue integrity

If the colorectal segment has severe disease, the tissue may not have enough integrity to hold and heal a staple line. In these circumstances, the surgeon may bring the proximal end of the Hartman pouch to the level of the skin as a matured mucus fistula, above the fascia as a possible fistula if the staple line fails within the subcutaneous tissue, or the surgeon may suture the rectosigmoid closed and place a Malecot drain into the rectal lumen for decompression and distal drainage.

Indeterminate colitis

In 10% of patients who undergo total abdominal colectomy for acute severe or fulminant colitis, a definite diagnosis of Crohn versus UC cannot be made. Patients with indeterminate colitis have a higher rate of future Crohn's disease, perineal complications, pouchitis, and eventual IPAA loss. Patients with indeterminate colitis should be counseled regarding these increased risks before reconstructive surgery. Use of serologic markers to identify patients with indeterminate colitis who are at increased risk for these complications may inform individual patient decision making.[25]

ELECTIVE SURGICAL TECHNIQUES
Total Proctocolectomy with End Ileostomy

Patients who require elective surgery for UC may undergo a TPC with end ileostomy. This procedure has less associated morbidity because of the lack of an intestinal anastomosis. This procedure should be considered in patients with UC with impaired sphincter function, low rectal cancer, significant comorbid conditions, or patients who do not wish to assume the additional risk with restorative procedures.

Follow steps previously described for total abdominal colectomy but do not transect the colon at the rectosigmoid junction.

Rectal dissection

The small bowel should be retracted into the upper abdomen. The left ureter is identified as it crosses over the iliac vessels. The peritoneal reflection overlying the rectum is incised bilaterally, and the presacral space is entered. Blunt dissection is performed beneath the superior hemorrhoidal vessels posterior to the mesorectal plane and in the areolar tissue until both sides meet (**Fig. 6**). The superior hemorrhoidal vessels

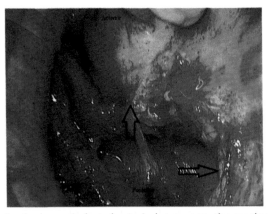

Fig. 6. The rectum is raised superiorly and anteriorly to expose the areolar plane posterior to the mesorectum and inferior to the superior hemorrhoidal vessels (*right arrow*). The up arrow marks the peritoneal refection over the left mesorectum, which must be incised to further mobilize the rectum.

are ligated with an energy device or suture ligation. The hypogastric nerves can be identified and swept posteriorly away from the mesorectum in order to preserve their function. Using a St Mark retractor, the mesorectum is retracted anteriorly while the avascular areolar plane is dissected. Care must be taken to follow the areolar plane as it meets the mesorectum anteriorly in order to avoid entry into the posterior presacral fascia and venous plexus, which can cause troublesome bleeding (**Fig. 7**). The plane is followed until the levators can be visualized within the posterior pelvic floor distal to the coccyx. Division of the lateral stalks on the right and left sides of the rectum is taken in a semicircular fashion. The areolar plane of the lateral stalks is exposed by retracting the rectum superiorly and placing the St Mark retractor on the rectum with medial force (**Fig. 8**). The surgeon can then incise lateral stalks as they course anteriorly. The anterior peritoneal plane is then incised with cautery and the areolar plane closest to the rectum is cauterized to preserve the parasympathetic plexus and avoid injury to the seminal vesicles, prostate, and vagina. Visualization of the anterior plane is best with superior and posterior retraction of the rectum and the St Mark retractor placed just above the plane of dissection and retracted anteriorly (**Fig. 9**). The dissection is complete when the rectum is fully mobilized to the levator ani muscles circumferentially.

Pitfalls
Dissection in the presacral plane away from the posterior mesorectum or failure to adequately replace the St Mark retractor as the dissection proceeds more distally on the rectum may lead to bleeding within the presacral space. This bleeding is most common in the distal third portion of the rectum as it begins to lie more anteriorly and horizontally within the pelvis compared with the more vertically oriented proximal rectum.

Anorectal dissection
The distal rectum and anal canal are removed from a perineal approach. For patients with UC with no malignancy, an intersphincteric proctectomy can be performed to preserve skeletal muscle and facilitate perineal wound closure and healing. However, in patients with UC who have distal rectal cancer and require a clear circumferential margin, an extrasphincteric perineal dissection should be performed.

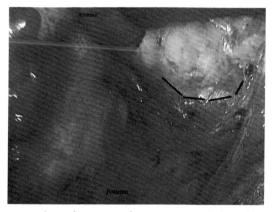

Fig. 7. A St Mark retractor is used to retract the rectum superiorly and anteriorly and expose the areolar plane between the presacral fascia and the mesorectum. The dotted line marks the plane of dissection.

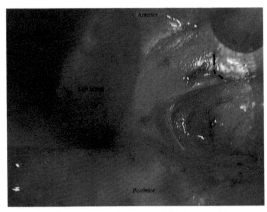

Fig. 8. The left lateral stalk of the rectum is exposed before incision. The rectum is retracted to the right and superiorly with the St Mark retractor. The left ureter and ovary are protected from injury with a malleable retractor. The dotted line marks the plane of dissection from posterior to anterior around the rectum.

Intersphincteric proctectomy

Eversion of the anal canal is performed by placing a self-retaining anal retractor (Lone Star anal retractor) or with 2 Gelpis. The intersphincteric plane is identified by palpation and injected with local anesthetic with epinephrine to facilitate hemostasis and plane dissection. The anoderm overlying the intersphincteric plane is incised. The plane is developed between the white-appearing internal anal sphincter and the red external anal sphincter. Initially, dissection is performed in the posterior plane more proximally toward the abdominal dissection. An assistant at the abdomen can assist with retraction of a Deaver placed within the intersphincteric plane as the perineal surgeon approaches the levator ani. Using the second hand, the abdominal surgeon palpates the plane between the levators and rectum posteriorly within the pelvis. The perineal surgeon then can palpate the abdominal surgeon's fingers to identify the plane through the levator ani. Once the abdominal and perineal planes are connected, the perineal surgeon follows the same planes circumferentially around the distal rectum and anal

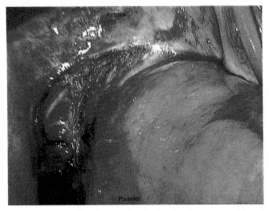

Fig. 9. The anterior peritoneal reflection to be incised using a semicircular extension of the plane exposed during lateral stalk division.

canal. In the anterior plane, the perineal surgeon must avoid straying away from the intersphincteric plane into the vagina or prostate anteriorly or the cervix and seminal vesicles superiorly. Placement of a finger with the vagina by the perineal surgeon and assistance from the abdominal surgeon to identify the plane used for pelvic dissection of the rectum away from the vagina or prostate is helpful to avoid injury (**Fig. 10**).

Extrasphincteric proctectomy

Patients with UC with distal rectal cancer require a clear circumferential margin to provide oncologic control. This margin requires resection of the entire sphincter complex. A self-retraining anal retractor is placed to evert the anal canal. A circumferential incision is made outside the anoderm and to include a portion of perianal skin. The dissection proceeds proximally outside the external sphincter within the ischioanal fossa laterally, anterior to the coccyx posteriorly and at the peroneus muscle anteriorly. The perineal surgeon then dissects in the posterior plane between the coccyx posteriorly and external sphincter anteriorly. Once dissection is proximal to the coccyx, the abdominal surgeon guides the perineal surgeon through the levator ani via palpation of the posterior dissection plane within the pelvis. Continued proximal dissection by the perineal surgeon allows connection of the perineal and abdominal surgical planes. Once this is achieved, the perineal surgeon can hook a finger along the levator ani muscles bilaterally, which allows the perineal surgeon to safely cauterize the ischioanal fat and levator ani posterolaterally. The anterior dissection should be performed carefully to prevent intrusion into the vagina and prostate, which can bleed, or even more anterior intrusion into the membranous urethra. Placement of a finger around the anterior tissue still requiring dissection at the level of the distal pelvic dissection can help guide the perineal surgeon to stay anterior to the Denonvilliers fascia along the rectovaginal septum and posterior to the prostate.

End ileostomy creation

Same as previously described.

Procedure completion

Complete circumferential excision of the anorectum allows removal of the colon and rectum from the abdominal incision. The midline incision is closed after abdominopelvic irrigation and assurance of hemostasis. A drain is placed in the posterior pelvis to

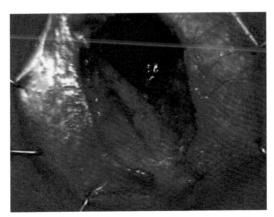

Fig. 10. The intersphincteric dissection is complete with exposure of the incised levator muscles and the retained external anal sphincter.

prevent fluid accumulation, abscess formation, and breakdown of the perineal closure. The perineal incision is closed in an interrupted fashion with 0 Vicryl sutures by first closing the levator ani from posterior to anterior. The external anal sphincter muscle or ischioanal fat from proximal to distal is also loosely approximated. Because of the propensity of this wound to become infected and break down, the skin is left opened and packed with damp to dry Kerlix gauze.

Additional Considerations

Long-term complications
Although the risk of postoperative complications is lower with this procedure, patients remain at risk for parastomal hernia, stomal prolapse, pouching difficulties, small bowel obstruction, and/or delayed healing of the perineal wound. In addition, the pelvic dissection puts patients at risk for pelvic nerve damage with impairment of sexual or urinary function.

Delayed intersphincteric proctectomy
Patients who are severely malnourished or steroid dependent may benefit from a delayed intersphincteric proctectomy. Placement of a low staple line at the anorectal junction within the pelvis allows the anal canal to be removed at a later date from a perineal approach.

Total Proctocolectomy with Ileal Pouch–Anal Anastomosis

TPC-IPAA was developed in the early 1980s and is the procedure of choice for many patients with UC, because it eliminates all active disease and eventually leaves the patient stoma free.

Preoperative considerations
Patients who undergo TPC-IPAA have multiple semisolid bowel movements per day. Thus, it is crucial that patients have adequate sphincter function in order to maintain continence. Patients with poor preoperative fecal continence have poor functional outcomes after this surgery and should instead undergo proctocolectomy with end ileostomy. It is controversial whether an ileal pouch should be created in patients with middle or distal rectal cancers because this may not leave adequate cancer resection margins above the dentate line. In addition, patients with locally advanced rectal cancer should receive radiation treatment before surgical treatment and formation of an ileal pouch in order to avoid direct radiation injury to the small intestinal pouch. Ultimately radiation exposure leads to radiation enteritis, poor pouch function, and pouch failure. Patients with a cecal cancer may require resection of distal ileum and its associated mesenteric vessels to obtain adequate margins, and thus may not allow the formation of a tension-free IPAA.[26]

Staged procedures
Proctectomy with formation of an ileal pouch may follow an earlier total colectomy in patients with severe malnutrition, chronic steroid use or dependency, or need for emergent surgery. For these high-risk patients, avoidance of proctectomy and ileal pouch formation avoids pelvic sepsis and higher risk of pouch failure.

Perform a total proctocolectomy to the point of circumferential rectal dissection to the level of the levator ani.

Separation of distal colon and rectum A digital rectal examination is performed to confirm the level of rectal transection at the top of the anal canal. The rectum is amputated transversely with various techniques (**Fig. 11**). A transverse stapler is used across

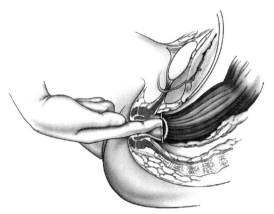

Fig. 11. Transanal digital assessment to mark the level of planned stapled anastomosis. (*From* Kirat HT, Remzi FH. Ileal pouch-anal anastomosis: indications and technique. Semin Colon Rectal Surg 2009;20(2):82–7; with permission; and *Courtesy of* CCF, 2003.)

the distal rectum if a double-stapled approach is used. Alternatively, a purse-string suture is placed at the anorectal junction and a right-angled bowel clamp placed across the distal rectum. The rectum is then sharply amputated above the purse-string suture.

Mobilization of distal ileum An energy device or cautery is used to mobilize the mesentery of the distal terminal ileum to the mesenteric root above the third portion of the duodenum. This method allows the ileal pouch to reach the anal canal without tension.

Formation of J pouch The distal 30 to 40 cm of ileum is folded back on itself, approximating the antimesenteric sides, and creating a 15-cm J pouch (**Fig. 12**). The reach of this pouch to the anal canal is typically adequate if the base of the J pouch reaches

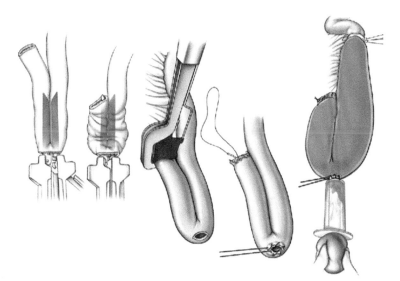

Fig. 12. Creation of J pouch. (*From* Kirat HT, Remzi FH. Ileal pouch-anal anastomosis: indications and technique. Semin Colon Rectal Surg 2009;20(2):82–7; with permission; and *Courtesy of* CCF, 2003.)

below the pubic symphysis. If the approximated base of the J pouch does not reach, further mobilization maneuvers must be performed before pouch creation. For J-pouch formation, an enterotomy is made at the base of the J pouch on the antimesenteric border. A linear 75-mm or 100-mm stapler is fired through the enterotomy after ensuring no small bowel mesentery is included with the staple line, which can be confirmed by medial rotation of the antimesenteric boundaries of the 2 small intestinal limbs toward the posterior aspect of the pouch before stapler closure. The surgeon can also place a finger between the mesentery of the pouch and the anterior stapler to ensure that there is no mesenteric impingement. A second or third reload may necessary to achieve a pouch of 15 to 20 cm in length.

Further mobilization if the pouch does not reach

A. The ileocolic vessels can be excised at the proximal and distal takeoff to allow the distal apex of the pouch more mobility (**Fig. 13**).
B. Peritoneal tissue superior to the third portion of the duodenum and to the right of the superior mesenteric artery can be dissected.
C. Transverse linear incisions along the peritoneum overlying the mesentery or vascular pedicles of the small intestine can be incised in a stepladder approach from distal to proximal. Care should be taken to only incise the peritoneal reflection overlying the mesentery because deeper dissection can cause bleeding that requires vascular ligation and possible pouch ischemia and necrosis.
D. A bulldog over distal branches of the ileal pouch to further release the mesentery and test for pouch ischemia before vessel ligation can be used when small increments of mobility are needed. Again, the risk of pouch ischemia and necrosis is present when this approach is undertaken.
E. Ileal pouch creation in an S configuration can achieve up to an additional 4 cm of reach to the anal canal. The S pouch is created by using three 12-cm to 15-cm limbs of small intestine, which are approximated with seromuscular stay sutures and a 2-cm afferent distal limb on the third arm of the pouch. An S-shaped enterotomy is made on the antimesenteric side of the pouch. Two running seromuscular suture lines are placed on the shared wall of the small intestinal limbs located on the posterior aspect of the S pouch. A continuous anterior seromuscular suture line between the 2 lateral limbs is used to close the anterior portion of the pouch (**Fig. 14**).

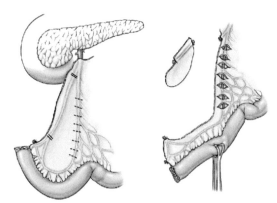

Fig. 13. Maneuvers for pouch to reach the level of the levator floor. (*From* Kirat HT, Remzi FH. Ileal pouch-anal anastomosis: indications and technique. Semin Colon Rectal Surg 2009;20(2):82–7; with permission; and *Courtesy of* CCF, 1998.)

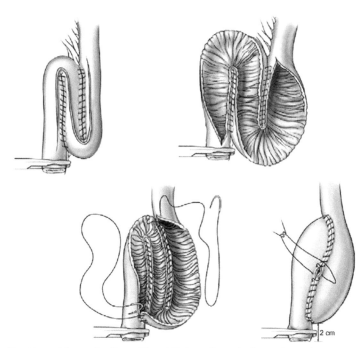

Fig. 14. Creation of S pouch. (*From* Kirat HT, Remzi FH. Ileal pouch-anal anastomosis: indications and technique. Semin Colon Rectal Surg 2009;20(2):82–7; with permission; and *Courtesy of* CCF, 2003.)

Formation of anal anastomosis A purse-string suture is placed within the enterotomy used to create the J pouch in order to secure the anvil of a circular stapling device. An assistant then goes to the perineum to place the stapler through the anal canal. Care should be taken to control the stapler placement through the anus so as not to rip the apex of the short anal canal. The abdominal and perineal surgeons work together to place the base of the stapler so that the trocar of the stapler, once advanced, passes through the distal rectum posterior to the staple line (double-stapled technique) or through the purse-string suture, which is then tied around the trocar. The trocar of the stapler is inserted into the anvil. As the stapler is closed, the ileal pouch is advanced to the anal canal. The ileal pouch tends to rotate and the abdominal surgeon should ensure that the mesentery of the ileal pouch is maintained in an untwisted posterior position. Before complete closure of the circular stapler, the abdominal surgeon must ensure that neither the vaginal cuff nor the anal sphincter is included in the stapling device. The circular stapler is then fired (**Fig. 15**). Proximal and distal tissue donuts are inspected for continuity and the integrity of the IPAA can be tested by air insufflation through the pouch, which is submerged under pelvic irrigation.

Diverting loop ileostomy creation An area of ileum is identified approximately 20 cm proximal to the pouch. This area should be freely mobile and able to be brought up through the abdominal wall rectus muscle without tension. A loop ileostomy is formed through the ileostomy orifice described earlier.

Procedure completion A closed suction drain is placed in the pelvis posterior to the ileal pouch. The incisions are closed and the loop ileostomy is matured. A loop ostomy

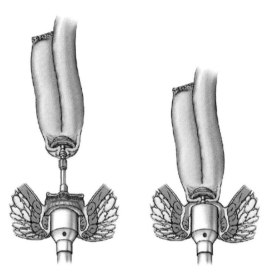

Fig. 15. Creation of double-stapled anastomosis. (*From* Kirat HT, Remzi FH. Ileal pouch-anal anastomosis: indications and technique. Semin Colon Rectal Surg 2009;20(2):82–7; with permission; and *Courtesy of* CCF, 2003.)

bar may be used to assist with abdominal wall fixation. However, in obese patients or patients with a foreshortened mesentery in which a mobile ileal segment cannot be identified, an end ileostomy can be fashioned by an additional stapler transection of the small intestine.

Additional Considerations

Laparoscopic versus open approach
Studies comparing laparoscopic versus open IPAA have shown lower morbidity with a laparoscopic approach and equivalent long-term function and quality of life.[27]

Surveillance
TPC-IPAA greatly reduces the long-term risk for carcinoma in patients with UC. However, the rectal mucosa left behind must be monitored, because a small risk for carcinoma still exists. Flexible fiberoptic pouchoscopy with surveillance biopsies of the ileal pouch should be performed approximately every 5 years.

Long-term outcomes
Pouchitis is the most common long-term complication after an IPAA, and represents a nonspecific inflammation of the ileal reservoir. Pouchitis can be seen in 23% to 46% of patients and significantly affects their quality of life by causing symptoms such as increased stool frequency, urgency, incontinence, nocturnal seepage, abdominal cramping, pelvic discomfort, and arthralgias.[28] Other complications associated with IPAA include strictures, cuffitis, Crohn's disease of the pouch, and neoplasia.

S-pouch function
The S-pouch configuration of an ileoanal pouch may over time cause elongation of the afferent limb causing the patient to have obstructive defecation. This condition may require catheterization of the S pouch to allow evacuation or, in refractory patients, surgical revision of the ileoanal pouch if technically possible.

Total Proctocolectomy and Ileal Pouch–Anal Anastomosis with Mucosectomy and Hand-sewn Anastomosis

In patients with midrectal dysplasia or carcinoma, mucosectomy with hand-sewn IPAA is performed to obtain adequate oncologic margins. In this procedure, the mucosa from the distal rectum is removed transanally. This procedure is more technically difficult to perform than the previously described stapled anastomosis.

Steps of a TPC with IPAA are followed up to but not including creation of the anal anastomosis.

Perineal dissection
After formation of the ileal pouch, the surgeon performs a perineal dissection. A self-retaining anal retractor is placed to evert the anal canal. Local anesthetic is injected in the submucosal plane at the dentate line to facilitate dissection of the anorectal mucosa off the sphincter complex. The mucosal dissection can be performed circumferentially or in quadrants to lift the mucosa from the dentate line to the level of the anorectal transection. Mucosal dissection must be complete so no islands of mucosa remain deep to the hand-sewn anastomosis. Four Vicryl stay sutures are placed through the anal canal wall and including a small portion of internal anal sphincter. Anterior sutures should be placed with care to avoid inclusion of the vaginal wall.

Hand-sewn anastomosis
The ileal J pouch is then brought down to the anus by placing a Babcock through the anal canal and onto the base of the ileal pouch. The abdominal surgeon places a hand posterior to the pouch and guides the pouch movement through the pelvis to avoid pouch rotation or trauma. The 4 stay sutures are placed full thickness through the enterotomy at the base of the ileal pouch and secured. Additional full-thickness interrupted sutures are placed circumferentially to complete the anastomosis (**Fig. 16**).

Ostomy creation
A diverting loop ileostomy is then created in the right lower quadrant as previously described.

Additional Considerations

Hand-sewn versus double-stapled technique
There is debate as to which anastomotic technique provides better functional results and long-term outcomes.

The hand-sewn technique involves anastomosis of the J pouch to the dentate line after endoanal mucosectomy, which has the advantage of removing all potential disease-bearing mucosa. However, this technique may result in higher risk of anal sphincter damage caused by stretching of the anal canal at the time of surgery.[29] In the double-stapled technique, an ileoanal anastomosis is created 1 to 2 cm above the dentate line. The disadvantage of this technique is that the transitional mucosa is left in situ so the potential for cancer in the retained rectal mucosa still exists. Annual surveillance of this transition zone is required, although the incidence of rectal cancer is small.[30] The advantage of a double-stapled technique is an improved ability to achieve a tension-free anastomosis, decreased risk of anal sphincter damage, and maintained anorectal sensation by maintenance of the anal transition zone.[29] In a meta-analysis of patients with IPAA, Lovegrove and colleagues[31] showed that patients with double-stapled anastomoses experienced higher resting sphincter pressures and less nighttime incontinence and seepage than their counterparts with hand-sewn anastomosis. In addition, a large prospective study of patients with IPAA followed long term showed that the double-stapled technique resulted in fewer

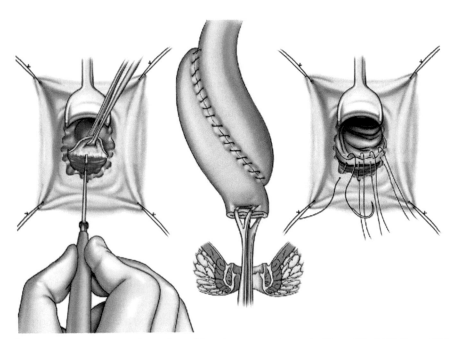

Fig. 16. Mucosectomy and creation of hand-sewn anastomosis. (*From* Kirat HT, Remzi FH. Ileal pouch-anal anastomosis: indications and technique. Semin Colon Rectal Surg 2009;20(2):82–7; with permission; and *Courtesy of* CCF, 2003.)

postoperative anastomotic strictures, septic complications, intestinal obstructions, reservoir failures, and permanent ileostomies than the hand-sewn anastomotic technique.[32] However, these results are not consistent across the literature, and another meta-analysis, by Schuendler and colleagues,[33] showed no statistically significant differences in functional outcome or manometric sphincter continence between hand-sewn versus double-stapled techniques. At present, surgeons should perform the technique with which they are most comfortable unless mucosectomy is needed to obtain oncologic margins for rectal malignancy or dysplasia at the time of pouch formation.[34]

Ileal pouch–anal anastomosis in patients with rectal cancer Patients who undergo proctectomy according to oncologic principles and preservation of the anal canal and sphincter can have ileoanal pouch reconstruction. However, radiation should be performed before surgery in locally advanced rectal cancers to avoid direct radiation exposure of the ileal pouch. In addition, patients should be counseled that pelvic radiation exposure with ileal pouch formation can cause a chronic decrement in pouch function compared with patients with no radiation exposure. A loop ileostomy should be maintained during chemotherapy treatments to help with quality-of-life issues that can be associated with chemotherapy-induced diarrhea.[35]

Surveillance Because rectal mucosa is left behind with either double-stapled anastomosis or mucosectomy, long-term annual examinations via pouchoscopy and biopsies of any retained rectal cuff or suspicious areas in the ileal pouch are recommended for all patients with IPAA regardless of the anastomotic technique.

Elective Total Abdominal Colectomy with Ileoproctostomy

This technique is rarely performed in patients with UC but may be considered in patients with minimal rectal involvement, good rectal compliance, and normal sphincter tone.[36] It can additionally be considered in young women of childbearing age who want to preserve fertility, because the lack of pelvic dissection reduces the risk of pelvic nerve damage and sexual dysfunction. Perform a total abdominal colectomy without ileostomy creation.

Ileorectal anastomosis

The terminal ileum is identified and the mesentery is inspected to ensure it is not twisted. The surgeon may choose to proceed with a hand-sewn or stapled anastomosis at this time. A stapled anastomosis is described. An enterotomy is made in the antimesenteric border of the ileum and an end to end anastomosis (EEA) anvil is secured with a purse-string suture. An assistant then advances the EEA stapler through the rectal stump. The 2 ends are joined, tightened appropriately, and the stapler is fired. The anastomosis can be tested for air leak under pelvic irrigation with proctoscope insufflation through the rectum. All incisions are then closed, sterile dressings applied, and the patient is awoken from anesthesia.

Pitfalls

Ability to advance the EEA stapler may require posterior rectal mobilization to straighten the rectum or hand-sewn anastomosis.

Additional Considerations

Persistent proctitis

Although functional outcome and quality of life after ileorectal have been shown to be comparable with IPAA, these patients have more urgency affecting work and diet restrictions than their IPAA cohorts.[37] Ileoproctostomy is not a definitive operation for all patients with UC; approximately 25% of these patients eventually require a proctectomy because of severe proctitis. If rectal resection is later required, these patients can undergo an IPAA, Brooke ileostomy, or a continent ileostomy. Most of these patients are able to undergo completion proctectomy and conversion to an IPAA if they wish to avoid a stoma.[37]

Rectal cancer risk

Close mucosal surveillance with rectal biopsies is recommended every 6 to 12 months following ileoproctostomy. Approximately 10% of patients develop malignant disease of the rectum.[38]

Elective Kock and Barnett Continent Ileostomies

Dr Nils Kock, a Swedish surgeon, developed the first continent intestinal reservoir (ie, the Kock pouch). Continent ileostomies allow patients to avoid wearing an ostomy appliance by way of a nipple valve that is created with intussusception of a portion of ileum into the planned reservoir. When this procedure is performed, approximately 60 cm (2 feet) of distal ileum is used to create the continent ileostomy and reservoir. The distal ileum is intussuscepted into a pouch constructed of more proximal bowel in order to form a continent nipple. The stoma can then be flush with the skin of the abdominal wall. However, this procedure has a high failure rate, mostly because of valve slippage and subsequent bowel obstruction.[39,40] Dr William Barnett developed the Barnett Continent Intestinal Reservoir, which modified the Koch pouch by adjusting the length of the valve and developing a collar to keep the valve from slipping.[41]

At present, these procedures are performed infrequently because of the excellent long-term outcomes with the ileal J pouch and the high complication rate associated with continent ileostomies. Continent ileostomy is a reasonable option for patients who are not candidates for IPAA because of poor sphincter function, previously having failed IPAA, or wanting to avoid an ileostomy.[42] Patients are not candidates for a continent ileostomy if they have Crohn's disease, obesity, or advanced age. For most patients, a continent ileostomy is not a permanent surgical treatment because complications from these procedures include intestinal obstruction from nipple valve slippage, pouchitis, stenosis, and incontinence.[40]

SUMMARY

Emergent surgical therapy with subtotal colectomy and end ileostomy is recommended in patients with UC who develop fulminant colitis, toxic megacolon, colonic perforation, or life-threatening hemorrhage. This procedure is the safest option and these patients can undergo later conversion to restorative procedures such as IPAA. Elective surgical therapy is indicated in patients with UC who do not tolerate medical therapy or who have failed medical management, or in patients with dysplasia or malignancy. Proctocolectomy with end ileostomy remains the safest procedure with the fewest complications and is a good option for patients who are not candidates for restorative procedures. Proctocolectomy with IPAA has been shown to be a safe and effective treatment of patients with good sphincter function because it eliminates the source of disease and does not require a permanent stoma. Mucosectomy can be performed in patients with rectal dysplasia or carcinoma to extend distal margins and achieve appropriate oncologic control. Total colectomy with ileoproctostomy is rarely performed because of the amount of residual disease left behind. Continent ostomies can be created in patients with UC. However, these are much less popular because of a high associated complication and failure rate compared with the proven long-term success and higher quality of life seen with restorative IPAA procedures.

REFERENCES

1. Hendrickson BA, Gokhale R, Cho JH. Clinical aspects and pathophysiology of inflammatory bowel disease. Clin Microbiol Rev 2002;15(1):79–94.
2. Kappelman MD, Rifas-Shiman SL, Kleinman K, et al. The prevalence and geographic distribution of Crohn's disease and ulcerative colitis in the United States. Clin Gastroenterol Hepatol 2007;5(12):1424–9.
3. Moum B, Vatn MH, Ekbom A, et al, Southeastern Norway IBD Study Group of Gastroenterologists. Incidence of inflammatory bowel disease in southeastern Norway: evaluation of methods after 1 year of registration. Digestion 1995; 56(5):377–81.
4. Langholz E, Munkholm P, Davidsen M, et al. Course of ulcerative colitis: analysis of changes in disease activity over years. Gastroenterology 1994;107(1):3–11.
5. Langholz E, Munkholm P, Davidsen M, et al. Changes in extent of ulcerative colitis: a study on the course and prognostic factors. Scand J Gastroenterol 1996; 31(3):260–6.
6. Kuriyama M, Kato J, Fujimoto T, et al. Risk factors and indications for colectomy in ulcerative colitis patients are different according to the patient's clinical background. Dis Colon Rectum 2006;49(9):1307–15.
7. Eaden JA, Abrams KR, Mayberry JF. The risk of colorectal cancer in ulcerative colitis: a meta-analysis. Gut 2001;48(4):526–35.

8. Itzkowitz SH, Harpaz N. Diagnosis and management of dysplasia in patients with inflammatory bowel disease. Gastroenterology 2004;126:1634–48.
9. Winawer S, Fletcher R, Rex D, et al, Gastrointestinal Consortium Panel. Colorectal cancer screening and surveillance: clinical guidelines and rationale-update based on new evidence. Gastroenterology 2003;124(2):544–60.
10. Cohen JL, Strong SA, Hyman NH, et al. Practice parameters for the surgical treatment of ulcerative colitis. Dis Colon Rectum 2005;48:1997–2009.
11. Ross H, Steele SR, Varma M, et al. Practice parameters for the surgical treatment of ulcerative colitis. Dis Colon Rectum 2014;57:5–22.
12. Gumaste V, Sachar DB, Greenstein AJ. Benign and malignant colorectal strictures in ulcerative colitis. Gut 1992;33:938–41.
13. Weiser JR, Waye JD, Janowitz HD, et al. Adenocarcinoma in strictures of ulcerative colitis without antecedent dysplasia by colonoscopy. Am J Gastroenterol 1994;89:119–22.
14. Hanauer SB. Inflammatory bowel disease. N Engl J Med 1996;334:841–8.
15. Dayan B, Tumer D. Role of surgery in severe ulcerative colitis in the era of medical rescue therapy. World J Gastroenterol 2012;18(29):3833–8.
16. Gan SI, Beck PL. A new look at toxic megacolon: an update and review of incidence, etiology, pathogenesis, and management. Am J Gastroenterol 2003; 98(11):2363–71.
17. Greenstein AJ, Barth JA, Sachar DB, et al. Free colonic perforation without dilation in ulcerative colitis. Am J Surg 1986;152:272–5.
18. Heppell J, Farkouh E, Dube S, et al. Toxic megacolon. An analysis of 70 cases. Dis Colon Rectum 1986;29:789–92.
19. Juviler A, Hyman N. Ulcerative colitis: the fate of the retained rectum. Clin Colon Rectal Surg 2004;17:29–34.
20. Munie S, Hyman N, Osler T. Fate of the rectal stump after subtotal colectomy for ulcerative colitis in the era of ileal pouch-anal anastomosis. JAMA Surg 2013; 148(5):408–11.
21. Gu J, Stocchi L, Geisler DP, et al. Staged restorative proctocolectomy: laparoscopic or open completion proctectomy after laparoscopic subtotal colectomy? Surg Endosc 2011;25:3294–9.
22. Holubar SD, Larson DW, Dozois EJ, et al. Minimally invasive subtotal colectomy and ileal pouch-anal anastomosis for fulminant ulcerative colitis: a reasonable approach? Dis Colon Rectum 2009;52:187–92.
23. Fowkes L, Krishna K, Menon A, et al. Laparoscopic emergency and elective surgery for ulcerative colitis. Colorectal Dis 2007;10:373–8.
24. Lo S, Zaidel O, Tabibzadeh S, et al. Utility of wireless capsule enteroscopy and IBD serology in re-classifying indeterminate colitis. Gastroenterology 2003;124: A-192.
25. Metcalf AM. Elective and emergent operative management of ulcerative colitis. Surg Clin North Am 2007;87:633–41.
26. Larson DW, Dozois EJ, Piotrowicz K, et al. Laparoscopic-assisted vs open ileal pouch-anal anastomosis: functional outcomes in a case-matched series. Dis Colon Rectum 2005;48:1845–50.
27. Shen B, Fazio VW, Remzi FH, et al. Comprehensive evaluation of inflammatory and noninflammatory sequelae of ileal pouch-anal anastomoses. Am J Gastroenterol 2005;100(1):93–101.
28. Fazio VW, Ziv Y, Church JM, et al. Ileal pouch-anal anastomoses complications and function in 1005 patients. Ann Surg 1995;222(2):120–7.

29. Litzendorf ME, Stucchi AF, Wishnia S, et al. Completion mucosectomy for retained rectal mucosa following restorative proctocolectomy with double-stapled ileal pouch-anal anastomosis. J Gastrointest Surg 2010;14:562–9.

30. Slors JF, Ponson AE, Taat CW, et al. Risk of residual rectal mucosa after procto-colectomy and ileal pouch-anal reconstruction with the double-stapling tech-nique. Postoperative endoscopic follow-up study. Dis Colon Rectum 1995;8:207–10.

31. Lovegrove RE, Constantinides VA, Heriot AG, et al. A comparison of hand-sewn versus stapled ileal pouch-anal anastomosis following proctocolectomy: a meta-analysis of 4183 patients. Ann Surg 2006;244:18–26.

32. Kirat HT, Remzi FH, Kiran RP, et al. Comparison of outcomes after hand-sewn versus stapled ileal pouch-anal anastomosis in 3109 patients. Surgery 2009;146:723–9.

33. Schluender SJ, Mei L, Yang H, et al. Can a meta-analysis answer the question: is mucosectomy and hand-sewn or double-stapled anastomosis better in ileal pouch-anal anastomosis? Am Surg 2006;72:912–6.

34. Dignass A, Lindsay JO, Sturm A, et al. Second European evidence-based consensus on the diagnosis and management of ulcerative colitis part 2: current management. J Crohns Colitis 2012;6:991–1030.

35. Wu X, Kiran RP, Remzi FH, et al. Preoperative pelvic radiation increases the risk for ileal pouch failure in patients with colitis-associated colorectal cancer. J Crohn's Colitis 2013;7:e419–26.

36. Da Luz Moreira A, Lavery IC. Ileorectal anastomosis and proctocolectomy with end ileostomy for ulcerative colitis. Clin Colon Rectal Surg 2010;23:269–73.

37. Da Luz Moreira A, Kiran RP, Lavery I. Clinical outcomes of ileorectal anastomosis for ulcerative colitis. Br J Surg 2010;97(1):65–9.

38. Johnson WR, McDermott FT, Hughes ES, et al. The risk of rectal carcinoma following colectomy in ulcerative colitis. Dis Colon Rectum 1983;26(1):44–6.

39. Beck DE. Clinical aspects of continent ileostomies. Clin Colon Rectal Surg 2004;17(1):57–63.

40. Litle VR, Barbour S, Schrock TR, et al. The continent ileostomy; long-term dura-bility and patient satisfaction. J Gastrointest Surg 1999;3:625–32.

41. Mullen P, Behrens D, Chalmers T, et al. Barnett continent intestinal reservoir. Multi-center experience with an alternative to the Brooke ileostomy. Dis Colon Rectum 1995;38(6):573–82.

42. Kornbluth A, Sachar DB, Practice Parameters Committee of the American Col-lege of Gastroenterology. Ulcerative colitis practice guidelines in adults: American College of Gastroenterology, Practice Parameters Committee. Am J Gastroenterol 2010;105(3):501–23.

Challenges in the Medical and Surgical Management of Chronic Inflammatory Bowel Disease

Ellen H. Bailey, MD, Sean C. Glasgow, MD*

KEYWORDS

- Crohn's disease • Ulcerative colitis • Intestinal fistula • Intestinal failure
- Intestinal pouch complications • Venothromboembolism

KEY POINTS

- Inflammatory bowel disease is often a chronic relapsing medical condition requiring a multidisciplinary team and thoughtful surgical approach for optimal outcomes.
- Intestinal fistula is a devastating but well-recognized complication of Crohn's disease, and the management approach involves nutritional optimization, wound containment, and careful operative planning.
- Crohn's disease after multiple resections or long segment involvement can result in short bowel syndrome, and the challenges of ongoing nutritional support are discussed.
- Intestinal pouches are a popular alternative to permanent stoma after total proctocolectomy, and this article addresses several common complications and management strategies.
- Increasing awareness of elevated venous thromboembolic events in the inflammatory bowel disease population mandates mention and aggressive prophylaxis during hospitalization and postoperatively.

INTRODUCTION

An estimated 1.6 million Americans are living today with inflammatory bowel disease, and as many as 70,000 new cases are diagnosed annually.[1] About half of all individuals with ulcerative colitis achieve remission, but recurrence is not uncommon after cessation of medical therapy, and up to 35% will require re-treatment within

Disclosure Statement: The authors have nothing to disclose.
Section of Colon & Rectal Surgery, Department of Surgery, Washington University School of Medicine, 660 South Euclid Avenue, Campus Box 8109, St Louis, MO 63110, USA
* Corresponding author.
E-mail address: GLASGOWS@WUDOSIS.WUSTL.EDU

Surg Clin N Am 95 (2015) 1233–1244
http://dx.doi.org/10.1016/j.suc.2015.08.003
0039-6109/15/$ – see front matter Published by Elsevier Inc.

1 year.[2] At any given time, 50% of Crohn patients are in remission with medical therapy, but maintenance of treatment is recommended for several years.[3] Unfortunately, recurrences are frequent in Crohn's disease, with relapse rates of 20% at 1 year, 40% at 2 years, 67% at 5 years, and 79% at 10 years.[4] This patient population faces an increasing number of medical therapies with frequent changes in regimens. The side-effect profiles and cumulative costs are not insignificant.

About 20% of patients with ulcerative colitis will require surgery during their lifetime, and up to 80% of individuals with Crohn's disease will undergo operative intervention.[5] Crohn's disease recurs in nearly 30% of people within 3 years after resection and 60% at 10 years after resection.[6] Up to 70% of patients are estimated to need repeat resections for Crohn.[7] Surgeries performed for inflammatory bowel disease are not without complications and require careful, multidisciplinary approaches for best outcomes. Several specific and challenging complications arising from long-term inflammatory bowel disease and its surgical management are discussed.

INTESTINAL FISTULA

By definition, this process involves only those patients with Crohn's disease, because ulcerative colitis does not demonstrate transmural inflammation except in the acute setting when perforation is more likely than fistulization. An estimated 5% to 15% of Crohn patients will experience this disease-related complication during their lifetime.[8] A fistula is a connection between 2 epithelialized surfaces and is commonly identified by the 2 involved organs (ie, enterocolonic or colovaginal). Enteroenteric fistulas can present on a spectrum from asymptomatic and an incidental finding at the time of exploration or imaging to debilitating and lifestyle limiting. For the purpose of this review, only the symptomatic variety is addressed, beginning with the troublesome and morbid enterocutaneous fistula.

The acute management of an enterocutaneous fistula in a patient with inflammatory bowel disease is focused on stabilizing the individual because they often present with sepsis, volume depletion, and malnutrition.[9] This process involves a several-pronged approach (**Box 1**) that is largely preserved since the original publication of management guidelines in 1964 by Chapman and colleagues.[10] The key elements include draining intra-abdominal sepsis, correcting volume depletion, and managing the effluent by protecting the skin. Measurements such as body mass index (BMI) and serum albumin can help estimate the degree of malnutrition.[11] Nutritional support should be initiated when the resuscitation is complete, and the enteral route is preferred if feasible to maintain the intestinal lining and use hormonal and absorptive functions. Patients with daily fistula output greater than 1500 mL typically require intravenous fluid replacement. Malnourishment due to proximal fistula losses can be subtle and requires close surveillance with serial nutrition laboratory tests (serum albumin, prealbumin, iron studies, electrolyte panels). Enteral feeding may not be tolerated if it significantly increases fistula output, and total parenteral nutrition (TPN) is another viable option.[12] Complications related to long-term TPN use are well established and are discussed in more detail later in the section on short bowel syndrome.

For ongoing patient support with fluids and nutrition as well as surgical planning, it is useful to define the fistula based on anatomic location and volume of output. Proximal small bowel fistulae are commonly high output (>500 mL/d) and less likely to close when compared with colonic or low output fistulae (<200 mL/d). Spontaneous closure of fistulae is rarely seen in Crohn's disease because ongoing inflammation or distal obstruction is usually present.[13] The amount of residual uninvolved bowel must be noted in this patient population for surgical planning. Antitumor necrosis factor therapy

---

Box 1
Approach to inflammatory bowel disease–related enterocutaneous fistula

Stabilize the patient

- Manage sepsis
  - Empiric systemic antibiotics as indicated
  - Remove infected central lines
  - Radiologic drainage of intra-abdominal fluid collections
  - Avoid acute operative intervention if possible
- Restore intravascular volume status
- Control wound effluent and protect abdominal skin

Optimize the patient

- Assess nutritional status objectively
- Enteral (preferred) or parenteral nutrition
- Measure daily wound effluent
- Manage abdominal wound
  - Negative pressure wound therapy
  - Ostomy appliance or large wound manager
  - Avoid simple gauze dressings
- Stop corticosteroids if possible

Surgical planning

- Quantify length of remaining bowel
- Localize enteric fistula
- Define remaining active inflammatory bowel disease (if any)
- Determine need for complex abdominal wall reconstruction

---

has shown modest success in perianal fistula closure but has not demonstrated similar results in enterocutaneous fistulae.[14] Wound management is often problematic in these patients (**Fig. 1**). Generally, routine wet-to-dry dressings with cotton gauze should be avoided because they poorly control effluent and serve no function for wound

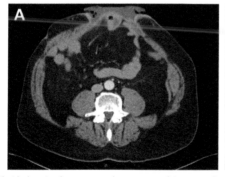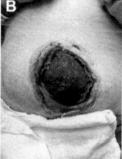

Fig. 1. (*A*) Abdominal computed tomographic scan showing open wound with underlying enteric fistula that occurred following reoperative ileocolic resection and subsequent dehiscence. (*B*) Clinical appearance of same patient. Note the previously placed polypropylene mesh at the edges of the open wound.

debridement. When possible, negative pressure wound therapy is used to speed development of granulation tissue, accelerate wound edge contraction, and control drainage.[15] Effort is required to avoid applying the vacuum dressing to the actual fistula, because this may overwhelm the collecting system and prevent adequate sealing. Creative techniques for wound management are described in the literature.[16,17]

A variety of medical therapies exist to aid in managing the patient with an enterocutaneous fistula. Most patients will require antidiarrheals to reduce fluid losses. Loperamide primarily inhibits μ-opioid signaling in the myenteric plexus (parasympathetic system) of the gastrointestinal tract, thereby impairing smooth muscle contractions and slowing intestinal transit. Patients may also benefit from reducing gastric acid and fluid secretion through the routine use of a proton pump inhibitor such as pantoprazole. Octreotide, a somatostatin analogue, has not shown efficacy in decreasing need for surgery in Crohn-associated enterocutaneous fistulae.[18] Antibiotic therapy for intestinal fistulae is limited to scenarios with sepsis or small bowel overgrowth.[19] The nonspecific signs and symptoms of small intestine bacterial overgrowth include diarrhea, abdominal pain, and bloating and overlap broadly with other pathologic conditions. No gold-standard diagnostic test exists, so empiric antibiotic therapy (frequently rifaximin) is often initiated, and clinical improvement supports this diagnosis.[20,21] Evidence exists to suggest that steroids worsen outcomes in complex Crohn's disease including those patients with internal fistulae,[19] and immunologics, particularly infliximab, likely do not have a role in the treatment of enterocutaneous fistulae.[22] Mahadevan and colleagues[23] demonstrated some improvement in CD fistulae with methotrexate in a small case series. In general, the diseased segment of bowel resulting in the fistula requires surgical resection.

Operative therapy for enterocutaneous fistulae begins with stabilization of the patient as described above and also a period of watchful waiting for the inflammatory intra-abdominal process to improve. The ideal duration of expectant management is widely accepted to be at least 6 months due to the associated obliterative peritonitis.[24] The need for patience in treating Crohn-related enterocutaneous fistulas cannot be overemphasized and must be reinforced to the patient, their family, and other consulting physicians. Before operative intervention, a complete radiographic "road map" is useful. The authors typically use magnetic resonance enterography to evaluate for other areas of active disease (aside from the fistula itself). Water-soluble contrast enemas may also aid in establishing the length of remaining distal bowel and to ensure prior ileocolonic anastomoses have not strictured. The procedure begins with a carefully planned incision with forethought given toward performing an abdominal closure with well-vascularized tissue. The intra-abdominal anatomy is well defined with a meticulous lysis of adhesions from the ligament of Treitz to the rectum if necessary to delineate the involved segment.[25] Following restoration of gastrointestinal continuity, complex abdominal wall reconstruction is frequently required. Unilateral or bilateral component separation should be performed to reduce tension on the midline closure. Ideally, bridging the gap between rectus muscles should be avoided. When bridging with mesh is required, the authors favor using biological mesh such as Strattice (LifeCell, Bridgewater, NJ, USA), with the understanding that subsequent incisional hernia repair may be needed.

SHORT BOWEL SYNDROME

Classically short bowel is defined by loss of absorptive surface to the degree that patients demonstrate dehydration and malnutrition necessitating supplementation for health maintenance. This complication is usually observed when less than 200 cm of small bowel remain proximal to a stoma or less than 100 cm of small bowel remain proximal to an enterocolostomy, although every patient responds differently, and long-term adaptations can lead to recovery of bowel function. A longer segment of diseased bowel in situ may demonstrate worse function than a shorter length of healthy intestine. Multiple bowel resections in Crohn's disease remain the number one cause of short bowel syndrome.[26]

A recent retrospective study from Watanabe and colleagues[27] showed increasing incidence of intestinal failure (defined as dependence on intravenous infusional therapy at least twice weekly for a year or more) with time since initial operation. In this study group, 8.5% of Crohn's disease patients had developed short bowel syndrome by 20 years after their first resection, and the individuals experiencing intestinal failure averaged 3.3 operations over their lifetime. For this reason, the surgical principles of bowel conservation in the Crohn patient population are mandatory. These measures include bowel-sparing procedures such as stricturoplasty when appropriate as well as minimization of gross resection margins and maximizing medical management before undertaking surgery.[28]

Medical optimization of patients with intestinal failure focuses on avoiding dehydration, acid/base disturbances, vitamin deficiencies (especially fat-soluble vitamins A, D, E, and K), and malnutrition. TPN is often used in the acute phase of postoperative intestinal failure, but with the adaptations of crypts and villi hypertrophy, this may be discontinued or at least weaned over time.[29] Although intestinal adaptation is more common in children, diseased remaining bowel in Crohn patients may adapt more slowly or not at all. Life-long parenteral nutrition may be necessary in a subset of patients with intestinal failure, along with associated hazards such as bloodstream infections and thromboembolic risks due to the required indwelling central venous catheter and multifactorial hepatic dysfunction.[30]

Various pharmacologic agents, supplements, and growth factors have shown promise in the support of patients with intestinal failure. Antimotility agents effectively slow intestinal transit time in many patients with proximal stomas.[26] Somatostatin analogues such as octreotide act globally to reduce all digestive secretions, thereby decreasing excreted fluid load. However, octreotide seems to lose efficacy and is not a long-term therapy in this patient population.[31] A landmark randomized, controlled, double-blind study by Byrne and colleagues[32] examining the use of human growth hormone (somatropin (rDNA); Zorbtive) with or without supplemental oral glutamine found a decrease in the need for parenteral calories and fluid volume after 4 weeks of treatment. However, on pooled analysis of several studies, durable benefits have not been demonstrated with either therapy in short bowel syndrome.[33]

In late 2012, the US Food and Drug Administration approved teduglutide (Gattex) injections for the treatment of short bowel syndrome secondary to many causes, including because of Crohn's disease. This glucagon-like peptide-2 analogue promotes structural adaptation such as lengthening villi and increasing crypt depth, as well as functional adaptation by slowing intestinal transit.[34] Several prospective studies demonstrated reduction in parenteral caloric and fluid volume requirements, with some patients experiencing sustained benefit after stopping treatment. The estimated annual cost of the medication is $300,000[35]; pharmacoeconomics analyses are needed to determine the role of this therapeutic.

Surgical therapies for short bowel syndrome range from restoration of intestinal continuity if the colon remains in situ, stricturoplasties, lengthening procedures, segmental reversals, and small bowel transplant. The common tenets used in these operations are increasing or maintaining absorptive area and slowing transit.[26] Intact colon has benefits including increased absorptive capacity for liquid and nutrients, but also downsides such as increased bile salt deconjugation leading to watery diarrhea.[30] Lengthening procedures are uncommon in the adult population because the mesenteric leaves are fused and very difficult to separate while maintaining blood supply, and this technique requires dilated bowel.[36] Segmental reversal techniques can be used in normal caliber bowel and lead to decreased parenteral nutrition dependence in intestinal failure populations.[37] Stricturoplasty, a well-described and conservative surgical technique commonly used in Crohn's disease, leads to resolution of obstructive symptoms and weight gain secondary to improved oral intake (**Fig. 2**).[38] The length of involved bowel dictates the type of stricturoplasty with Heineke-Mickulicz used for short segment (<10 cm) narrowing, Finney for medium length (10–20 cm) diseased regions, and the side-to-side isoperistaltic stricturoplasty used in long strictures. Short bowel syndrome secondary to Crohn's disease is an indication for intestinal transplantation, although fewer than 50 patients worldwide have undergone transplant for failure due to inflammatory bowel disease, and long-term survival may be worse than maintenance on parenteral nutrition.[39]

Depending on the distribution of inflammation and regions of intestinal resections, patients with inflammatory bowel disease display several well-described malabsorption syndromes. The distal 100 cm of the terminal ileum performs critical functions in water-soluble vitamin (absorption, especially B12), and inflammatory disease or surgical absence of this segment can lead to megaloblastic anemia and neurologic symptoms. Health maintenance in patients with inflammatory bowel disease includes daily multivitamin with iron supplementation, vitamin D, and calcium, as well as vitamin B12 and folate serum level monitoring.[11] Height, weight, and BMI measurements are crucial components of outpatient visits especially in children, adolescents, and young adults because protein loss in chronic diarrhea can lead to growth disturbances.[40] In a recent European case control study, BMI and serum albumin level were the 2 patient characteristics most associated with malnutrition, and recent unintentional weight loss can also indicate a significant ongoing nutritional disturbance.[41]

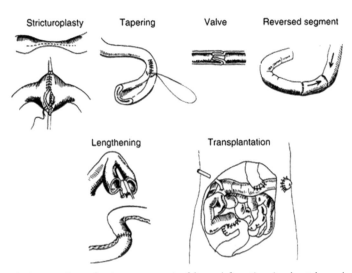

Fig. 2. Surgical procedures for improvement of bowel function in short bowel syndrome. (*From* Thompson JS, Langnas AN, Pinch LW, et al. Surgical approach to short-bowel syndrome. Experience in a population of 160 patients. Ann Surg 1995;222(4):602; [discussion: 605–7]; with permission).

POUCH COMPLICATIONS

For patients with a diagnosis of ulcerative colitis who desire restoration of intestinal continuity after proctocolectomy, the ileal pouch anal anastomosis (IPAA) is performed. This procedure was first described by Sir Alan Parks and Nicholls in 1978[42] and is now commonly offered to individuals with good sphincter function as an alternative to a permanent stoma. Despite a low mortality, there are several unique complications arising from this restorative proctocolectomy.

Pelvic sepsis results from a presumed pouch leak in 3 of 4 cases, and the specific location of the leak is usually the pouch-anal anastomosis (56%).[43] A leak is identified from the tip of the pouch more rarely (7% in Heuschen series), but based on the small case series published by Kirat and colleagues,[44] this complication often mandates an abdominal approach for management with either pouch repair or re-creation for pouch salvage. These leaks are extremely rare and notoriously difficult to diagnose; they require a high index of suspicion in patients presenting with a chronic, indolent course of pelvic sepsis or a fistula.

Anastomotic stricture can be observed after resolution of pelvic sepsis and may require repeated dilations[45] or even pouch advancement to achieve acceptable function.[46] At the first postoperative visit, patients undergo a digital rectal examination to break the filmy adhesions that commonly form over the defunctionalized distal anastomosis and also to identify an early anastomotic stricture. Before reversing a diverting ileostomy, the patient should again be examined for any evidence of a distal narrowing that would render pouch function unacceptable; serial dilations may be initiated at this time. Routine retrograde contrast study of the pouch before ostomy takedown may not increase the diagnosis of occult leaks or routinely alter management.[47]

Pouch vaginal fistulas are a devastating complication observed in 2% to 6% of cases following IPAA.[48] Often these are located at the pouch-anal anastomosis and have high recurrence rates up to 70% following attempted primary repair.[49] Those fistulas presenting within 6 months of surgery are thought to be secondary to pelvic sepsis and seem to be more successfully repaired than later fistulas that are more suggestive of previously undiagnosed Crohn's disease.[50] A transanal or transvaginal approach is often used for fistulae originating at or distal to the anastomosis[49,50] and both yield a fistula closure rate of 50%. It is the authors' opinion that almost all symptomatic pouch-vaginal fistulas require loop ileostomy creation before (or concurrent with) fistula repair in order to optimize healing conditions at the initial attempt.

Nonspecific inflammation of the ileal pouch is known as pouchitis, and the incidence increases over time from surgery, with one recent series reporting at least one episode in 70% of patients at 20-year follow-up.[51] Patients will often describe fever, pelvic pain, increase in defecation, and cramping. Index presentation with these symptoms should prompt endoscopic evaluation of the pouch, with random biopsies to evaluate for other causes, such as undiagnosed Crohn's disease. The cause remains uncertain but is thought to be related to overgrowth of anaerobic bacteria. Because of uncertainty of the true cause, many systemic and intraluminal therapies have been examined (**Box 2**). Currently, first-line treatment is primarily with antibiotics such as rifaximin or ciprofloxacin with or without metronidazole.[52] A *Cochrane Review* of 11 randomized controlled trials suggested budesonide enemas and probiotics were more effective than placebo at inducing remission.[53] Cuffitis refers to inflammation of the 1 to 4 cm of remnant rectal mucosa after the double stapled technique of IPAA. It presents in similar fashion to pouchitis, although only 10% of patients are symptomatic.[54] Treatment of cuffitis includes topical steroids or 5-aminosalicylic preparations with an excellent response rate of greater than 90%.[55] If cuffitis or

---

Box 2
Treatment options for acute and chronic pouchitis

Systemic

- Antibiotics such as rifaximin, ciprofloxacin, metronidazole
- Probiotics such as VSL3
- Oral 5-aminosalicylic acid (5-ASA) agents
- Absorbant spherical carbon
- Infliximab

Intraluminal/topical

- 5-ASA agent enemas
- Budesonide enemas or by mouth
- Bismuth carbomer foam enemas
- Tacrolimus enemas
- Hydrocortisone suppositories
- Glutamine suppositories
- Butyrate suppositories

Surgical

- Pouch excision with end ileostomy

---

pouchitis fails to improve with established therapies, the clinician must rule out other causes of bowel habit changes, such as infection with *Clostridium difficile* or cytomegalovirus, Crohn's disease, and other more unusual cause such as ischemic pouchitis or autoimmune disorders.[56] Fecal transplantation may be a successful management strategy in patients with refractory pouchitis or *C difficile* colonization, leading to pouch dysfunction, although evidence to support this practice is currently lacking.[57]

Overall pouch failure rate ranges from 3% to as high as 48% in the literature due to differing definitions and length of follow-up.[51,58] Many patient and technical factors are associated with pouch failure, but pelvic sepsis and Crohn's disease remain the most consistently identified.[56] Salvage surgery for pouch dysfunction after septic complications seems to lead to reasonable long-term function with up to an 86% success rate.[59] In patients who do require a permanent stoma for pouch failure, the current literature supports pouch excision with end ileostomy rather than diverting stoma (and leaving the pouch in situ) when feasible due to improved quality of life.[60]

DEEP VENOUS THROMBOSIS

Individuals with inflammatory bowel disease exhibit increased rates of venous thromboembolic events (VTE) during hospitalizations and especially after intestinal resection.[61] Sites of involvement range from extremity deep venous thrombosis to pulmonary embolism, mesenteric and portal venous thrombosis, and thromboembolic phenomena and can occasionally result in death. Patients can experience VTE despite appropriate mechanical and pharmacologic prophylaxis so the provider's index of suspicion must remain high. Gross and colleagues[62] recently demonstrated that patients with inflammatory bowel disease are at higher risk for postoperative VTEs than patients with cancer. After operative resection, the National Comprehensive

Cancer Network recommends 4 weeks of out-of-hospital pharmacologic thromboprophylaxis for patients with colorectal cancer; individuals with inflammatory bowel disease would likely benefit from similar management.[63]

Portomesenteric vein thrombosis occurs in both patients with ulcerative colitis and patients with Crohn's disease, and its occurrence is likely underestimated. Symptoms of acute thrombosis include nonspecific abdominal pain, fevers, and inflammatory symptoms. Forty percent of patients remain asymptomatic, and the thrombus is found incidentally.[64] Hyperhomocysteinemia and other known prothrombotic disorders should be sought, although a firm diagnosis occurs in the minority. Risk factors for portal thrombosis in this population include active inflammatory bowel disease, tobacco use, underlying malignancy or hepatic disease (eg, nonalcoholic steatohepatitis or hepatitis), and recent abdominal surgery.[64–66] Although the natural history of this thrombus is uncertain, systemic anticoagulation should be initiated if not otherwise contraindicated. Successful recanalization of the portomesenteric venous system is more likely in the acute setting (65% vs 37% for chronic thrombosis).[64]

SUMMARY

Inflammatory bowel disease affects a significant portion of the American population and frequently follows a chronic clinical course with episodic flares and periods of remission. Many patients with Crohn's disease and ulcerative colitis will ultimately come to surgical resection, and these individuals require an organized operative approach tailored to their anatomy and distribution of disease. Presented are several specific complications with unique implications in the inflammatory bowel disease population, and evidence-based techniques for management are discussed. Caring for this patient population often leads to the development of long-term clinical relationships, and a systematic approach toward treatment of ongoing disease-related complications will yield the best possible outcomes.

REFERENCES

1. Loftus CG, Loftus EV Jr, Harmsen WS, et al. Update on the incidence and prevalence of Crohn's disease and ulcerative colitis in Olmsted County, Minnesota, 1940–2000. Inflamm Bowel Dis 2007;13(3):254–61.
2. Farkas K, Lakatos PL, Nagy F, et al. Predictors of relapse in patients with ulcerative colitis in remission after one-year of infliximab therapy. Scand J Gastroenterol 2013;48(12):1394–8.
3. Affronti A, Orlando A, Cottone M. An update on medical management on Crohn's disease. Expert Opin Pharmacother 2015;16(1):63–78.
4. Lapidus A, Bernell O, Hellers G, et al. Clinical course of colorectal Crohn's disease: a 35-year follow-up study of 507 patients. Gastroenterology 1998;114(6): 1151–60.
5. Sica GS, Biancone L. Surgery for inflammatory bowel disease in the era of laparoscopy. World J Gastroenterol 2013;19(16):2445–8.
6. Larson DW, Pemberton JH. Current concepts and controversies in surgery for IBD. Gastroenterology 2004;126(6):1611–9.
7. Bernell O, Lapidus A, Hellers G. Risk factors for surgery and postoperative recurrence in Crohn's disease. Ann Surg 2000;231(1):38–45.
8. Michelassi F, Stella M, Balestracci T, et al. Incidence, diagnosis, and treatment of enteric and colorectal fistulae in patients with Crohn's disease. Ann Surg 1993; 218(5):660–6.

9. Schein M. What's new in postoperative enterocutaneous fistulas? World J Surg 2008;32(3):336–8.
10. Chapman R, Foran R, Dunphy JE. Management of intestinal fistulas. Am J Surg 1964;108:157–64.
11. Song HK, Buzby GP. Nutritional support for Crohn's disease. Surg Clin North Am 2001;81(1):103–15, viii.
12. Lloyd DA, Gabe SM, Windsor AC. Nutrition and management of enterocutaneous fistula. Br J Surg 2006;93(9):1045–55.
13. McIntyre PB, Ritchie JK, Hawley PR, et al. Management of enterocutaneous fistulas: a review of 132 cases. Br J Surg 1984;71(4):293–6.
14. Reenaers C, Belaiche J, Louis E. Impact of medical therapies on inflammatory bowel disease complication rate. World J Gastroenterol 2012;18(29):3823–7.
15. Terzi C, Egeli T, Canda AE, et al. Management of enteroatmospheric fistulae. Int Wound J 2014;11(Suppl 1):17–21.
16. Hoedema RE, Suryadevara S. Enterostomal therapy and wound care of the enterocutaneous fistula patient. Clin Colon Rectal Surg 2010;23(3):161–8.
17. de Leon JM. Novel techniques using negative pressure wound therapy for the management of wounds with enterocutaneous fistulas in a long-term acute care facility. J Wound Ostomy Continence Nurs 2013;40(5):481–8.
18. Draus JM Jr, Huss SA, Harty NJ, et al. Enterocutaneous fistula: are treatments improving? Surgery 2006;140(4):570–6 [discussion: 576–8].
19. Peter Irving DR, Shanahan F. Clinical dilemmas in inflammatory bowel disease. Malden (MA): Mass: Blackwell Pub. LTD; 2006.
20. Shah SC, Day LW, Somsouk M, et al. Meta-analysis: antibiotic therapy for small intestinal bacterial overgrowth. Aliment Pharmacol Ther 2013;38(8):925–34.
21. Grace E, Shaw C, Whelan K, et al. Review article: small intestinal bacterial overgrowth–prevalence, clinical features, current and developing diagnostic tests, and treatment. Aliment Pharmacol Ther 2013;38(7):674–88.
22. Miehsler W, Reinisch W, Kazemi-Shirazi L, et al. Infliximab: lack of efficacy on perforating complications in Crohn's disease. Inflamm Bowel Dis 2004;10(1):36–40.
23. Mahadevan U, Marion JF, Present DH. Fistula response to methotrexate in Crohn's disease: a case series. Aliment Pharmacol Ther 2003;18(10):1003–8.
24. Joyce MR, Dietz DW. Management of complex gastrointestinal fistula. Curr Probl Surg 2009;46(5):384–430.
25. Schecter WP, Hirshberg A, Chang DS, et al. Enteric fistulas: principles of management. J Am Coll Surg 2009;209(4):484–91.
26. Keller J, Panter H, Layer P. Management of the short bowel syndrome after extensive small bowel resection. Best Pract Res Clin Gastroenterol 2004;18(5):977–92.
27. Watanabe K, Sasaki I, Fukushima K, et al. Long-term incidence and characteristics of intestinal failure in Crohn's disease: a multicenter study. J Gastroenterol 2014;49(2):231–8.
28. Michelassi F, Sultan S. Surgical treatment of complex small bowel Crohn disease. Ann Surg 2014;260(2):230–5.
29. Lentze MJ. Intestinal adaptation in short-bowel syndrome. Eur J Pediatr 1989;148(4):294–9.
30. Sundaram A, Koutkia P, Apovian CM. Nutritional management of short bowel syndrome in adults. J Clin Gastroenterol 2002;34(3):207–20.
31. Harris AG. Somatostatin and somatostatin analogues: pharmacokinetics and pharmacodynamic effects. Gut 1994;35(3 Suppl):S1–4.

32. Byrne TA, Wilmore DW, Iyer K, et al. Growth hormone, glutamine, and an optimal diet reduces parenteral nutrition in patients with short bowel syndrome: a prospective, randomized, placebo-controlled, double-blind clinical trial. Ann Surg 2005;242(5):655–61.

33. Wales PW, Nasr A, de Silva N, et al. Human growth hormone and glutamine for patients with short bowel syndrome. Cochrane Database Syst Rev 2010;(6):CD006321.

34. Wilhelm SM, Lipari M, Kulik JK, et al. Teduglutide for the treatment of short bowel syndrome. Ann Pharmacother 2014;48(9):1209–13.

35. Herper M. Inside the pricing of a $300,000-a-year drug. New York: Pharma & Healthcare; 2013. Available at: http://www.forbes.com/sites/matthewherper/2013/01/03/inside-the-pricing-of-a-300000-a-year-drug/. Accessed March 1, 2013.

36. Carlson GL. Surgical management of intestinal failure. Proc Nutr Soc 2003;62(3):711–8.

37. Beyer-Berjot L, Joly F, Maggiori L, et al. Segmental reversal of the small bowel can end permanent parenteral nutrition dependency: an experience of 38 adults with short bowel syndrome. Ann Surg 2012;256(5):739–44 [discussion: 744–5].

38. Yamamoto T, Fazio VW, Tekkis PP. Safety and efficacy of strictureplasty for Crohn's disease: a systematic review and meta-analysis. Dis Colon Rectum 2007;50(11):1968–86.

39. Harrison E, Allan P, Ramu A, et al. Management of intestinal failure in inflammatory bowel disease: small intestinal transplantation or home parenteral nutrition? World J Gastroenterol 2014;20(12):3153–63.

40. Rufo PA, Denson LA, Sylvester FA, et al. Health supervision in the management of children and adolescents with IBD: NASPGHAN recommendations. J Pediatr Gastroenterol Nutr 2012;55(1):93–108.

41. Mijac DD, Jankovic GL, Jorga J, et al. Nutritional status in patients with active inflammatory bowel disease: prevalence of malnutrition and methods for routine nutritional assessment. Eur J Intern Med 2010;21(4):315–9.

42. Parks AG, Nicholls RJ. Proctocolectomy without ileostomy for ulcerative colitis. Br Med J 1978;2(6130):85–8.

43. Heuschen UA, Allemeyer EH, Hinz U, et al. Outcome after septic complications in J pouch procedures. Br J Surg 2002;89(2):194–200.

44. Kirat HT, Kiran RP, Oncel M, et al. Management of leak from the tip of the "J" in ileal pouch-anal anastomosis. Dis Colon Rectum 2011;54(4):454–9.

45. Lewis WG, Kuzu A, Sagar PM, et al. Stricture at the pouch-anal anastomosis after restorative proctocolectomy. Dis Colon Rectum 1994;37(2):120–5.

46. Fazio VW, Tjandra JJ. Pouch advancement and neoileoanal anastomosis for anastomotic stricture and anovaginal fistula complicating restorative proctocolectomy. Br J Surg 1992;79(7):694–6.

47. Kalady MF, Mantyh CR, Petrofski J, et al. Routine contrast imaging of low pelvic anastomosis prior to closure of defunctioning ileostomy: is it necessary? J Gastrointest Surg 2008;12(7):1227–31.

48. Johnson PM, O'Connor BI, Cohen Z, et al. Pouch-vaginal fistula after ileal pouch-anal anastomosis: treatment and outcomes. Dis Colon Rectum 2005;48(6):1249–53.

49. Heriot AG, Tekkis PP, Smith JJ, et al. Management and outcome of pouch-vaginal fistulas following restorative proctocolectomy. Dis Colon Rectum 2005;48(3):451–8.

50. Shah NS, Remzi F, Massmann A, et al. Management and treatment outcome of pouch-vaginal fistulas following restorative proctocolectomy. Dis Colon Rectum 2003;46(7):911–7.

51. Hahnloser D, Pemberton JH, Wolff BG, et al. Results at up to 20 years after ileal pouch-anal anastomosis for chronic ulcerative colitis. Br J Surg 2007;94(3): 333–40.
52. Shen B, Achkar JP, Lashner BA, et al. A randomized clinical trial of ciprofloxacin and metronidazole to treat acute pouchitis. Inflamm Bowel Dis 2001;7(4):301–5.
53. Holubar SD, Cima RR, Sandborn WJ, et al. Treatment and prevention of pouchitis after ileal pouch-anal anastomosis for chronic ulcerative colitis. Cochrane Database Syst Rev 2010;(6):CD001176.
54. Thompson-Fawcett MW, Mortensen NJ, Warren BF. "Cuffitis" and inflammatory changes in the columnar cuff, anal transitional zone, and ileal reservoir after stapled pouch-anal anastomosis. Dis Colon Rectum 1999;42(3):348–55.
55. Shen B, Lashner BA, Bennett AE, et al. Treatment of rectal cuff inflammation (cuffitis) in patients with ulcerative colitis following restorative proctocolectomy and ileal pouch-anal anastomosis. Am J Gastroenterol 2004;99(8):1527–31.
56. Francone TD, Champagne B. Considerations and complications in patients undergoing ileal pouch anal anastomosis. Surg Clin North Am 2013;93(1):107–43.
57. Allegretti JR, Hamilton MJ. Restoring the gut microbiome for the treatment of inflammatory bowel diseases. World J Gastroenterol 2014;20(13):3468–74.
58. Fazio VW, Ziv Y, Church JM, et al. Ileal pouch-anal anastomoses complications and function in 1005 patients. Ann Surg 1995;222(2):120–7.
59. Fazio VW, Wu JS, Lavery IC. Repeat ileal pouch-anal anastomosis to salvage septic complications of pelvic pouches: clinical outcome and quality of life assessment. Ann Surg 1998;228(4):588–97.
60. Kiran RP, Kirat HT, Rottoli M, et al. Permanent ostomy after ileoanal pouch failure: pouch in situ or pouch excision? Dis Colon Rectum 2012;55(1):4–9.
61. Dwyer JP, Javed A, Hair CS, et al. Venous thromboembolism and underutilisation of anticoagulant thromboprophylaxis in hospitalised patients with inflammatory bowel disease. Intern Med J 2014;44(8):779–84.
62. Gross ME, Vogler SA, Mone MC, et al. The importance of extended postoperative venous thromboembolism prophylaxis in IBD: a National Surgical Quality Improvement Program analysis. Dis Colon Rectum 2014;57(4):482–9.
63. Vedovati MC, Becattini C, Rondelli F, et al. A randomized study on 1-week versus 4-week prophylaxis for venous thromboembolism after laparoscopic surgery for colorectal cancer. Ann Surg 2014;259(4):665–9.
64. Landman C, Nahon S, Cosnes J, et al. Portomesenteric vein thrombosis in patients with inflammatory bowel disease. Inflamm Bowel Dis 2013;19(3):582–9.
65. Leung GG, Sivasankaran MV, Choi JJ, et al. Risk factors of portal vein thrombosis in Crohn's disease patients. J Gastrointest Surg 2012;16(6):1199–203.
66. Fichera A, Cicchiello LA, Mendelson DS, et al. Superior mesenteric vein thrombosis after colectomy for inflammatory bowel disease: a not uncommon cause of postoperative acute abdominal pain. Dis Colon Rectum 2003;46(5):643–8.

Extraintestinal Manifestations Associated with Inflammatory Bowel Disease

Shaun R. Brown, DO[a,b], Lisa C. Coviello, DO[c,d],*

KEYWORDS

- Inflammatory bowel disease • Multiple organ systems
- Extraintestinal manifestations

KEY POINTS

- Inflammatory bowel disease (IBD) affects multiple organ systems outside of the gastrointestinal tract.
- The clinician treating patients with IBD should be acutely aware of the diagnosis and treatment of extraintestinal manifestations in order to decrease morbidity.
- The management can be difficult and often times requires a multidisciplinary approach.
- Future research investigating the pathophysiology, diagnosis, and treatment is needed to further the care of these patients.

INTRODUCTION

Extraintestinal manifestations (EIMs) associated with inflammatory bowel disease (IBD) are conditions commonly seen in patients who suffer from ulcerative colitis (UC) or Crohn's disease (CD). These manifestations can involve several organ systems and may develop before the onset of gastrointestinal symptoms. In this article, the major EIMs of IBD affecting the musculoskeletal, dermatologic, hepatobiliary, ocular, renal, and pulmonary system are reviewed, as well as current treatment options (**Table 1**).

The underlying pathophysiology related to the development of EIM associated with IBD remains uncertain. Several hypotheses have been proposed, including genetic susceptibility, abnormal self-recognition, and autoantibodies against organ-specific cellular antigens shared by the gastrointestinal tract and other organ systems[1]; this

[a] Department of Colorectal Surgery, Oschner Clinic Foundation, New Orleans, LA, USA; [b] Department of Surgery, Uniformed Services University of Health Sciences, Bethesda, MD 20814, USA; [c] Department of Surgery, National Capital Region Medical Directorate, Fort Belvoir, VA 22060, USA; [d] Department of Surgery of the Uniformed Services University of Health Sciences and the Walter Reed National Military Medical Center, Bethesda, MD 20814, USA
* Corresponding author.
E-mail address: lccovi@gmail.com

Surg Clin N Am 95 (2015) 1245–1259
http://dx.doi.org/10.1016/j.suc.2015.08.002
0039-6109/15/$ – see front matter Published by Elsevier Inc.

surgical.theclinics.com

Table 1 Extraintestinal manifestations associated with inflammatory bowel disease	
Musculoskeletal	Pauciarticular arthritis AS/axial arthropathies
Dermatologic	EN PG Apthous ulcers Sweets syndrome
Ocular	Uveitis Episcleritis
Hepatobiliary	PSC Cholelithiasis PVT
Pulmonary	Large and small airway disease Chronic bronchitis Bronchiectasis
Renal	Nephrolithiasis Obstructive uropathy Fistulization

has been demonstrated in patients with primary sclerosing cholangitis (PSC) wherein autoantibodies to the colon cross-react with the biliary epithelium.[2]

EIMs can be classified into 3 groups, based on the association with intestinal disease activity (Box 1).[1] The first group has a direct relationship with intestinal disease and parallels the disease process. These EIMs include episcleritis, erythema nodosum (EN), oral apthous ulcers, and pauciarticular arthritis.[3] The second group of EIMs seems to develop and progress independent from intestinal disease activity and may simply reflect the susceptibility of these patients to autoimmune disorders. This group includes ankylosing spondylitis (AS) and uveitis.[3] The third group consists of

Box 1 Association between inflammatory bowel disease and extraintestinal manifestations
Group I: EIMs that parallel disease activity of IBD
Oral aphthous ulcers
Erythema nodosum
Pauciarticular arthritis
Episcleritis
Group II: EIMs with independent course from IBD activity
Ankylosing spondylitis
Uveitis
Group III: EIMs and IBD activity unclear
Primary sclerosing cholangitis
Pyoderma gangrenosum
(*From* Trikudanathan G, Venkatesh PG, Navaneethan U. Diagnosis and therapeutic management of extra-intestinal manifestations of inflammatory bowel disease. Drugs 2012;72(18): 2333–49; with permission.)

EIMs that have an unclear relationship with intestinal inflammation. This group includes pyoderma gangrenosum (PG) and PSC, which may or may not be related to intestinal inflammation[3] (see **Box 1**).

MUSCULOSKELETAL MANIFESTATIONS

Musculoskeletal manifestations are the most common EIM seen in IBD and are present in 20% to 30% of patients.[4] Joint involvement can be classified as either peripheral or axial, and men and women appear to have a similar risk of developing joint involvement.[5]

Peripheral Arthropathies

Peripheral arthropathies (PA) are divided into 2 subgroups, according to the classification of Orchard and colleagues.[6] Type 1 (pauciarticular) arthritis is an acute, self-limiting arthropathy that typically affects fewer than 5 large joints. It occurs in approximately 5% to 10% of UC and 10% to 20% of CD patients, respectively.[6] Type 1 PA is unique from other forms of arthritis in that there is little to no joint destruction, and patients are serologically negative for rheumatoid factor and antinuclear antibody.[7] Thus, PA is a seronegative arthritis. The risk of developing peripheral arthritis increases with the extent of IBD activity. In addition, the presence of complications related to IBD activity, such as abscess, perianal disease, or other EIM, also appears to be associated with an increased risk of PA.[5]

In contrast, type 2 (polyarticular) arthritis is a chronic, often bilateral, symmetric, polyarticular arthropathy affecting 5 or more small joints. Often, type 2 arthritis flares occur independent from IBD activity, with a prevalence of 2% to 4% in both CD and UC.[8] It may persist before surgery for IBD or present years later after a total abdominal proctocolectomy with ileopouch anal anastomosis.[9] In addition, type 2 arthritis is associated with an increased risk of uveitis.[10]

The diagnosis of PA is made clinically, given that radiologic imaging fails to show any erosions or deformities. Treatment recommendations for IBD-related arthropathies are based on the treatment of other forms of arthritis/spondyloarthropathy.[11] Because type I PA is linked with IBD activity, treatment is aimed at addressing the underlying intestinal inflammation. Symptoms usually resolve within 8 to 10 weeks after successful treatment of an IBD flare.[12] Nonsteroidal anti-inflammatory drugs (NSAIDs) may be used, but with caution due to the risk of exacerbating the underlying IBD. Selective cyclo-oxygenase (COX)-2 inhibitors have been used with improvement in symptoms in up to 60% of patients; however, clinical relapse of IBD requiring discontinuation of therapy was seen within the first few days of treatment in 25% of patients.[13] Although a recent *Cochrane Review* failed to show an increased risk of IBD exacerbation with the use of COX-2 inhibitors, the investigators thought that due to the small sample size and short follow-up, no definitive conclusion could be made.[14] Thus, more trials with COX-2 inhibitors are needed to determine the safety and provide further recommendations for their use. Treatment of type 2 arthritis is different in that it does not simply mirror the underlying bowel activity. Sulfasalazine is the first-line treatment. However, methotrexate may be used when sulfasalazine is not effective and should be started at 7.5 mg weekly along with folic acid to decrease side effects.[5] In addition, biologic therapy may be used in those patients that continue to suffer from refractory disease. Kaufman and colleagues[15] demonstrated an improvement in symptoms of 7 of 11 arthralgia patients after a single dose of infliximab 5 mg/kg. However, this improvement in symptoms may be short lived. A randomized prospective study, which included 487 patients, confirmed that infliximab therapy is a valid option for refractory disease, but concluded that this treatment must be weighed against the absence of clinical differences at 24 months and an increase in treatment cost.[16]

Axial Arthropathies

Axial arthropathies occur in 3% to 5% of patients with IBD, with men being affected more commonly than women.[17] Axial arthropathies are categorized into AS and sacroiliitis. Axial arthropathies do not parallel IBD activity. AS occurs in up to 10% of patients with IBD, which is 20-fold higher than the general population. Most patients are HLA-B27 positive. The disease course is usually progressive and often results in spinal destruction. Clinically, patients often experience severe back pain that is aggravated by periods of rest. On physical examination, there is limited spinal mobility and reduced chest expansion. Advanced cases are characterized by squaring of vertebral bodies, and bony proliferation and ankylosis, classically known as "bamboo spine." Although plain films may demonstrate abnormal findings, MRI is now the gold standard for diagnosis.[18] Management of IBD-related AS is similar to non-IBD patients. Physical therapy and exercise regimens, such as deep breathing, spinal exercises, and swimming, are essential to retain spine mobility and minimize disability.[19] NSAIDs may aid in symptom relief but they do not have an effect on underlying spinal destruction. Similarly, local corticosteroid injections may provide symptom improvement, but their effects are fleeting. Sulfasalazine, methotrexate, and azathioprine are generally ineffective in the treatment of AS. Biologic therapy, including both infliximab and adalimumab, has been well studied in several placebo-controlled trials in AS patients without IBD and have demonstrated efficacy.[20,21] In a controlled trial of 36 patients with both IBD and spondyloarthropathy, 24 patients were treated with infliximab versus 12 patients treated with steroids, azathioprine, antibiotics, and salicylates. The infliximab arm showed a rapid and continued improvement in disease activity with an improvement in the Bath Ankylosing Spondylitis Disease Activity Index at 1 year compared with the control group.[22]

Unlike AS, sacroiliitis is usually asymptomatic and non-progressive. Most patients with sacroiliitis are HLA-B27 negative and do not progress to AS.[1] Plain radiographs may show unilateral or bilateral sclerosis along with evidence of erosion. Unfortunately, patients with radiographic evidence of sacroiliitis are more likely to progress to AS.[5] MRI has a high sensitivity to detect sacroiliitis and is regarded as the gold standard.

DERMATOLOGIC MANIFESTATIONS

Skin manifestations are common EIMs associated with IBD. The 2 most recognized examples are EN and PG, although the incidence varies, widely affecting 3% to 20%, and 0.5% to 20% of patients, respectively.[17,23] At the time of diagnosis of IBD, up to 10% of patients may already be suffering from cutaneous manifestations.[24] The diagnosis of cutaneous EIM is often made based on clinical examination, specifically, the characteristic features associated with each manifestation.

Erythema Nodosum

EN has been reported to occur in up to 15% of patients with CD and 10% of patients with UC.[25] EN is classically described as raised, red, tender inflammatory nodules of 1 to 5 cm in diameter. The lesions are usually on the anterior, extensor surface of the lower extremities, but can affect the face and trunk.[25] The lesions usually heal without ulceration, and the prognosis is good.[26] EN flares often reflect underlying intestinal activity and improve with treatment of IBD. Histologically, EN demonstrates nonspecific focal panniculitis and can develop anywhere subcutaneous fat is present; the anterior tibial area is the most common site. EN exacerbations have been associated with infections to include tuberculosis, coccidioidomycosis, histoplasmosis, blastomycosis, and sarcoidosis.[27–30] In addition, medications such as sulfonamides, iodides, bromides, and estrogens have been associated with EN.[26] Symptoms usually mimic intestinal activity; therefore, treatment is aimed at the underlying bowel disease. However, EN may precede intestinal activity and in these cases oral corticosteroids may be required for treatment.[26]

Pyoderma Gangrenosum

PG is a severe, debilitating EIM that is more commonly associated with UC than with CD.[31] Patients with more severe disease or colonic involvement are more likely to develop PG.[31] PG begins with discrete pustules than contain purulent material. These pustules are often sterile unless they become secondarily infected. They then evolve into deep evacuating ulcerations. The most common sites include the shins and peristomal skin, but can occur anywhere. Similar to EN, the diagnosis is made on clinical examination, but cultures and biopsy may be taken to exclude other diagnoses. Histologic examination generally reveals diffuse neutrophilic infiltration and dermolysis. PG lesions are usually preceded by trauma through a phenomenon known as pathergy. Because of this, aggressive surgical debridement is strongly discouraged. Local wound care should follow the tenets of common ulcer treatment and consists of topical compresses, enzymatic ointments, and clean dressings. Peristomal PG is especially problematic given the difficulties with appliance application (**Fig. 1**). Unfortunately, PG often recurs at the area of a new stoma; therefore, stomal relocation is often reserved as a last resort after all other measures have been exhausted.[32] Management of PG is usually begun with high-dose prednisone with tapering or intralesional injections. Funayama and colleagues[33] found that patients with peristomal PG treated with early systemic prednisone, a dose 20 mg to 40 mg, was affective in healing the ulcerations. In more severe cases, cyclosporine or tacrolimus may be effective. Topical tacrolimus has also emerged as a treatment option.[34] Compared with the numerous TNF inhibitor-joint disease trials, very few rigorous studies have been performed to investigate the effectiveness of adalimumab and infliximab for cutaneous EIM associated with IBD. However, there is evidence to support the use of biologic therapy. Brooklyn and colleagues[35] performed a multicenter, randomized, placebo-controlled trial of 30 patients with PG, 19 of which had IBD. Patients were given infliximab 5 mg/kg or placebo infusions at week 0 and were evaluated for response. At week 2, subjects in both arms were offered open-label infliximab 5 mg/kg. Two weeks after the initial infusion, 6 of 13 (46%) patients treated with infliximab had a response compared with 1 of 17 (6%) in the control group ($P = .025$). Most patients (69%) who received open-label infusions of infliximab had a positive response by week 6. There was no difference in response between patients with underlying IBD compared with non-IBD patients.

Aphthous Ulcers

Oral apthous ulcers occur in approximately 10% of patients with UC and 20% to 30% of patients with CD. Ulcers tend to rapidly resolve once remission is achieved in patients with active CD. Ulcer patients with other EIMs are more likely to develop recurrent episodes. Treatment consists of addressing the underlying bowel disease, but symptomatic relief may be achieved with the use of 2% viscous lidocaine along with 0.1% triamcinolone topically.[36]

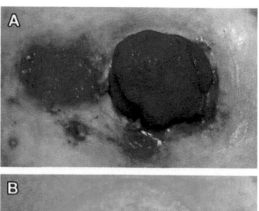

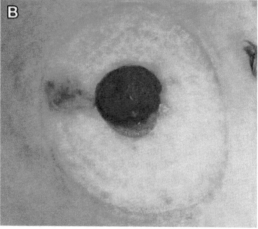

Fig. 1. Peristomal PG (*A*) before and (*B*) after treatment. (*From* Poritz LS, Lebo MA, Bobb AD, et al. Management of peristomal pyoderma gangrenosum. J Am Coll Surg 2008;206(2):313; with permission.)

Sweet Syndrome

Sweet syndrome is a rare EIM that is best described as a neutrophilic dermatosis characterized by painful erythematous plaques or nodules on the face, neck, and extremities. It is often accompanied by fever and leukocytosis.[37] It has been suggested that Sweet syndrome may be part of the spectrum of diseases related to PG.[38] Sweet syndrome is more common in women (87%) and in patients with colonic involvement (100%).[9] Patients usually respond well to corticosteroids, and there are some case reports demonstrating success with biologic therapy.[37,39,40]

Other cutaneous manifestations have been associated with IBD. Acrodermatitis enteropathica is a rare skin disorder that manifests as psoriasiform erythema with vesicles, pustules, and crusts around orifices (perioral, perigenital, perianal) or on extensor surfaces. It is often associated with zinc-deficient diets and malabsorption.[38] In addition, psoriasis has been observed in patients suffering from IBD. Psoriasis occurs in about 1% to 2% of the population, but affects 7% to 11% of patients with IBD. There is no correlation between the course of psoriasis and the activity of intestinal disease.[24]

OCULAR MANIFESTATIONS

Ocular complications are involved in 4% to 10% of IBD patients,[41] which include scleritis, episcleritis, and uveitis. Most patients will already carry the diagnosis of

IBD when they develop ocular symptoms, but a minority of patients will manifest symptoms before the diagnosis of IBD.[42] The ophthalmic complications are usually of inflammatory origin; however, some of these complications may reflect overall disease activity.[25,43]

Episcleritis and Scleritis

Episcleritis is defined as painless hyperemia of the conjunctiva and sclera with no visual deficits (**Fig. 2**). Episcleritis may be unilateral or bilateral and is more common in women.[43] Episcleritis usually mirrors acute flares of IBD, with resolution of symptoms following the use of anti-inflammatory medications. Scleritis is a chronic, painful, and potentially blinding inflammatory process characterized by edema and cellular infiltration of the scleral tissues. It is often classified into anterior and posterior. The initial therapy consists of NSAIDs, followed by corticosteroids if needed.[44,45] In cases refractory to therapy, methotrexate or cyclosporine may be helpful.

Uveitis

Uveitis is the most commonly diagnosed ocular manifestation of IBD. Uveitis is an acute painful condition with associated blurred vision and photophobia. Uveitis may look very similar to episcleritis on gross examination. However, this is a serious condition that must be treated immediately with corticosteroids, because it can progress to blindness if left untreated. Similar to PG, uveitis flares may not be associated exacerbation of IBD or be an indicator of active disease. In addition, uveitis refractory to steroids has been successfully treated with cyclosporine A.[46]

Biologic therapy has shown promising results in treating ocular EIM associated with IBD. Infliximab seems to be effective for acute and chronic uveitis, specifically for patients with ocular disease refractory to other immunosuppressants.[47] Currently, there are more than 65 publications on the use of infliximab for uveitis patients.[48] Suhler and colleagues[49] performed a prospective trial investigating the use of infliximab for the treatment of refractory autoimmune uveitis. In 23 cases of uveitis given a loading dose regimen of infliximab, 18 patients had responded to treatment within 10 weeks based on a composite clinical assessment. In addition, 7 of 14 patients who went on to receive infliximab for 1 year continued to benefit from therapy. In another study, Kahn and colleagues[50] observed that 17 children with refractory uveitis had favorable responses to infliximab, with 13 of the 17 patients having no ocular inflammation after only 2 infusions.

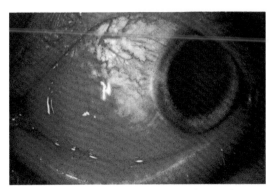

Fig. 2. Slit-lamp view of left eye shows nodular episcleritis. (*From* Hegde V, Mitrut I, Bennett H, et al. Episcleritis: an association with IgA nephropathy. Cont Lens Anterior Eye 2009;32(3):141; with permission.)

HEPATOBILIARY MANIFESTATIONS

Hepatobiliary manifestations are common among patients with IBD. Although PSC is the most recognized, others include cholelithiasis, portal vein thrombosis (PVT), drug-induced hepatotoxicity, and acute and chronic idiopathic pancreatitis.

Primary Sclerosing Cholangitis

PSC is the most recognized biliary EIM of IBD, with a prevalence of 1.4% to 7%.[51] PSC is a chronic, progressive, nonreversible cholestatic disorder that results in fibrosis of the biliary system. Clinical symptoms include fatigue, pruritus, jaundice, abdominal pain, and weight loss. PSC is characterized by progressive inflammation, destruction of the intrahepatic, extrahepatic, or both resulting in obliterative fibrosis.[52] These pathologic changes lead to biliary cirrhosis and in some cases hepatic failure.[53] The pathogenesis of PSC is unclear, but multiple genetic factors associated with susceptibility have been reported.[54] Autoantibodies and bacterial translocation have been hypothesized to be related to PSC in IBD patients; however, these theories have been challenged by recent studies.[55–58]

The prevalence of PSC ranges from 2% to 7.5% in patients with UC and from 1.4% to 3.4% in patients with CD.[59–61] In patients with PSC-IBD, 85% to 90% have UC and the remaining patients have Crohn colitis or Crohn ileocolitis.[62]

The development of cholestasis in any IBD patient should prompt an evaluation for PSC. Jaundice may arise at any time due to biliary strictures. Laboratory abnormalities show an elevated alkaline phosphatase level, whereas aspartate aminotransferase and alanine aminotransferase levels are typically normal. Albumin and prothrombin times are typically normal until the development of cirrhosis. Approximately 33% of patients have an elevated antinuclear antibody level, and 80% will have a positive antineutrophil cytoplasmic antibody level.[63,64] Visualization of the biliary tree is essential to confirm the diagnosis of PSC. The typical findings include multifocal strictures of both the intrabiliary and the extrabiliary system, which results in the classic "bead-on-a-string" pattern (**Fig. 3**). Magnetic resonance cholangiopancreatography is the initial imaging study of choice, with endoscopic retrograde cholangiopancreatography being reserved for those patients that require stenting or biopsy of lesions that are concerning for malignancy due to the risk of cholangitis with instrumentation.[5]

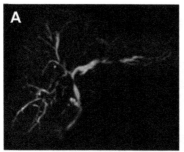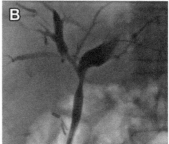

Fig. 3. Typical cholangiographic findings of PSC. (*A*) Magnetic resonance cholangiopancreatography shows multiple strictures and dilatations of the biliary tree, affecting the intrahepatic and extrahepatic biliary tree. (*B*) Endoscopic retrograde cholangiopancreatography with typical findings of pruning and beaded appearance of the biliary tree. (*From* Singh S, Talwalkar JA. Primary sclerosing cholangitis: diagnosis, prognosis, and management. Clin Gastroenterol Hepatol 2013;11(8):899; with permission.)

PSC-IBD patients appear to have a unique form of IBD. UC associated with PSC has a higher prevalence of rectal sparing, backwash ileitis, and colorectal neoplasia.[65] In addition, new onset PSC may be diagnosed years after UC diagnosis with or without proctocolectomy.[5] PSC-IBD patients often have a more quiescent course of colitis than UC patients without PSC.[5]

The presence of PSC is associated with an increased risk for UC-associated dysplasia.[66] This risk continues even after orthotopic liver transplant.[67] Because of this increased risk, it is recommended that patients with PSC-IBD receive annual surveillance colonoscopy once the PSC diagnosis is made,[68] and this surveillance program has been shown to have a survival advantage.[69] In addition, PSC patients have a higher prevalence of cholangiocarcinoma with an annual incidence of 0.6% to 1%.[70] Cholangiocarcinoma may present as an intraductal mass or liver lesion.[71] Although it is clear that PSC is a risk factor for cholangiocarcinoma, it is less clear if there is a link to IBD.

Currently, no medical therapies have been effective at preventing the progression of PSC. Ursodeoxycholic acid (UDCA) has been extensively studied, and the utility of this drug for the treatment of PSC is unclear. In addition, although initially thought to decrease the risk of colorectal neoplasia associated with IBD,[72] UDCA may actually increase that risk.[73] Endoscopic intervention is often needed in patients with progressive disease, increasing jaundice, cholangitis, or suspicion of cholangiocarcinoma. Endoscopic treatments with balloon dilation of strictures and stent placement are required for strictures.[74]

Cholelithiasis

Cholelithiasis is common in IBD patients, specifically in CD patients with ileal disease. Abnormal bile salt absorption and metabolism may result in an increased incidence of gallstone formation in CD patients, ranging from 13% to 38%. Recent studies demonstrated that CD patients have an increased level of both conjugated and unconjugated bilirubin in bile and that an increased enterohepatic circulation of bilirubin was a contributing factor for cholelithiasis formation.[75,76] In addition, CD patients have a decreased gallbladder motility; therefore, the development of cholelithiasis seems to be multifactorial.[77–79]

Portal Vein Thrombosis

PVT is a rare complication in the nonsurgical setting that has been association with coagulation abnormalities; however, the incidence seems to be higher in IBD compared with the general population.[80] It also occurs more frequently in IBD patients with recent abdominal surgery.[80] Venkatesh and colleagues[81] demonstrated that the incidence of PVT in IBD patients was higher (odds ratio [OR] 1.7; 95% confidence interval [CI] 1.01–2.8), which persisted after being adjusted for hypercoagulable disorders. Younger patients (18–39 years) and women had the highest risk compared with control (OR 4.1; 95% CI 1.87–8.9) and (OR 10.9; 95% CI 4.62–25.7).[82]

RENAL

EIM of IBD associated with the renal collecting system includes nephrolithiasis, obstructive uropathy, and fistulization of the urinary tract.[83] Such symptoms may occur in 4% to 23% of IBD patients.[84] Nephrolithiasis, which is more prevalent in CD than UC, is primarily composed of calcium oxalate and urate crystals. Ileocolonic resection in patients with CD and colectomy in UC patients may accelerate the formation of oxalate stones.[84] Another renal EIM associated with IBD is a rare condition known as secondary amyloidosis. Patients may present with proteinuria, renal failure, and uremia. This condition more commonly affects men and CD patients with a 3-fold and 10-fold increased risk, respectively.[85] The diagnosis is made via liver, rectal, or renal biopsy, because this is a systemic disease. Treatment is aimed at the systemic nature of the disease; although biologic therapy has some proven benefit, some patients may progress to requiring renal transplantation.[86]

PULMONARY

IBD patients commonly suffer from subclinical EIM involving the pulmonary system.[87] The spectrum of respiratory manifestations reported includes both small and large airway disease. Specifically, conditions include chronic bronchitis, subglottic stenosis, bronchiectasis, and bronchiolitis.[88,89] It is important to mention that pulmonary symptoms in IBD patients may be secondary to the treatment of the underlying intestinal disease. Although drug-related conditions are not normally considered EIM of IBD, it is important to remember that nearly all of the proposed treatments for IBD may have some pulmonary side effects.[90] Pulmonary manifestations can occur in nonsmokers, and in general, follow the onset of bowel disease, but in rare cases may precede the onset of intestinal symptoms.[91] Bronchoalveolar lavage demonstrates alveolitis in up to 50% of CD patients without pulmonary symptoms, and pulmonary function testing is abnormal in up to 42% of asymptomatic patients.[87] Lung biopsy often shows nonspecific inflammation, small airway fibrosis, and occasionally, granulomatous bronchiolitis.[5] IBD-related pulmonary disease is difficult to manage and is treated similarly to non-IBD patients for the specific conditions. Improvement following oral steroid therapy may be slight to modest, and lung transplantation may be required for extreme cases.

SUMMARY

IBD affects multiple organ systems outside of the gastrointestinal tract. The clinician treating patients with IBD should be acutely aware of the diagnosis and treatment of EIM in order to decrease morbidity. The management can be difficult and often times requires a multidisciplinary approach. Future research investigating the pathophysiology, diagnosis, and treatment is needed to further the care of these patients.

REFERENCES

1. Trikudanathan G, Venkatesh PGK, Navaneethan U. Diagnosis and therapeutic management of extra-intestinal manifestations of inflammatory bowel disease. Drugs 2012;72(18):2333–49.
2. Chapman RW, Cottone M, Selby WS, et al. Serum autoantibodies, ulcerative colitis and primary sclerosing cholangitis. Gut 1986;27(1):86–91.
3. Loftus EV Jr. Management of extraintestinal manifestations and other complications of inflammatory bowel disease. Curr Gastroenterol Rep 2004;6(6):506–13.
4. Bernstein CN, Wajda A, Blanchard JF. The clustering of other chronic inflammatory diseases in inflammatory bowel disease: a population-based study. Gastroenterology 2005;129(3):827–36.
5. Rothfuss KS, Stange EF. Extraintestinal manifestations and complications in inflammatory bowel diseases. World J Gastroenterol 2006;12(30):4819–31.
6. Orchard TR, Wordsworth BP, Jewell DP. Peripheral arthropathies in inflammatory bowel disease: their articular distribution and natural history. Gut 1998;42(3):387–91.

7. Schorr-Lesnick B, Brandt LJ. Selected rheumatologic and dermatologic mani-festations of inflammatory bowel disease. Am J Gastroenterol 1988;83(3): 216–23.
8. Lakatos PL, Lakatos L, Kiss LS, et al. Treatment of extraintestinal manifestations in inflammatory bowel disease. Digestion 2011;86(Suppl 1):28–35.
9. Ardizzone S, Puttini PS, Cassinotti A. Extraintestinal manifestations of inflamma-tory bowel disease. Dig Liver Dis 2008;40(Suppl 2):S253–9.
10. Williams H, Walker D, Orchard TR. Extraintestinal manifestations of inflammatory bowel disease. Curr Gastroenterol Rep 2008;10(6):597–605.
11. Juillerat P, Mottet C, Pittet V, et al. Extraintestinal manifestations of Crohn's dis-ease. Digestion 2005;71:31–6.
12. Scarpa R, Puente AD, D'arienzo A. The arthritis of ulcerative colitis: clinical and genetic aspects. J Rheumatol 1992;19(3):373–7.
13. Reinisch W, Miehsler W, Dejaco C. An open-label trial of the selective cyclo-oxygenase-2 inhibitor, rofecoxib, in inflammatory bowel disease-associated pe-ripheral arthritis and arthralgia. Aliment Pharmacol Ther 2003;17(11):1371–80.
14. Miao XP, Li JS, Ouyang Q, et al. Tolerability of selective cyclooxygenase 2 inhib-itors used for the treatment of rheumatological manifestations of inflammatory bowel disease. Cochrane Database Syst Rev 2014;(10):CD007744.
15. Kaufman I, Caspi D, Yeshurun D, et al. The effect of infliximab on extraintestinal manifestations of Crohn's disease. Rheumatol Int 2005;25(6):406–10.
16. Vollenhoven RFV, Geborek P, Forslind K. Conventional combination treatment versus biological treatment in methotrexate-refractory early rheumatoid arthritis: 2 year follow-up of the randomised, non-blinded, parallel-group Swefot trial. Lancet 2012;379(9827):1712–20.
17. Su CG, Judge TA, Lichtenstein GR. Extraintestinal manifestations of inflammatory bowel disease. Gastroenterol Clin North Am 2002;31(1):307–27.
18. Braun J, Heijde DVD. Imaging and scoring in ankylosing spondylitis. Best Pract Res Clin Rheumatol 2002;16(4):573–604.
19. Dignass A, Assche GV, Lindsay JO. The second European evidence-based consensus on the diagnosis and management of Crohn's disease: current man-agement. J Crohns Colitis 2010;4(1):28–62.
20. Rosman Z, Shoenfeld Y, Zandman-Goddard G. Biologic therapy for autoimmune diseases: an update. BMC Med 2013;11:88.
21. Zochling J, Heijde DVD, Dougados M. Current evidence for the management of ankylosing spondylitis: a systematic literature review for the ASAS/EULAR man-agement recommendations in ankylosing spondylitis. Ann Rheum Dis 2006; 65(4):423–32.
22. Generini S, Giacomelli R, Fedi R, et al. Infliximab in spondyloarthropathy associ-ated with Crohn's disease: an open study on the efficacy of inducing and main-taining remission of musculoskeletal and gut manifestations. Ann Rheum Dis 2004;63(12):1664–9.
23. Bodegraven AAV, Peña AS. Treatment of extraintestinal manifestations in inflam-matory bowel disease. Curr Treat Options Gastroenterol 2003;6(3):201–12.
24. Veloso FT. Skin complications associated with inflammatory bowel disease. Aliment Pharmacol Ther 2004;20(Suppl 4):50–3.
25. Greenstein AJ, Janowitz HD, Sachar DB. The extra-intestinal complications of Crohn's disease and ulcerative colitis: a study of 700 patients. Medicine (Balti-more) 1976;55(5):401–12.
26. Levine JS, Burakoff R. Extraintestinal manifestations of inflammatory bowel dis-ease. Gastroenterol Hepatol 2011;7(4):235–41.

27. Saslaw S, Beman FM. Erythema nodosum as a manifestation of histoplasmosis. J Am Med Assoc 1959;170(10):1178–9.
28. Löfgren S, Wahlgren F. On the histo-pathology of erythema nodosum. Acta Derm Venereol 1949;29:1–13.
29. Hannuksela M. Erythema nodosum. Clin Dermatol 1986;4(4):88–95.
30. Soderstrom RM, Krull EA. Erythema nodosum. A review. Cutis 1978;21(6): 806–10.
31. Orchard TR, Chua CN, Ahmad T, et al. Uveitis and erythema nodosum in inflammatory bowel disease: clinical features and the role of HLA genes. Gastroenterology 2002;123(3):714–8.
32. Kiran RP, O'Brien-Ermlich B, Achkar JP. Management of peristomal pyoderma gangrenosum. Dis Colon Rectum 2005;48(7):1397–403.
33. Funayama Y, Kumagai E, Takahashi K. Early diagnosis and early corticosteroid administration improves healing of peristomal pyoderma gangrenosum in inflammatory bowel disease. Dis Colon Rectum 2009;52(2):311–4.
34. Chiba T, Isomura I, Suzuki A. Topical tacrolimus therapy for pyoderma gangrenosum. J Dermatol 2005;32(3):199–203.
35. Brooklyn TN, Dunnill MGS, Shetty A, et al. Infliximab for the treatment of pyoderma gangrenosum: a randomised, double blind, placebo controlled trial. Gut 2006;55(4):505–9.
36. Larsen S, Bendtzen K, Nielsen OH. Extraintestinal manifestations of inflammatory bowel disease: epidemiology, diagnosis, and management. Ann Med 2010;42(2): 97–114.
37. Kemmett D, Hunter JAA. Sweet's syndrome: a clinicopathologic review of twenty-nine cases. J Am Acad Dermatol 1990;23(3 Pt 1):503–7.
38. Ochsendorf FR. Cutaneous manifestations of IBD and IBD-associated inflammatory lesions. 1998. Falk symposium Titisee. Germany, May 25–26, 1997.
39. Rochet NM, Chavan RN, Cappel MA, et al. Sweet syndrome: clinical presentation, associations, and response to treatment in 77 patients. J Am Acad Dermatol 2013;69(4):557–64.
40. Foster EN, Nguyen KK, Sheikh RA. Crohn's disease associated with Sweet's syndrome and Sjögren's syndrome treated with infliximab. Clin Dev Immunol 2005; 12(2):145–9.
41. Knox DL, Schachat AP, Mustonen E. Primary, secondary and coincidental ocular complications of Crohn's disease. Ophthalmology 1984;91(2):163–73.
42. Soukiasian SH, Foster CS, Raizman MB. Treatment strategies for scleritis and uveitis associated with inflammatory bowel disease. Am J Ophthalmol 1994; 118(5):601–11.
43. Hopkins DJ, Horan E, Burton IL, et al. Ocular disorders in a series of 332 patients with Crohn's disease. Br J Ophthalmol 1974;58(8):732–7.
44. Galor A, Jabs DA, Leder HA, et al. Comparison of antimetabolite drugs as corticosteroid-sparing therapy for noninfectious ocular inflammation. Ophthalmology 2008;115(10):1826–32.
45. Sobrin L, Christen W, Foster CS. Mycophenolate mofetil after methotrexate failure or intolerance in the treatment of scleritis and uveitis. Ophthalmology 2008; 115(8):1416–21, 1421.e1.
46. Barrie A, Regueiro M. Biologic therapy in the management of extraintestinal manifestations of inflammatory bowel disease. Inflamm Bowel Dis 2007;13(11): 1424–9.
47. Hale S, Lightman S. Anti-TNF therapies in the management of acute and chronic uveitis. Cytokine 2006;33(4):231–7.

48. Schwartzman S, Schwartzman M. The use of biologic therapies in uveitis. Clin Rev Allergy Immunol 2014. [Epub ahead of print].
49. Suhler EB, Smith JR, Wertheim MS. A prospective trial of infliximab therapy for refractory uveitis: preliminary safety and efficacy outcomes. Arch Ophthalmol 2005;123(7):903–12.
50. Kahn P, Weiss M, Imundo LF, et al. Favorable response to high-dose infliximab for refractory childhood uveitis. Ophthalmology 2006;113(5):860–4.e2.
51. Fausa O, Schrumpf E, Elgjo K. Relationship of inflammatory bowel disease and primary sclerosing cholangitis. Semin Liver Dis 1991;11(1):31–9.
52. Chapman RW, Arborgh BA, Rhodes JM. Primary sclerosing cholangitis: a review of its clinical features, cholangiography, and hepatic histology. Gut 1980;21(10): 870–7.
53. Lee YM, Kaplan MM. Primary sclerosing cholangitis. N Engl J Med 1995;332(14): 924–33.
54. Farrant JM, Doherty DG, Donaldson PT. Amino acid substitutions at position 38 of the DRβ polypeptide confer susceptibility to and protection from primary sclerosing cholangitis. Hepatology 1992;16(2):390–5.
55. O'Mahony CA, Vierling JM. Etiopathogenesis of primary sclerosing cholangitis. Semin Liver Dis 2006;26(1):3–21.
56. Worthington J, Cullen S, Chapman R. Immunopathogenesis of primary sclerosing cholangitis. Clin Rev Allergy Immunol 2005;28(2):93–103.
57. Hatano H, Nakajima Y, Sugita S. Experimental portal fibrosis produced by intraportal injection of killed nonpathogenic Escherichia coli in rabbits. Gastroenterology 1988;94(3):787–96.
58. Björnsson ES, Kilander AF, Olsson RG. Bile duct bacterial isolates in primary sclerosing cholangitis and certain other forms of cholestasis–a study of bile cultures from ERCP. Hepatogastroenterology 2000;47(36):1504–8.
59. Schrumpf E, Elgjo K, Fausa O, et al. Sclerosing cholangitis in ulcerative colitis. Scand J Gastroenterol 1980;15(6):689–97.
60. Shepherd HA, Selby WS, Chapman RWG, et al. Ulcerative colitis and persistent liver dysfunction. Q J Med 1983;52(208):503–13.
61. Rasmussen HH, Fallingborg JF. Hepatobiliary dysfunction and primary sclerosing cholangitis in patients with Crohn's disease. Scand J Gastroenterol 1997;32(6): 604–10.
62. Olsson R, Danielsson A, Jarnerot G, et al. Prevalence of primary sclerosing cholangitis in patients with ulcerative colitis. Gastroenterology 1991;100(5 Pt 1):1319–23.
63. Mulder AH, Horst G, Haagsma EB, et al. Prevalence and characterization of neutrophil cytoplasmic antibodies in autoimmune liver diseases. Hepatology 1993;17(3):411–7.
64. Bansi DS, Fleming KA, Chapman RW. Importance of antineutrophil cytoplasmic antibodies in primary sclerosing cholangitis and ulcerative colitis: prevalence, titre, and IgG subclass. Gut 1996;38(3):384–9.
65. Vries BAD, Janse M, Blokzijl H, et al. Distinctive inflammatory bowel disease phenotype in primary sclerosing cholangitis. World J Gastroenterol 2015;21(6): 1956–71.
66. Soetikno RM, Lin OS, Heidenreich PA. Increased risk of colorectal neoplasia in patients with primary sclerosing cholangitis and ulcerative colitis: a meta-analysis. Gastrointest Endosc 2002;56(1):48–54.
67. Bleday R, Lee E, Jessurun J, et al. Increased risk of early colorectal neoplasms after hepatic transplant in patients with inflammatory bowel disease. Dis Colon Rectum 1993;36(10):908–12.

68. Kornbluth A, Sachar DB. Ulcerative colitis practice guidelines in adults. American College of Gastroenterology, Practice Parameters Committee. Am J Gastroenterol 1997;92(2):204–11.

69. Rutter MD, Saunders BP, Wilkinson KH, et al. Cancer surveillance in longstanding ulcerative colitis: endoscopic appearances help predict cancer risk. Gut 2004; 53(12):1813–6.

70. Bergquist A, Ekbom A, Olsson R, et al. Hepatic and extrahepatic malignancies in primary sclerosing cholangitis. J Hepatol 2002;36(3):321–7.

71. Fevery J, Verslype C, Lai G, et al. Incidence, diagnosis, and therapy of cholangio-carcinoma in patients with primary sclerosing cholangitis. Dig Dis Sci 2007; 52(11):3123–35.

72. Pardi DS, Loftus EV, Kremers WK, et al. Ursodeoxycholic acid as a chemopreven-tive agent in patients with ulcerative colitis and primary sclerosing cholangitis. Gastroenterology 2003;124(4):889–93.

73. Eaton JE, Silveira MG, Pardi DS, et al. High-dose ursodeoxycholic acid is asso-ciated with the development of colorectal neoplasia in patients with ulcerative colitis and primary sclerosing cholangitis. Am J Gastroenterol 2011;106(9): 1638–45.

74. Baluyut AR, Sherman S, Lehman GA, et al. Impact of endoscopic therapy on the survival of patients with primary sclerosing cholangitis. Gastrointest Endosc 2001;53(3):308–12.

75. Brink MA, Slors JFM, Keulemans YCA, et al. Enterohepatic cycling of bilirubin: a putative mechanism for pigment gallstone formation in ileal Crohn's disease. Gastroenterology 1999;116(6):1420–7.

76. Parente F, Pastore L, Bargiggia S, et al. Incidence and risk factors for gallstones in patients with inflammatory bowel disease: a large case-control study. Hepatol-ogy 2007;45(5):1267–74.

77. Damiao A, Sipahi AM, Vezozzo DP, et al. Gallbladder hypokinesia in Crohn's dis-ease. Digestion 1997;58(5):458–63.

78. Annese V, Vantrappen G. Gall stones in Crohn's disease: another hypothesis. Gut 1994;35(11):1676.

79. Pitt HA, King W, Mann LL, et al. Increased risk of cholelithiasis with prolonged total parenteral nutrition. Am J Surg 1983;145(1):106–12.

80. Jackson LM, O'Gorman PJ, O'connell J. Thrombosis in inflammatory bowel dis-ease: clinical setting, procoagulant profile and factor V Leiden. QJM 1997; 90(3):183–8.

81. Venkatesh PGK, Navaneethan U, Shen B. Hepatobiliary disorders and complica-tions of inflammatory bowel disease. J Dig Dis 2011;12(4):245–56.

82. Sridhar ARM, Parasa S, Navaneethan U. Comprehensive study of cardiovascular morbidity in hospitalized inflammatory bowel disease patients. J Crohns Colitis 2011;5(4):287–94.

83. Banner MP. Genitourinary complications of inflammatory bowel disease. Radiol Clin North Am 1987;25(1):199–209.

84. McConnell N, Campbell S, Gillanders I. Risk factors for developing renal stones in inflammatory bowel disease. BJU Int 2002;89(9):835–41.

85. Wester AL, Vatn MH, Fausa O. Secondary amyloidosis in inflammatory bowel dis-ease: a study of 18 patients admitted to Rikshospitalet University Hospital, Oslo, from 1962 to 1998. Inflamm Bowel Dis 2001;7(4):295–300.

86. Kuroda T, Tanabe N, Kobayashi D, et al. Treatment with biologic agents improves the prognosis of patients with rheumatoid arthritis and amyloidosis. J Rheumatol 2012;39(7):1348–54.

87. Herrlinger KR, Noftz MK, Dalhoff K, et al. Alterations in pulmonary function in inflammatory bowel disease are frequent and persist during remission. Am J Gastroenterol 2002;97(2):377–81.
88. Camus PH, Colby TV. The lung in inflammatory bowel disease. Eur Respir J 2000; 15(1):5–10.
89. Spira A, Grossman R, Balter M. Large airway disease associated with inflammatory bowel disease. Chest 1998;113(6):1723–6.
90. Casella G, Villanacci V, Bella CD, et al. Pulmonary diseases associated with inflammatory bowel diseases. J Crohns Colitis 2010;4(4):384–9.
91. Kelly MG, Frizelle FA, Thornley PT, et al. Inflammatory bowel disease and the lung: is there a link between surgery and bronchiectasis? Int J Colorectal Dis 2006;21(8):754–7.

Colorectal Neoplasia and Inflammatory Bowel Disease

Jamie Cannon, MD

KEYWORDS

- Colorectal cancer • Inflammatory bowel disease • Neoplasia • Crohn's disease
- Ulcerative colitis

KEY POINTS

- Ulcerative colitis and Crohn's colitis are associated with a 2- to 5-fold increased risk of colorectal cancer.
- Patients with ulcerative colitis and Crohn's colitis should undergo surveillance colonoscopy to detect dysplasia, and if detected, should generally undergo prophylactic surgical resection.
- Patients that have undergone restorative proctocolectomy should have their ileal pouch and the anal transition zone surveyed via endoscopy.
- Patients with Crohn's disease are at increased risk of developing small bowel and anal cancers.

INTRODUCTION

Crohn's disease and ulcerative colitis are significant risk factors for the development of gastrointestinal neoplasias.[1] The association between ulcerative colitis and colorectal cancer has long been recognized, and surveillance protocols to detect neoplasia in the setting of ulcerative colitis are well established. Engaging in surveillance has been shown to decrease the risk of death from colorectal cancer among ulcerative colitis patients. Although the cancer risk related to Crohn's disease is not as well defined, all inflamed segments of bowel are at increased risk for the development of neoplasia. Crohn's colitis is associated with a risk of colorectal cancer similar to that of ulcerative colitis, and the risk of small bowel adenocarcinoma in patients with Crohn's enteritis is greatly elevated compared with that of the general population.

Department of Surgery, University of Alabama at Birmingham, 1720 2nd Ave S, Birmingham, AL 35294-0016, USA
E-mail address: jacannon@uab.edu

Surg Clin N Am 95 (2015) 1261–1269
http://dx.doi.org/10.1016/j.suc.2015.08.001
0039-6109/15/$ – see front matter © 2015 Elsevier Inc. All rights reserved.

MECHANISM OF ACTION OF INCREASED RISK

Sporadic colorectal cancers develop via the classic adenoma-dysplasia-carcinoma sequence. The development of colorectal cancer in the setting of colitis also progresses from dysplasia to carcinoma, although the process appears to be different and the progression is accelerated. It is thought that the inflammatory process leads to oxidative stress-induced DNA damage of the affected mucosa. Loss of p53 function is seen early in this sequence, unlike in sporadic cancers wherein this is usually a late finding.[2,3] Constant attempts at regeneration provide more opportunities for transcription errors and the subsequent development of neoplasia via activation of procarcinogenic genes and inhibition of tumor suppressor genes. Alteration in the colonic flora has also been proposed as a mechanism to increase the cancer risk. Altered flora may increase the degree of inflammation, or possibly produce procarcinogenic substances. *Bacteroides fragilis* and *Enterococcus feacalis* have been implicated as procarcinogens.

The use of immunosuppression to treat inflammatory bowel disease plays a role as well. Optimal control of inflammation is important, because the degree of inflammation correlates with the cancer risk.[4] However, immunosuppression may also allow neoplasia to advance at a faster rate. 5-Aminosalicylic acid drugs, on the other hand, have been shown to have a protective effect.[5] Cancers that arise in the setting of inflammatory bowel disease are more likely to be poorly differentiated,[2] although whether this portends a poorer prognosis is not clear. Studies have been contradictory, with some showing similar overall survival to sporadic cancers,[6,7] and others showing a poorer stage-for-stage survival.[8,9] As the increased risk is a field effect to all areas of inflamed bowel, inflammatory bowel disease–related cancers are also associated with a higher risk of both synchronous (12.4%) and metachronous (14.3%) cancers.[8]

ULCERATIVE COLITIS AND COLORECTAL CANCER

Ulcerative colitis is associated with a 2- to 5-fold risk for the development of colorectal cancer,[10–12] although the reported increased risk varies widely from study to study. The incidence has been estimated as approximately 1% per year, or 30% at 35 years.[13] Alternatively, Choi and colleagues[14] found the incidence of colorectal cancer to be only 10% at 40 years. Those who also have primary sclerosing cholangitis are at an even greater risk for colorectal cancer, and that increased risk is present at the onset of disease.[15]

SURVEILLANCE

Prophylactic total proctocolectomy is the recommended surgical treatment option for those at greatest risk of colorectal cancer. As the risk of developing neoplasia increases with the duration of disease, prophylactic surgery used to be recommended after 10 years of active disease to reduce cancer risk. The current trend is toward a more individualized approach, with surveillance recommended for most patients. Multiple societies have published recommended surveillance guidelines, although they are all quite similar. National Comprehensive Cancer Network (NCCN) guidelines recommend beginning surveillance after 8 to 10 years of pancolitis[16] with colonoscopies performed every 1 to 2 years, because the incidence of colorectal cancer increases after 8 years of disease.[1,17] Biopsies should be taken in 4 quadrants every 10 cm, resulting in more than 30 biopsy specimens for pathology. The chance of a false-negative surveillance colonoscopy decreases with the more biopsies that are taken.

It has been estimated that it is necessary to take 33 biopsies to achieve a 90% sensitivity for the detection of dysplasia.[3] Many authors have recommended using chromoendoscopy rather than standard white light colonoscopy to perform targeted rather than random biopsies. Chromoendoscopy allows for the identification of abnormal-appearing mucosa and has been demonstrated to detect neoplasia at double the rate of standard white-light colonoscopy.[14,18] However, a recent review by Mooiweer and colleagues[19] did not find that chromoendoscopy improved the detection of dysplasia.

Surveillance colonoscopy is less effective in those who have continuing active disease and abnormal-appearing colonic mucosa. If possible, surveillance colonoscopies should be performed when disease is in remission. The presence of active inflammation interferes with the pathologist's ability to accurately diagnose dysplasia on biopsy specimens. In addition, cancers in the presence of abnormal colonic mucosa can be difficult to detect. A reactive pseudopolyposis of the colon can very easily hide a colon cancer, as can tissue bridges and active ulceration. If medical therapy does not render the colon easier to survey, consideration should be given to prophylactic surgery. Even in the absence of active inflammation, advanced cancers develop in patients undergoing a surveillance program. Cancers that develop in the setting of ulcerative colitis are more likely to be flat cancers without significant mass effect than cancers that arise spontaneously. They also have more extensive submucosal spread and advance more quickly.

MANAGEMENT OF DYSPLASIA

The goal of a surveillance program is to identify those with dysplasia that are at greatest risk for having or developing colorectal cancer. The presence of high-grade dysplasia (HGD) in normal appearing mucosa is widely accepted as an indication for prophylactic surgery. When HGD is detected on random biopsies, there is a high incidence of occult colorectal cancer in the resected specimen. Most studies estimate the risk of occult cancer to be from 36% to 71%.[14,20–24] Choi and colleagues[14] reviewed 40 years of a surveillance program from the United Kingdom and found that among patients who had HGD on their surveillance colonoscopies, 55% were found to have occult cancer in their colon resection specimens. The high rate of occult cancer clearly demonstrates that the presence of HGD warrants proctocolectomy.

The management of low-grade dysplasia (LGD) is a continued area of controversy. The same study from the United Kingdom found a 28% incidence of occult cancer in the surgical resection specimens of patients who were preoperatively found to have LGD on their surveillance colonoscopy. Among patients that did not have a colectomy for LGD, 32% progressed to more advanced neoplasia (HGD or adenocarcinoma). These findings suggest that even LGD should be managed with prophylactic surgery. However, a recent study by Murphy and colleagues[25] found drastically different results. This study showed only a 2% incidence of occult colorectal cancer when biopsies showed LGD, and 3% when they showed HGD. **Table 1** summarizes the incidence of occult colorectal cancer from numerous studies. These contradictory results present a challenge when counseling patients concerning prophylactic surgery. NCCN guidelines recommend surgical consultation for resection when LGD is detected.[16] The approach should be individualized, and consideration should be given to the patient's disease state, likelihood of follow-up for continued surveillance, and acceptance of prophylactic surgery versus cancer risk. **Fig. 1** provides a proposed algorithm for the management of endoscopically detected neoplasia.

Table 1
Incidence of occult colorectal cancer after dysplasia is detected on surveillance colonoscopy

Study	LGD on Biopsy	HGD on Biopsy
Choi et al,[14] 2015	9/32 (28%)	16/29 (55%)
Murphy et al,[25] 2014	3/141 (2%)	1/33 (3%)
Bernstein et al,[20] 1994	3/16 (19%)	10/24(42%)
Nugent et al,[21] 1991	—	7/18 (39%)
Kewenter et al,[22] 1982	—	5/14 (36%)
Fuson et al,[23] 1980	—	5/7 (71%)
Lennard-Jones et al,[24] 1977	—	4/7 (57%)

Data from Refs.[14,20–25]

DYSPLASIA-ASSOCIATED LESION OR MASS

A patient with ulcerative colitis can develop a sporadic adenoma with HGD, as can any other patient. The challenge to the physician is determining if the HGD is related to a global effect caused by the inflammatory state, in which case proctocolectomy would be recommended. If the lesion is truly sporadic and not related to the patient's inflammatory bowel disease, resection of the lesion alone with close surveillance should be sufficient. Therefore, whenever an actual mass or polyp is identified and removed from a patient with inflammatory bowel disease, biopsies of normal-appearing mucosa around the lesion should be obtained. If the lesion is able to be completely resected, and surrounding mucosal biopsies are normal without evidence of dysplasia, the lesion may be considered more likely to be sporadic and managed in a fashion similar to that of a healthy individual. However, if there is any dysplasia surrounding the lesion, this would be an indication for proctocolectomy. A dysplasia-associated lesion or mass that cannot be completely resected endoscopically requires surgical intervention and is associated with a 43% to 58% cancer risk.[20,26]

NEOPLASIA FOLLOWING PROCTOCOLECTOMY WITH ILEAL POUCH-ANAL ANASTOMOSIS

Most patients undergoing surgical treatment of ulcerative colitis undergo total proctocolectomy with ileal pouch-anal anastomosis reconstruction. When ileal pouch reconstruction was first introduced, the resection was described as being performed along with a mucosectomy of the anal canal. This resection was thought to eliminate all of the colorectal mucosa, and thus, the concern for development of colorectal cancer. More recent studies, however, have shown that there is still a risk of neoplasia even after mucosectomy. In addition, mucosectomy was also associated with high rates of anal stenosis, and this technique has for the most part been replaced with a double-stapled technique. The double-stapled technique is generally preferred because it provides better bowel function, has fewer complications, and is easier to perform.[27,28] With this operation, the proximal bowel is divided at the level of the pelvic floor and the anastomosis is constructed at this level. The bowel mucosa between the dentate line and the pelvic floor represents the transition zone and is left in place. This 1- to 2-cm remnant of colorectal mucosa is still at risk for the development of colorectal cancer. The incidence of dysplasia in the transition zone has been estimated to be 3% to 4%.[29] Although progression to invasive cancer in this region is very rare, it has been reported in multiple case series,[30–32] and this area should therefore continue to be surveyed. Although some have argued that the low incidence of cancer

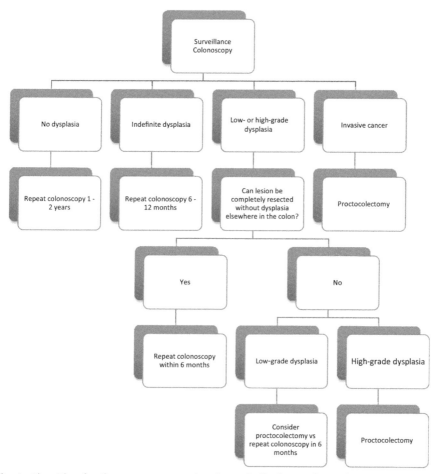

Fig. 1. Algorithm for the management of endoscopically detected neoplasia.

does not warrant surveillance, annual endoscopic examination of the transition zone is generally recommended[33] and widely practiced. Some authors have also promoted random biopsies of the transition zone[29] to identify occult dysplasia.

In addition to neoplasia of the transition zone, cancer can develop within the ileal pouch. Although this is rare, it occurs at a much greater rate than one would expect for a sporadic small bowel cancer. The incidence of pouch neoplasia has been reported to be similar to that in the transition zone, from 0% to 18.5%. A meta-analysis by Scarpa and colleagues[33] estimated the risk to be 1.13%. The most significant risk factor for pouch dysplasia was a diagnosis of dysplasia or cancer at the time of proctocolectomy. Kariv and colleagues[34] grouped pouch and anal transition zone neoplasia together and demonstrated that the risk increases over time, with a 5.1% incidence of neoplasia at 25 years. Options for management of LGD include continued surveillance versus resection. HGD should be treated with resection. The location of the dysplasia determines the surgical management, which is either mucosectomy with pouch advancement or excision and re-creation of the ileal pouch. If re-creation of a pouch-anal anastomosis is not technically feasible, an end ileostomy may be necessary.

CROHN'S DISEASE

Like ulcerative colitis, Crohn's colitis is associated with increased rates of colorectal cancer. In the presence of colitis, the risk is similar to that of ulcerative colitis, with an estimated 8% incidence after 20 years of disease.[35] Therefore, patients with Crohn's colitis should undergo a surveillance regimen of the colon and rectum identical to that of patients with ulcerative colitis. The findings of neoplasia should be managed in a similar fashion, although segmental colectomy can be considered. The at-risk bowel should in theory be the segments of colon that have been affected by inflammation, and not necessarily the entire colon. However, if a segmental resection is performed, close surveillance should continue, because there is a high rate of metachronous cancers.

Because Crohn's disease also affects the small intestine, Crohn's is associated with increased rates of small bowel adenocarcinoma. Fortunately, this more aggressive cancer is not common in the general population, but patients with Crohn's disease have a 20- to 30-fold risk of development of small bowel cancer.[36,37] No specific surveillance is recommended other than the standard management of active Crohn's disease. It seems reasonable, however, to examine as much of the terminal ileum as possible during surveillance colonoscopies. In a patient undergoing surgery for small bowel Crohn's disease, the possibility of neoplasm should be kept in mind at the time of the operation. Although mesenteric dissection can be difficult in the setting of active Crohn's disease, if there is concern for malignancy, an attempt should be made to include the mesentery of the affected and surrounding small bowel.

CANCER IN A FISTULA

The presence of fistulizing anorectal disease is a risk factor for development of rectal/anal adenocarcinoma and squamous cell cancer. Although this is not common, it is a hard condition to treat and is associated with very high mortality. Treatment of the cancer is also complicated by the fact that it occurs in the presence of active Crohn's disease, which may limit treatment options. Fistulizing tracts throughout the perirectal tissues result in the loss of normal anatomic barriers, which allows for easier and earlier spread of neoplasia, making local control a challenge. This disease process is associated with high rates of local recurrence. When possible, these patients should be treated with neoadjuvant chemoradiation in order to maximize local control. The extent of perianal sepsis, however, may preclude the ability to provide neoadjuvant treatment and mandate surgery as the initial management. Surgical therapy is an abdominal perineal resection with wide margins to include all fistula tracts. Reconstruction with myocutaneous rectus abdominus flaps is often necessary given the extent of resection required. Despite aggressive therapy, these cancers are associated with very poor 5-year survival. Devon and colleagues[38–42] reported 14 patients with this diagnosis. With a mean follow-up of 42 months, only 5 patients were without evidence of disease. This study also found that none of the patients' malignancies were detected on preoperative imaging. Therefore, when operating on perianal Crohn's disease, the surgeon must maintain a high index of suspicion and be liberal with biopsies of concerning areas.

SUMMARY

Inflammatory bowel disease is associated with increased rates of gastrointestinal neoplasia. Ulcerative colitis and Crohn's colitis increase the risk of colorectal cancer, and patients with these conditions should be monitored via an intensive surveillance program. This intensive surveillance program should include colonoscopies every 1 to 2 years with multiple biopsies of the colon taken. The presence of dysplasia should warrant referral for consideration of prophylactic proctocolectomy. Crohn's disease is also associated with an increased risk of small bowel and anal cancers.

REFERENCES

1. Eaden JA, Abrams KR, Mayberry JF. The risk of colorectal cancer in ulcerative colitis: a meta-analysis. Gut 2001;48:526–35.
2. Harpaz N, Peck AL, Yin J, et al. p53 protein expression in ulcerative colitis-associated colorectal dysplasia and carcinoma. Hum Pathol 1994;25:1069–74.
3. Cohen RD, Hanauer SB. Surveillance colonoscopy in ulcerative colitis: is the message loud and clear. Am J Gastroenterol 1995;90:2090–2.
4. Rubin DT, Huo D, Kinnucan JA, et al. Inflammation is an independent risk factor for colonic neoplasia in patients with ulcerative colitis: a case-control study. Clin Gastroenterol Hepatol 2013;11(12):1601–8.e1–4.
5. Lyakhovich A, Gasche C. Systematic review: molecular chemoprevention of colorectal malignancy by mesalazine. Aliment Pharmacol Ther 2010;31:202–9.
6. Delaunoit T, Limburg PJ, Goldberg RM, et al. Colorectal cancer prognosis among patients with inflammatory bowel disease. Clin Gastroenterol Hepatol 2006;4:335–42.
7. Kiran R, Khoury W, Church J, et al. Colorectal cancer complicating inflammatory bowel disease. Ann Surg 2010;252:330–5.
8. Gearhart SL, Nathan H, Pawlik TM, et al. Outcomes from IBD-associated and non-IBD associated colorectal cancer: a surveillance epidemiology and end results medicare study. Dis Colon Rectum 2012;55(3):270–7.
9. Jensen A, Larsen M, Gislum M, et al. Survival after colorectal cancer in patients with ulcerative colitis: a nationwide population-based Danish study. Am J Gastroenterol 2006;101:1283–7.
10. Herrinton LJ, Liu L, Levin TR, et al. Incidence and in persons with inflammatory bowel disease from 1998 to 2010. Gastroenterology 2012;143:382–9.
11. Efthymiou M, Taylor AC, Kamm MA. Cancer surveillance strategies in ulcerative colitis: the need for modernization. Inflamm Bowel Dis 2011;17:1800–13.
12. Bernstein CN, Blanchard JF, Kliewer E, et al. Cancer risk in patients with inflammatory bowel disease: a population-based study. Cancer 2001;91:854–62.
13. Ekbom A, Helmick C, Zack M, et al. Ulcerative colitis and colorectal cancer: a population based study. N Engl J Med 1990;323:1228–33.
14. Choi CH, Rutter MD, Askari A, et al. Forty-year analysis of colonoscopic surveillance program for neoplasia in ulcerative colitis: an updated overview. Am J Gastroenterol 2015;110(7):1022–34.
15. Jess T, Simonsen J, Jorgensen KT, et al. Decreasing risk of colorectal cancer in patients with inflammatory bowel disease over 30 years. Gastroenterology 2012;143(2):375.
16. NCCN Guidelines Version 1. 2014 Colorectal Cancer Screening.
17. Lutgens MW, van Oijen MG, van der Heijden GJ, et al. Declining risk of colorectal cancer in inflammatory bowel disease: an updated meta-analysis of population-based cohort studies. Inflamm Bowel Dis 2013;19:789–99.
18. Annese V, Daperno M, Rutter MD, et al. European evidence based consensus for endoscopy in inflammatory bowel disease. J Crohn's Colitis 2013;7:982–1018.
19. Mooiweer E, van der Meulen-de Jong AE, Ponsioen CY, et al. Chromoendoscopy for surveillance in inflammatory bowel disease does not increase neoplasia

detection compared with conventional colonoscopy with random biopsies: results from a large retrospective study. Am J Gastroenterol 2015;110(7):1014–21.

20. Bernstein C, Shanahan F, Weinstein W. Are we telling patients the truth about surveillance colonoscopy in ulcerative colitis? Lancet 1994;343:71–5.

21. Nugent FW, Haggitt RC, Gilpin PA. Cancer surveillance in ulcerative colitis. Gastroenterology 1991;100(5 pt 1):1241–8.

22. Kewenter J, Hultén L, Ahrén C. The occurrence of severe epithelial dysplasia and its bearing on treatment of longstanding ulcerative colitis. Ann Surg 1982;195:209–13.

23. Fuson JA, Farmer RG, Hawk A, et al. Endoscopic surveillance for cancer in chronic ulcerative colitis. Am J Gastroenterol 1980;73:120–6.

24. Lennard-Jones JE, Morson BC, Ritchie JK, et al. Cancer in colitis: assessment of the individual risk by clinical and histological criteria. Gastroenterology 1977;73:1280–9.

25. Murphy J, Kalkbrenner KA, Pemberton JH, et al. Dysplasia in ulcerative colitis as a predictor of unsuspected synchronous colorectal cancer. Dis Colon Rectum 2014;57(8):993–8.

26. Blackstone MO, Riddell RH, Rogers BH, et al. Dysplasia-associated lesion or mass (DALM) detected by colonoscopy in long-standing ulcerative colitis: an indication for colectomy. Gastroenterology 1981;80:366–74.

27. Lovegrove RE, Constantinides VA, Heriot AG, et al. A comparison of hand-sewn versus stapled ileal pouch anal anastomosis (IPAA) following proctocolectomy: a meta-analysis of 4183 patients. Ann Surg 2006;244:18–26.

28. Lavery IC, Tuckson WB, Easley KA. Internal anal sphincter function after total abdominal colectomy and stapled ileal pouch-anal anastomosis without mucosal proctectomy. Dis Colon Rectum 1989;32:950–3.

29. Silva-Velazco J, Stocchi L, Wu XR, et al. Twenty-year-old stapled pouches for ulcerative colitis without evidence of rectal cancer: implications for surveillance strategy? Dis Colon Rectum 2014;57:1275–81.

30. Um JW, M'Koma AE. Pouch-related dysplasia and adenocarcinoma following restorative proctocolectomy for ulcerative colitis. Tech Coloproctol 2011;15:7–16.

31. Sequens R. Cancer in the anal canal (transitional zone) after restorative proctocolectomy with stapled ileal pouch–anal anastomosis. Int J Colorectal Dis 1997;12:254–5.

32. Rotholtz NA, Pikarsky AJ, Singh JJ, et al. Adenocarcinoma arising from along the rectal stump after double-stapled ileorectal J-pouch in a patient with ulcerative colitis: the need to perform a distal anastomosis. Report of a case. Dis Colon Rectum 2001;44:1214–7.

33. Scarpa M, van Koperen PJ, Ubbink DT, et al. Systematic review of dysplasia after restorative proctocolectomy for ulcerative colitis. Br J Surg 2007;94:534–45.

34. Kariv R, Remzi FH, Lian L, et al. Preoperative colorectal neoplasia increases risk for pouch neoplasia in patients with restorative proctocolectomy. Gastroenterology 2010;139:806–12.

35. Gillen CD, Andrews HA, Prior P, et al. Crohn's disease and colorectal cancer. Gut 1994;35:651–5.

36. Jess T, Gamborg M, Matzen P, et al. Increased risk of intestinal cancer in Crohn's disease: a meta-analysis of population-based cohort studies. Am J Gastroenterol 2005;100:2724–9.

37. von Roon AC, Reese G, Teare J, et al. The risk of cancer in patients with Crohn's disease. Dis Colon Rectum 2007;50(6):839–55.

38. Devon KM, Brown CJ, Burnstein M, et al. Cancer of the anus complicating perianal Crohn's disease. Dis Colon Rectum 2009;52(2):211–6.

39. Wu XR, Remzi FH, Liu XL, et al. Disease course and management strategy of pouch neoplasia in patients with underlying inflammatory bowel diseases. Inflamm Bowel Dis 2014;20(11):2073–82.
40. Rosenstock E, Farmer RG, Petras R, et al. Surveillance for colonic carcinoma in ulcerative colitis. Gastroenterology 1985;89:1342–6.
41. von Herbay A, Herfarth C, Otto HF. Cancer and dysplasia in ulcerative colitis: a histologic study of 301 surgical specimen. Z Gastroenterol 1994;32:382–8.
42. Beaugerie L, Itzkowitz SH. Cancers complicating inflammatory bowel disease. N Engl J Med 2015;372(15):1441–52.

Nutritional Support of Patient with Inflammatory Bowel Disease

 CrossMark

Stephanie C. Montgomery, MD[a],*, Cayla M. Williams, MD[b],
Pinkney J. Maxwell IV, MD[c]

KEYWORDS

- Nutrition • Inflammatory bowel disease • Crohn's disease • Ulcerative colitis

KEY POINTS

- The overwhelming majority of patients with inflammatory bowel disease (IBD) have some degree of malnutrition.
- IBD can lead to specific nutrient deficiencies.
- There can be significant microbial alteration in intestinal flora in patients with IBD.
- Nutritional support is a critical aspect of the overall care of patients with IBD.
- Patients with IBD require special perioperative nutritional support.

INTRODUCTION

Ulcerative colitis (UC) and Crohn's disease (CD) are the 2 most prevalent chronic inflammatory disorders of the digestive tract and affect approximately 1 million Americans. They have common clinical and pathologic features, but each is a distinct condition requiring individual approaches to management. CD can occur at any part of the gastrointestinal tract and may cause transmural tissue damage, whereas UC affects only the superficial mucosal layer of the colon and rectum. In both of these conditions, there is an activation of the immune system that results in chronic inflammation and ulceration. The underlying cause of inflammatory bowel disease (IBD) has not been completely elucidated, but it is thought to be multifactorial, with both genetic and environmental factors playing a role.

The authors have nothing to disclose.
[a] Department of Surgery, Saint Francis Hospital and Medical Center, 114 Woodland Street, Hartford, CT 06105, USA; [b] Department of Emergency Medicine Western Michigan University Homer Stryker M.D. School of Medicine, 1000 Oakland Drive Kalamazoo, MI 49008, USA; [c] Department of Surgery, Medical University of South Carolina, Ashley River Tower, 25 Courtenay Drive, Charleston, SC 29425, USA
* Corresponding author.
E-mail address: scmontgo@stfranciscare.org

Surg Clin N Am 95 (2015) 1271–1279
http://dx.doi.org/10.1016/j.suc.2015.08.006
0039-6109/15/$ – see front matter © 2015 Elsevier Inc. All rights reserved.

The incidence and prevalence of UC and CD continue to rise in the developing world.[1] The observed differences in the disease incidence across age, time, and geographic region suggest that environmental factors may significantly modify the expression of CD and UC.[1] This continuing increase in the number of patients diagnosed with IBD strongly suggests an environmental trigger that may be related to dietary patterns.[2]

EFFECT OF INFLAMMATORY BOWEL DISEASE ON DIET, NUTRITION, AND METABOLISM

Studies have shown that up to 92.1% of patients with IBD are considered malnourished and many factors can contribute to their overall nutritional state (**Table 1**).[3] Recent evidence suggests that even patients who appear clinically to be well nourished may harbor baseline vitamin and mineral deficiencies, even during periods of disease remission.[4,5] Patients with IBD frequently ask their physicians for recommendations regarding diet to improve or even cure their gastrointestinal symptoms while obtaining the appropriate quantities of both micronutrients and macronutrients. Despite data that suggest dietary factors may play a role in the onset and course of IBD, there is very limited information regarding specific foods to avoid or include in a patient's diet. Currently, the only recommendation most health care providers can offer is to adhere to a healthy and varied diet.[6] To further confound the issue, important clinical trials on this topic have been limited by their inability to include a placebo control, contamination of study groups, and inclusion of patients receiving medical therapies.[7]

Dietary Intake in Patients with Inflammatory Bowel Disease

Studies have yet to reliably demonstrate an association between the Western diet rich in carbohydrates, starch, and sugar with worsening of IBD symptoms.[8] However, observations of detailed dietary journals reveal most patients with IBD continue to self-restrict their diet.[9] Pain and inflammatory mediators are known to induce anorexia and cachexia, thus a relationship between disease activity and nutrient intake exists in IBD. Patients admit to restricting certain foods to alleviate perceived symptoms or triggers for active disease. The most commonly avoided food groups among this patient population are dairy products and fiber-containing foods. Studies have shown that avoiding dairy is actually associated with an increase in severity of gastrointestinal symptoms, in addition to decreased levels of serum calcium and folate.[10] Fiber has been shown to play a role in decreasing inflammation systemically; however, there is limited evidence supporting supplementation or restriction of fiber-containing foods in patients with IBD.[11] Also of concern, the fat intake of the average patients with IBD is above current recommended values.[9]

Table 1 Etiologies of malnutrition in inflammatory bowel disease	
Drug Interactions	**Abdominal Pain**
Inflammation	Stricture formation
Fistula formation	Hypoalbuminemia
Short-gut syndrome	Diarrhea
Anorexia	Malabsorption
Altered bacterial flora	Disease chronicity
Nutrient losses from gut	Increased resting energy expenditure

Specific Nutrient Deficiencies in Inflammatory Bowel Disease

The pathophysiology of IBD predisposes patients to certain nutritional deficiencies (**Table 2**). To complicate matters further, the medications that are prescribed to treat these conditions can also negatively affect the nutritional state of this special patient population (**Table 3**).

Patients with IBD frequently exhibit calcium deficiencies due to the binding of calcium to unabsorbed fatty acids in the intestinal lumen, anatomically reduced absorptive surface area due to diseased tissue or secondary to intestinal resections, and patients' common practice of restricting dairy in their diets. The most common disease location in patients with CD is the terminal ileum, which causes distinct problems associated with bile acids, which are selectively reabsorbed in this region. As a result, these patients may experience fat-soluble vitamin deficiencies (vitamins A, D, E, and K) secondary to fat malabsorption. The use of medications such as sulfasalazine renders folate unavailable for absorption in the intestinal lumen. Therefore, folic acid supplementation is recommended if patients have low levels of serum folate. Zinc deficiency leads to increased apoptosis of intestinal cells and should be avoided in IBD.[12] Iron deficiency is common in patients with IBD and is a major concern for the development of anemia. The concurrent vitamin B12 deficiency that is observed in these patients can exacerbate this problem. Disease in the terminal ileum can further increase this prevalence as well as patients requiring resection of this important area of the bowel. Low circulating vitamin D levels have been reported as a risk factor for IBD and studies suggest that this associates with more severe disease.[13] Studies also suggest that adequate intake of nutrients is important to prevent bone loss. Not surprisingly, an increase in prevalence of decreased bone mineral density has been reported in patients with IBD.[14] Considering these circumstances, prescribing appropriate nutrient supplementation in early stages of disease is thought to decrease morbidity and mortality and should be considered.

Microbial Alterations in Inflammatory Bowel Disease

There is a symbiotic relationship between patients and their enteric community of microbes, referred to as the microbiota. This relationship provides nutritional optimization, protection against pathogenic organisms, and promotes immune homeostasis. Dysbiosis, or the imbalance of the normal enteric microbiota composition, along with altered mucosal immune response to luminal bacterial antigens, leads to the

Table 2
Nutrient deficiencies in inflammatory bowel disease

Nutrient Class	Specific Nutrient Deficiencies	Additional Considerations
Vitamins	Vitamins A, C, K, B12, D	International normalized ratio may be reduced due to low vitamin K levels
Electrolytes	Na, K, Cl	Most often occurs in patients with short bowel syndrome
Minerals	Magnesium, iron, zinc, calcium	Normal ferritin levels (acute phase reactant) do not exclude iron deficiency anemia Parathyroid hormone levels may be elevated due to low Ca levels
Protein	Serum albumin, total protein	50%–80% of patients with Crohn's disease and 25%–50% with ulcerative colitis have low levels

Table 3
Adverse effects of medications and their effect on nutrition

Drug	Adverse Effect	Etiology of Malnutrition
Aminosalicylates	Abdominal pain and cramping	Decreased intake
Immunomodulators	Intestinal ulceration (mercaptopurine)	Malabsorption
Corticosteroids	Alterations in metabolism, binding interactions	Decreased absorption, increased losses
Biologic agents	Dyspepsia, pancreatitis, abscess formation, intestinal perforation (infliximab)	Decreased intake

All medications used in the treatment of inflammatory bowel disease can cause nausea, vomiting, and diarrhea.

chronic inflammation seen in IBD.[15] Individual susceptibilities, genetic variants, and environmental factors, such as nutrition, medications, and smoking, can all modify one's luminal environment and microbiome.[16,17] Therapies targeted at restoration of enteric flora, including prebiotics, probiotics, and dietary polyphenols have been investigated with some encouraging results.[15] When used in conjunction with a nutritionally diverse diet, these therapies favorably affect the overall microbial balance and possess anti-inflammatory properties. The result is a more appropriate immune response, enhanced gut barrier function, and increased absorptive capacity.[18,19]

Pediatric Patients with Inflammatory Bowel Disease: A Special Patient Population

Children with IBD, especially CD, represent a special challenge to clinicians. Vitamin and nutritional deficiencies as a result of IBD confer consequences unique to children and adolescents, such as growth stunting, slower pubertal development, and delayed weight gain.[20] Up to 85% of patients with a childhood diagnosis of CD exhibit linear growth deficiency and delayed puberty.[21] The delay in growth observed in these children can be linked to malnutrition and the effects of the inflammatory process on the growth plate via the alterations in the growth hormone/insulinlike growth factor-1 axis.[22] Thus, long-term control of active inflammation and adequate intake of nutrients are both fundamental in promoting normal growth and puberty.[21] To further complicate the care of these patients, glucocorticoid therapy remains a mainstay for treatment for active disease, which clearly shows deleterious effects on growth in these children. Frequent and detailed nutritional assessments, including weight, height, and pubertal stage, should be considered critical in children and adolescents with any history of IBD.

DIAGNOSIS AND TREATMENT OF MALNUTRITION IN INFLAMMATORY BOWEL DISEASE
Nutritional Assessment

It is recognized that malnutrition is not readily diagnosable in early IBD, and even among experts there is no full agreement on the elements that define malnutrition.[23,24] In the past only low body mass index (BMI) was associated with malnutrition, but we now know patients can lack vital nutrients while maintaining a normal to even obese-range BMI. In a large prospective cohort of US women, measures of obesity were associated with an increased risk of CD, and dietary logs reported less than ideal diet habits among these individuals.[25] Given the high percentage of patients with IBD at risk for malnutrition, self-screening may increase the detection of nutritional deficiencies. Self-administered testing using the malnutrition universal screening tool has been shown to be reliable and easy to use and we should encourage patient involvement in self-screening.[26] Studies demonstrate that patient access to high-quality, written, IBD-specific information is variable, and nutritional software applications that are available for download onto electronic devices are an appropriate way to engage patients, especially those in the younger generations.[27,28] At the very least, a detailed dietary history is necessary to get an appropriate estimate of food intake and is recommended. Obtaining BMI, serial weights, and laboratory studies, such as albumin and iron studies, are useful information to follow to provide a trend for your patient's nutritional status. Muscle mass depletion, as well as fat mass depletion, were observed in patients with IBD and should be monitored.[29]

Nutritional Therapy

Although traditionally bowel rest was used in the treatment of IBD, it is no longer recommended.[30] Enteral nutrition is now considered a mainstay of treatment and should be considered. The exact mechanism by which enteral nutrition improves IBD remains unclear, but it is thought to decrease systemic inflammatory response and the subsequent hypermetabolic state during active disease.[31] Specific enteral diet compositions have not shown to confer any advantage over standard polymeric diets among these patients.[32,33] In addition to having the benefit of minimal adverse effects, enteral nutrition enhances mucosal healing, controls local inflammation, and confers benefits for growth and overall nutritional status.[32]

There is robust evidence of the effectiveness of enteral nutrition in patients with CD.[34] Randomized controlled trials estimate an overall remission rate of 60% in patients with CD with enteral nutrition alone.[35] Enteral nutrition has been to shown to decrease mesenteric adipose tissue hypertrophy and inflammation, a hallmark of active CD.[36] Stricture formation as a result of the inflammatory response to transmural intestinal edema is the most frequent complication of CD and a common indication for operative intervention in these patients. Exclusive enteral nutrition has been associated in studies with a 59% decrease in bowel wall thickness, as well as a 331% increase in luminal cross-sectional area.[37] Despite the usefulness of enteral nutrition, it is no panacea and corticosteroids continue to play a role in treating active CD with increased rates of remission.[33] Even with the robust evidence of the utility of exclusive enteral nutrition, there is a wide variability in its use. It is believed that monotony of the therapy would lead to poor patient compliance, but that has not been shown in studies and should be considered.[38]

In IBD, the use of total parenteral nutrition (TPN) should be restricted to those patients in whom enteral nutrition is contraindicated or only during special circumstances, such as patients with short-gut syndrome, high-output fistulas, or intolerance of enteral nutrition.[39] In these instances, TPN should be used as a short-term solution and conversion to enteral nutrition should begin as soon as appropriate. In addition to the higher risk of complications, a lower quality of life was reported by patients who were subjected to parenteral nutrition.[40]

PERIOPERATIVE CONSIDERATIONS

Surgery rates for patients with UC and CD have been declining recently, but remain very high compared with the general population. Recent population-based cohorts report surgery rates of 10% to 14% after 1 year and 18% to 35% after 5 years in patients with IBD.[41] More notably, up to 75% of patients with CD will require an operation at some point during the course of their disease.[42] Undergoing a surgical procedure induces a stress response in these patients, which has a catabolic effect on the body's substrate stores. Nutrients that are believed to have immune-enhancing effects, such as glutamine, arginine, and taurine, become rapidly deficient under this surgical stress. Interestingly, studies have suggested that the supplementation of these nutrients may counteract the negative effects of surgical injury and improve clinical outcomes post-operatively.[43] Additionally, nutritional therapy should be considered in these patients to reverse their catabolic state and provide the support for healing of operative wounds.

Research continues to demonstrate that disease-related malnutrition in patients with IBD is a serious clinical problem in both hospitalized and nonhospitalized patients.[44] A malnourished state is associated with increased inpatient length of stay, increased mortality, increased infection rates, and higher resource utilization.[23] Surgical site infections continue to be an important perioperative complication that can significantly contribute to this reported increase in duration of hospital stay and postoperative morbidity. Studies reveal that having a low preoperative nutritional index correlates with an increased incidence of surgical site infections after bowel resection in CD. Also of concern, postoperative intra-abdominal septic complications were demonstrated in 9% to 12% of patients with CD after surgery.[45] Preoperative exclusive enteral nutrition (EEN) may reduce these risks, as research has shown that patients who receive EEN suffer a lower risk of septic complications.[46] Furthermore, the risk of anastomotic leak is significantly increased in patients whose preoperative albumin levels are lower than 3.5 g/dL and low albumin levels may be associated with higher rates of abdominal septic complications after surgery in patients with CD.[47,48] Enterocutaneous fistulas (ECFs), highly morbid conditions that can lead to sepsis and death, remain a dreaded complication for surgeons. Aggressive nutritional support remains the most significant predictor of outcome with ECFs and cannot be overemphasized.[49] The elderly are a special population and are at an increased risk of hospital-related and therapy-related complications.[50] Despite this, some studies surprisingly demonstrate that they may have the same surgical complication rate as younger patients with IBD in the contemporary era.[51] Enteral nutrition optimization before elective surgery is therefore essential for all patients. Also notable for surgeons, preoperative fasting has a negative effect on the patient's condition and recovery after surgery and should be discouraged, if possible.[43]

SUMMARY

IBD remains a very complex issue that every surgeon will most likely encounter during his or her practice. The very nature of IBD lends itself to the development of nutritionally deficient states and the medications that are prescribed by physicians can further compound these nutritional problems. Surgeons must therefore be aware of the nutritional issues specific to this patient population and screen for underlying deficiencies that may be present, even in disease remission. Nutritional screening must be an integral part of the preoperative workup and postoperative plan, including supplementation where appropriate. Enteral nutrition should be encouraged and TPN should be used only in a small set of circumstances and only until enteral therapies can be instituted.

REFERENCES

1. Loftus EV Jr. Clinical epidemiology of inflammatory bowel disease: incidence, prevalence, and environmental influences. Gastroenterology 2004;126(6): 1504–17.

2. Hou JK, Lee D, Lewis J. Diet and inflammatory bowel disease: review of patient-targeted recommendations. Clin Gastroenterol Hepatol 2014;12(10):1592–600.

3. Sokulmez P, Demirbag AE, Arslan P, et al. Effects of enteral nutritional support on malnourished patients with inflammatory bowel disease by subjective global assessment. Turk J Gastroenterol 2014;25(5):493–507.

4. Vagianos K, Bector S, McConnell J, et al. Nutrition assessment of patients with inflammatory bowel disease. JPEN J Parenter Enteral Nutr 2007;31(4):311–9.

5. Filippi J, Al-Jaouni R, Wiroth JB, et al. Nutritional deficiencies in patients with Crohn's disease in remission. Inflamm Bowel Dis 2006;12(3):185–91.

6. Massironi S, Rossi RE, Cavalcoli FA, et al. Nutritional deficiencies in inflammatory bowel disease: therapeutic approaches. Clin Nutr 2013;32(6):904–10.

7. Lee D, Albenberg L, Compher C, et al. Diet in the pathogenesis and treatment of inflammatory bowel diseases. Gastroenterology 2015;148(6):1087–106.

8. Chan SS, Luben R, van Schaik F, et al. Carbohydrate intake in the etiology of Crohn's disease and ulcerative colitis. Inflamm Bowel Dis 2014;20(11):2013–21.

9. Walton M, Alaunyte I. Do patients living with ulcerative colitis adhere to healthy eating guidelines? A cross-sectional study. Br J Nutr 2014;112(10):1628–35.

10. Brasil Lopes M, Rocha R, Castro Lyra A, et al. Restriction of dairy products; a reality in inflammatory bowel disease patients. Nutr Hosp 2014;29(3):575–81.

11. Wedlake L, Slack N, Andreyev HJ, et al. Fiber in the treatment and maintenance of inflammatory bowel disease: a systematic review of randomized controlled trials. Inflamm Bowel Dis 2014;20(3):576–86.

12. Ranaldi G, Ferruzza S, Canali R, et al. Intracellular zinc is required for intestinal cell survival signals triggered by the inflammatory cytokine TNFalpha. J Nutr Biochem 2013;24(6):967–76.

13. O'Sullivan M. Vitamin D as a novel therapy in inflammatory bowel disease: new hope or false dawn? Proc Nutr Soc 2015;74(1):5–12.

14. Lim H, Kim HJ, Hong SJ, et al. Nutrient intake and bone mineral density by nutritional status in patients with inflammatory bowel disease. J Bone Metab 2014;21(3):195–203.

15. Chen WX, Ren LH, Shi RH. Enteric microbiota leads to new therapeutic strategies for ulcerative colitis. World J Gastroenterol 2014;20(42):15657–63.

16. Bringiotti R, Ierardi E, Lovero R, et al. Intestinal microbiota: the explosive mixture at the origin of inflammatory bowel disease? World J Gastrointest Pathophysiol 2014;5(4):550–9.

17. Scharl M, Rogler G. Inflammatory bowel disease pathogenesis: what is new? Curr Opin Gastroenterol 2012;28(4):301–9.

18. Guandalini S. Are probiotics or prebiotics useful in pediatric irritable bowel syndrome or inflammatory bowel disease? Front Med (Lausanne) 2014;1:23.

19. Tilg H, Moschen AR. Food, immunity, and the microbiome. Gastroenterology 2015;148(6):1107–19.

20. dos Santos GM, Silva LR, Santana GO. Nutritional impact of inflammatory bowel diseases on children and adolescents. Rev Paul Pediatr 2014;32(4):403–11 [in Portuguese].

21. Gasparetto M, Guariso G. Crohn's disease and growth deficiency in children and adolescents. World J Gastroenterol 2014;20(37):13219–33.

22. Ezri J, Marques-Vidal P, Nydegger A. Impact of disease and treatments on growth and puberty of pediatric patients with inflammatory bowel disease. Digestion 2012;85(4):308–19.

23. Nguyen GC, Munsell M, Harris ML. Nationwide prevalence and prognostic significance of clinically diagnosable protein-calorie malnutrition in hospitalized inflammatory bowel disease patients. Inflamm Bowel Dis 2008;14(8):1105–11.
24. Meijers JM, van Bokhorst-de van der Schueren MA, Schols JM, et al. Defining malnutrition: mission or mission impossible? Nutrition 2010;26(4):432–40.
25. Khalili H, Ananthakrishnan AN, Konijeti GG, et al. Measures of obesity and risk of Crohn's disease and ulcerative colitis. Inflamm Bowel Dis 2015;21(2):361–8.
26. Sandhu A, Mosli M, Yan B, et al. Self-screening for malnutrition risk in outpatient inflammatory bowel disease patients using the Malnutrition Universal Screening Tool (MUST). JPEN J Parenter enteral Nutr 2015. [Epub ahead of print].
27. Prince AC, Moosa A, Lomer MC, et al. Variable access to quality nutrition information regarding inflammatory bowel disease: a survey of patients and health professionals and objective examination of written information. Health Expect 2014. [Epub ahead of print].
28. Boyce B. Nutrition apps: opportunities to guide patients and grow your career. J Acad Nutr Diet 2014;114(1):13–5.
29. Rocha R, Santana GO, Almeida N, et al. Analysis of fat and muscle mass in patients with inflammatory bowel disease during remission and active phase. Br J Nutr 2009;101(5):676–9.
30. Wiese DM, Rivera R, Seidner DL. Is there a role for bowel rest in nutrition management of Crohn's disease? Nutr Clin Pract 2008;23(3):309–17.
31. Zhao J, Dong JN, Gong JF, et al. Impact of enteral nutrition on energy metabolism in patients with Crohn's disease. World J Gastroenterol 2015;21(4):1299–304.
32. Hartman C, Eliakim R, Shamir R. Nutritional status and nutritional therapy in inflammatory bowel diseases. World J Gastroenterol 2009;15(21):2570–8.
33. Zachos M, Tondeur M, Griffiths AM. Enteral nutritional therapy for induction of remission in Crohn's disease. Cochrane Database Syst Rev 2007;(1):CD000542.
34. Yamamoto T, Nakahigashi M, Saniabadi AR. Review article: diet and inflammatory bowel disease–epidemiology and treatment. Aliment Pharmacol Ther 2009;30(2):99–112.
35. Wahed M, Geoghegan M, Powell-Tuck J. Novel substrates. Eur J Gastroenterol Hepatol 2007;19(5):365–70.
36. Feng Y, Li Y, Mei S, et al. Exclusive enteral nutrition ameliorates mesenteric adipose tissue alterations in patients with active Crohn's disease. Clin Nutr 2014;33(5):850–8.
37. Hu D, Ren J, Wang G, et al. Exclusive enteral nutritional therapy can relieve inflammatory bowel stricture in Crohn's disease. J Clin Gastroenterol 2014;48(9):790–5.
38. Kansal S, Wagner J, Kirkwood CD, et al. Enteral nutrition in Crohn's disease: an underused therapy. Gastroenterol Res Pract 2013;2013:482108.
39. Goh J, O'Morain CA. Review article: nutrition and adult inflammatory bowel disease. Aliment Pharmacol Ther 2003;17(3):307–20.
40. Raczkowska A, Lawinski M, Gradowska A, et al. Quality of life considering patients with chronic inflammatory bowel diseases—natural and parenteral nutrition. Pol Przegl Chir 2014;86(9):410–7.
41. Burisch J, Munkholm P. The epidemiology of inflammatory bowel disease. Scand J Gastroenterol 2015;50(8):1–10.
42. Latella G, Papi C. Crucial steps in the natural history of inflammatory bowel disease. World J Gastroenterol 2012;18(29):3790–9.
43. Buijs N, Worner EA, Brinkmann SJ, et al. Novel nutritional substrates in surgery. Proc Nutr Soc 2013;72(3):277–87.

44. Elia M, Stratton RJ. How much undernutrition is there in hospitals? Br J Nutr 2000; 84(3):257–9.
45. Morar P, Hodgkinson J, Thalayasingam S, et al. Determining predictors for intra-abdominal septic complications following ileocolonic resection for Crohn's disease—considerations in pre-operative and peri-operative optimisation techniques to improve outcome. J Crohns Colitis 2015;9(6):483–91.
46. Li G, Ren J, Wang G, et al. Preoperative exclusive enteral nutrition reduces the postoperative septic complications of fistulizing Crohn's disease. Eur J Clin Nutr 2014;68(4):441–6.
47. Telem DA, Chin EH, Nguyen SQ, et al. Risk factors for anastomotic leak following colorectal surgery: a case-control study. Arch Surg 2010;145(4):371–6 [discussion: 376].
48. Huang W, Tang Y, Nong L, et al. Risk factors for postoperative intra-abdominal septic complications after surgery in Crohn's disease: a meta-analysis of observational studies. J Crohns Colitis 2015;9(3):293–301.
49. Polk TM, Schwab CW. Metabolic and nutritional support of the enterocutaneous fistula patient: a three-phase approach. World J Surg 2012;36(3):524–33.
50. Shung DL, Abraham B, Sellin J, et al. Medical and surgical complications of inflammatory bowel disease in the elderly: a systematic review. Dig Dis Sci 2015;60(5):1132–40.
51. Bautista MC, Otterson MF, Zadvornova Y, et al. Surgical outcomes in the elderly with inflammatory bowel disease are similar to those in the younger population. Dig Dis Sci 2013;58(10):2955–62.

Psychosocial Support of the Inflammatory Bowel Disease Patient

Abdul Alarhayem, MD*, Ebele Achebe, MS, Alicia J. Logue, MD

KEYWORDS

- Psychological impacts • Inflammatory bowel disease • Depression • Anxiety

KEY POINTS

- Inflammatory bowel disease (IBD) is a chronic, debilitating disease whose effects spread far beyond the gut.
- IBD does not generally result in excess mortality; health care providers should thus focus their efforts on improving health-related quality of life and minimizing associated morbidity.
- A bidirectional relationship exists between IBD and psychiatric conditions; chronic inflammation can produce neuromodulatory effects with resultant mood disorders, and the course of IBD is worse in patients with anxiety and depression.
- Screening for the early signs of depression or anxiety and initiating appropriate treatment can lead to improved functioning and positively impact disease course.

INTRODUCTION

Inflammatory bowel disease (IBD), namely Crohn's disease (CD) and ulcerative colitis (UC), afflicts 1.5 million people in the United States and 28 million worldwide.[1,2] The chronic, unpredictable, disabling, and progressively destructive nature of IBD gives rise to substantial psychosocial implications.[3]

There has been a great deal of speculation over the years on the importance of psychiatric and social factors in IBD; however, it is only in the last decade or so that studies with stronger designs have been available to clarify the nature of this relationship. And although there is no conclusive evidence for anxiety, depression, and psychosocial stress contributing to the risk for IBD onset, they have been found to impact the course of IBD patients, including risk of relapse.

The purpose of this review is to shed light on the complex relationship between mental health and IBD, highlighting the various associations and risk factors for

Department of Surgery, University of Texas Health Science Center in San Antonio, 7703 Floyd Curl Drive, San Antonio, TX 78229-3900, USA
* Corresponding author.
E-mail address: alarhayema@uthscsa.edu

Surg Clin N Am 95 (2015) 1281–1293
http://dx.doi.org/10.1016/j.suc.2015.08.005   surgical.theclinics.com
0039-6109/15/$ – see front matter Published by Elsevier Inc.

psychiatric disorders, and clinical recommendations for the detection, screening, and management of these conditions in patients with IBD, bolstering a more patient-centered approach with improving outcomes.[2,4–6]

PSYCHIATRIC DISORDERS IN INFLAMMATORY BOWEL DISEASE

Chronic medical conditions in general are associated with higher rates of anxiety and mood disorders compared with the general population; the stress associated with these conditions may trigger or intensify a psychiatric condition. Newer insight, however, has linked depression and anxiety specifically to inflammatory conditions, like IBD, possibly via induced immunoregulatory circuit dysfunction.[3] This section considers recent evidence on the prevalence of anxiety and depressive disorders in IBD, the role of these disorders as a risk factor for IBD onset, the degree to which they affect its course. Screening for psychiatric illness and management strategies is also discussed.

Four population-based studies consistently demonstrated a clear relationship between IBD and depression and higher levels of anxiety.[7–9] The largest of these studies found patients with CD to be 5 times more likely than controls to have anxiety or depression, whereas patients with UC were 4 times as likely to have anxiety and twice as likely to be depressed than matched controls.[7] Overall, the mean prevalence of depression in patients with IBD is estimated to be 20%,[10] and abnormal anxiety levels are found in up to 40% of patients with IBD.[11]

In an attempt to establish a temporal relationship between IBD and depression/anxiety, a prospective, population-based study found UC to be at least twice as common in patients with anxiety and depression compared with controls without these conditions years before the onset of IBD.[12] This, however, was likely reflective of reactive anxiety or depressive symptoms related to early signs of IBD. Also, increased levels of inflammatory mediators seen in patients before the onset of IBD symptoms may play a role in initiating mood disorders.

Currently, there is no conclusive evidence to suggest that anxiety, depression or psychosocial stress play an etiologic role in the onset of IBD.[4,5,13] Nevertheless, evidence does suggest that the course of IBD is worse in patients with anxiety and depression and that patients with active disease or symptoms demonstrate higher levels of anxiety or depression than those in remission.[14–16] A 2-year study that assessed a small sample of CD patients at 2- to 3-month intervals found that higher depression scores were associated with higher Crohn's Disease Activity Index scores in the subsequent time period. Mittermaier and colleagues[17] reported similar findings in patients with UC.[16] Severe active and aggressive disease seems to be the primary risk factor for depression and anxiety disorders.[18] Psychological stress, advancing age, surgery and stoma, and poor socioeconomic status have all been reported as well.

PATHOPSYCHOLOGY OF DEPRESSION AND ANXIETY DISORDERS IN INFLAMMATORY BOWEL DISEASE

The etiology of mood disorders in patients with IBD seems multifactorial. Recently, there has been considerable interest in the combined role of inflammatory and stress biomarkers to cause changes in brain structure and function, with resultant mood disorders.[6,19–21] Most of the evidence that links inflammation to depression comes from 3 observations:

- One-third of patients with major depression show elevated peripheral concentrations of inflammatory biomarkers, namely C-reactive protein, tumor necrosis factor-α and interleukin (IL)-6, even in the absence of medical illness.[22,23]

- Patients with IBD with higher levels of acute phase reactants have a higher incidence of depression compared with those with normal inflammatory marker levels. A recent metaanalysis found treatment with selective serotonin reuptake inhibitors produced a decrease in IL-1b and IL-6 levels that paralleled improvement in depressive symptoms.[24]
- Patients treated with cytokines are at greater risk of developing major depressive illness.[25]

Proposed mechanisms include the direct effects of proinflammatory cytokines on monoamine levels, dysregulation of the hypothalamic–pituitary–adrenal axis, pathologic microglial cell activation, impaired neuroplasticity, and structural and functional brain changes.[26]

Targeting specific immune markers, for example, tumor necrosis factor-α inhibitors, however, has had little effect on psychiatric morbidity. This is likely to the complex multifactorial nature of "brain–gut" interactions in IBD. A holistic approach would potentially target underlying inflammation, and in turn this would decrease the excitability of sensitized afferent pathways and alter emotional and/or cognitive functions, ultimately enabling more effective management of both inflammation and depression in patients with IBD.

Visceral hyperalgesia also seems to play a role in IBD associated mood disorders. Pain is the presenting symptom in up to 70% of patients with IBD.[27,28] The relationship between chronic pain and depression, like the brain–gut axis, is bidirectional. The brain–gut axis is a communication between the central and autonomic nervous system, the hypothalamic–pituitary–adrenal axis, and the intestinal response.[5,29,30] Depression can present itself as chronic abdominal pain, and patients with pain are at increased risk for depression independent of disease activity.[29,31]

Chronic inflammation, as seen in IBD, induces persistent sensitizing effects in the sensory afferent pathways and leads to an altered processing of pain by the central nervous system, with downstream alterations in the emotional and cognitive processing of this increased visceral input.[5,6,29]

Medications used in the treatment of IBD have also been linked to mood disorders. Results from -analyses have suggested that more than one-quarter of patients on corticosteroids may experience adverse psychiatric effects.[32,33] Fardet and colleagues[33] found that 10% of patients on greater than 20 mg of daily prednisone for 3 months required hospitalization for either mania or severe depression. In 1 survey, psychiatric symptoms were second only to "moon facies" as the most distressing side effect of corticosteroids. The incidence of psychiatric disorders seems to be related directly to medication dosage. Patients with a prior history of steroid-induced psychiatric symptoms are also at greater risk. With the widespread use of steroid alternatives, especially biologics, steroids now are relatively small contributors to the overall prevalence of psychiatric disorders in patients with IBD.

SCREENING FOR PSYCHIATRIC DISORDERS IN INFLAMMATORY BOWEL DISEASE

Given the frequency and impact of psychiatric disorders in IBD, updated consensus guidelines for the management of IBD have included a recommendation for routine screening for these disorders. Ensuring that patient are screened routinely for common psychiatric symptoms can help those patients most likely to benefit from assistance, especially considering that most patients are reluctant to voice such concerns.

Both anxiety disorders and depression are criterion-based diagnoses (**Table 1**). The former is characterized by symptoms of excessive fear and worry that are difficult to control, a state of hyperarousability, and resultant behavioral disturbances (typically,

Table 1
Anxiety and depression are criterion-based diagnoses

Depression	Anxiety
Persistently depressed mood[a]	Excessive anxiety or worry, difficult controlling worry
Diminished interest or pleasure[a]	—
Significant weight loss, or change in appetite[a]	—
Insomnia or hypersomnia	Sleep disturbance[b]
Psychomotor agitation or retardation[a]	Muscle tension[b], irritability[b]
Fatigue or loss of energy[a]	Fatigue or loss of energy[b]
Feelings of worthlessness or inappropriate guilt[a]	Feelings of restlessness, or keyed up or on edge[b]
Diminished ability to think or concentrate[a]	Diminished ability to think or concentrate[b]
Recurrent suicidal ideation[a]	—

[a] Five or more symptoms for 2 or more weeks.
[b] Three or more symptoms occurring more days than not for at least 6 months.
  Data from Diagnostic and statistical manual of mental disorders. 5th edition. Washington, DC: American Psychiatric Association; 2013.

avoidance of source of fear). Depression is characterized by a sad or depressed mood affect, with cognitive and somatic symptoms that cause significant distress or impairment in social, occupational, or other important areas of functioning. Symptoms of both disorders must be persistent and are not secondary to direct physiologic effects of a substance (eg, a drug of abuse, a medication) or a general medical condition.

Patient-based screening forms and health care provider administered brief standardized questions are simple, valid psychosocial screening instruments frequently used in patients with IBD.

The 5-item Anxiety and Depression Detector is an example of a self-report scale[34]; its questions focus on eliciting information regarding depression and anxiety. Its high sensitivity and specificity combined with its relative ease of use (yes/no responses, simple language, can be completed while patient is in the waiting room) make it favorable. Clinician-administered scales, such as the Luebeck Interview for Psychosocial Screening in Patients with IBD, are not only useful in identifying patients with manifestations of illness, but also help to identify social support mechanisms, distress caused by IBD, and the patients interest in receiving psychological care. It has shown good interobserver reliability and correlates with other psychometric measures. Two approaches have been used in the management of psychiatric conditions in IBD patients. This is usually done in collaboration with mental health professionals (**Table 2**).[5,6,13]

PHARMACOLOGIC TREATMENTS

Selective serotonin reuptake inhibitors, such as citalopram, fluoxetine, and sertraline, and serotonin norepinephrine reuptake inhibitors, such as venlafaxine, are both safe and effective in the treatment of anxiety and depressive disorders,[4,5,13] with a significant percentage of IBD patients with anxiety or depression reporting a favorable response. In addition to controlling symptoms of anxiety and depression, both selective serotonin reuptake inhibitors and serotonin norepinephrine reuptake inhibitors have been reported to decrease pain, gut irritability, and urgency of defecation.[35,36] Goodhand and colleagues[37] stated that patients reported fewer clinical IBD relapses

Table 2
Screening instruments for patients with IBD

The Anxiety and Depression Detector	LIPS – IBD*
Did you ever have a spell or an attack when all of a sudden you felt frightened, anxious, or very uneasy? Yes/No	With whom do you live together? Do you have children? Is anyone available for you who supports you with your problems? *Social support* 1 2 3 4 5
Would you say that you have been bothered by nerves or feeling anxious or on edge? Yes/No	During the last months, did you feel sad, depressed, or hopeless? Were you at least interested in activities you used to enjoy? *Depression* 1 2 3 4 5
Would you say that being anxious or uncomfortable around other people is a problem for you in your life? Yes/No	During the last months, did you often feel restless? Did you worry a lot? Did you sometimes experience sudden feelings of worry or anxiety? *Anxiety* 1 2 3 4 5
Did you have a period of 1 week or more when you lost interest in most things like work, hobbies, and other things you usually enjoyed? Yes/No	How much do you feel stressed by your IBD? *Impact of disease* 1 2 3 4 5
Some people have terrible experiences happen to them, like being attacked or threatened with a weapon, being in a fire or a bad traffic accident, being sexually assaulted, or seeing someone being badly injured or killed. Has anything like this ever happened to you? Yes/No	—

Abbreviation: IBD, inflammatory bowel disease; LIPS, Luebeck Interview for Psychosocial Screening.
Adapted from Means-Christensen AJ, Sherbourne CD, Roy-Byrne PP, et al. Using five questions to screen for five common mental disorders in primary care: diagnostic accuracy of the Anxiety and Depression Detector. Gen Hosp Psychiatry 2006;28(2):108–18; and Kunzendorf S, Jantschek G, Straubinger K, et al. The Luebeck interview for psychosocial screening in patients with inflammatory bowel disease. Inflamm Bowel Dis 2007;13(1):33–41.

after receiving antidepressants for 1 year. This may explained by the fact that patients in better psychological health report fewer functional gastrointestinal symptoms. A recent survey found almost 80% of gastrointestinal specialists had prescribed antidepressants as an adjunctive therapy, especially for pain and sleep difficulties. Patients should be made aware that clinical benefit is generally not seen for at least 2 to 4 weeks after start of treatment, and that side effects are not unusual and can be problematic (namely weight gain and sexual dysfunction). Up to 50% of patients discontinue treatment within the first weeks or months, often because of side effects, limiting the effectiveness of the treatment. The dose of these medications should be adjusted or altered to ensure maximum therapeutic benefit while minimizing side effects. Relapse is common after discontinuation of treatment; maintenance of treatment gains requires long-term treatment in patients who demonstrate a good response to therapy.

NONPHARMACOLOGIC PSYCHOTHERAPY

Cognitive–behavioral therapy has been found to be effective in the treatment of both anxiety and depression. In patients with IBD, a randomized controlled trial reported significantly decreased depression and improved global functioning after cognitive–behavioral therapy. For those who also had a comorbid anxiety disorder, there was a significant decrease in anxiety as well.[38,39] Similar findings were reported in adults in a Spanish randomized controlled trial after a structured cognitive–behavioral therapy program that included relaxation training, distraction, and cognitive restructuring.[40] The benefits in both studies were maintained at 12-month follow-up. A recent Cochrane review however found the evidence supporting psychological therapy in adult patients with IBD to be inconclusive.[41]

Psychological treatment, however, is not indicated for all patients with IBD. In patients with no evidence of depression or anxiety, evidence that psychological interventions help patients to cope with disease is lacking. In a large pooled analysis of unselected adult patients with IBD, psychotherapy was ineffective in improving quality of life (QOL), emotional problems, and disease activity.[41] Validated treatments should thus only be used in high-risk subgroups with comorbid psychiatric conditions. In addition, cognitive–behavioral therapy is less readily available, costlier, and more labor/time intensive than pharmacologic treatment.

Importantly, health care providers must be aware of compliance issues in patients with depression. Overall, the reported rate of non-compliance in patients with IBD was 30% in 1 report, comparable with that of patients with other chronic illnesses.[42] Depression and psychological distress are both predictors of nonadherence, with 1 series citing those with IBD and depression are 3 times less likely to comply with treatment compared with nondepressed counterparts.[13] Approaches such as improving the physician–patient relationship, individualized therapy, providing patient information and support, self-management programs and practical memory aids can increase the likelihood of adherence and prolonged remission rates.[43]

Last, physicians treating IBD patients should be vigilant about expressions of suicidal ideation or signs and symptoms of self-harm. Studies have demonstrated an increased rate of suicide among patients with CD and UC, even after adjusting for confounders.[44,45]

HEALTH-RELATED QUALITY OF LIFE

Health-related QOL (HRQoL) is defined as "a quantitative measurement of subjective perception of ones' health state, including physical, emotional and social functioning."[42] It provides important insight into patients' perception of their health and the effect of treatments. Various QOL measures have been developed and used by researchers and health care providers. These measures can be either generic or disease specific; the former being useful to compare HRQoL across different disease states, whereas disease specific measures are more sensitive to changes in a patient's health state.

A recent systematic review of HRQoL measures found the Inflammatory Bowel Disease Questionnaire (IBDQ) to be the most widely used IBD-specific measure of HRQoL.[46] Several studies have confirmed its reliability, validity, and internal consistency. The IBDQ questionnaire, originally composed of 32 items, has been shortened to 10 (Short IBDQ, **Box 1**) and 9 items (IBDQ-9).

In a recent survey by the European Federation of Crohn's and Ulcerative Colitis Associations (n = 5576 participants), 75% of patients reported symptoms affected their ability to enjoy leisure activities, and two-thirds felt that their symptoms affected their ability to perform at work. Interestingly, nearly one-half (n = 2666; 47.8%) reported that their doctor does not ask about the impact of symptoms on their QOL.[3] In another survey, almost 50% of patients reported IBD had negatively affected their performance in educational settings, and 24% had received unfair comments about their work performance, mainly owing to absenteeism.[47]

Box 1
Colitis: short Inflammatory Bowel Disease Questionnaire

Bowel

Frequency of bowel movements compared with when disease is stable

Frequency of distress from abdominal cramps

Systemic

Feelings of fatigue, or being "worn out"

Energy

Emotion

Worried about possibility of surgery

Fear of not finding a toilet

Free of tension

Mood irritability

Social

Limitation of leisure or sports activity secondary to disease

Limitation of sexual activity secondary to disease

DETERMINANTS OF HEALTH-RELATED QUALITY OF LIFE IN INFLAMMATORY BOWEL DISEASE

Numerous studies have found that patients with active disease have significantly impaired HRQoL compared with patients in remission.[6–8,48–51] This is owing to the fact that patients with active IBD tend to have more bowel symptoms that interfere with daily activities, as well as more disease-related worries, perceived stress, and emotional distress.[51] Conversely, achievement of disease remission in Crohn's disease, whether by pharmacologic or surgical means, is associated with improved HRQoL.[52] Importantly, poor HRQoL is not restricted to active episodes; rather, it persists even when the disease is inactive. Newer treatments have come with a greater ability to induce and maintain remission; this in turn has resulted in greater improvements in HRQoL. However, improving social support systems and even patient–physician interactions are necessary in view of their ability to positively impact HRQoL.[53–55] Treating concomitant anxiety and depression also seems to improve HRQoL, an added benefit of identifying those likely to benefit from psychiatric treatment of these conditions.[9]

Gender, socioeconomic status, and ethnicity have also been shown to be determinants of HRQoL. Several reports suggest that females report more disease-related concerns than males, particularly regarding self-image and relationships. In adults with CD, poorer HRQoL was reported in black compared with white patients. Self-esteem also was found to be a predictor of HRQoL.

Factors that are not direct effects of IBD can also diminish QOL in IBD patients, including stress, sleeping problems, depression, pain, and conflicts at work or home. Numerous studies have found unemployed people to exhibit poorer QOL; estimated unemployment rates among patients with IBD range from 25% to 39%.[55] One study found long-term active disease and the presence of psychiatric comorbidity, particularly depression, to be major determinants of work-related disability.[55] Even personality traits such as neuroticism and alexithymia (inability to describe feelings) have been reported to predict HRQoL, likely owing to effects on coping and adjustment.

COPING WITH INFLAMMATORY BOWEL DISEASE

The unpredictable, chronic, and debilitating nature of IBD gives rise to significant psychological concerns, including loss of control of bowel function, fatigue, impairment of body image, a fear of sexual inadequacy, feelings of social isolation, and dependency.

Table 3 Psychosocial factors shown to improve QOL	
Strategy	**Rationale**
Education/self-management	Having inadequate information about a patient's own disease process been found to result in poorer reported QOL.[59,60] Self-management training has also been shown to improve HRQoL.[61]
Exercise and sleep	Exercise may help counter stress and psychiatric disturbance associated with IBD. A randomized trial found significant improvement in QOL in IBD patients randomized to light exercise, with no adverse effect on disease activity.[62] A survey of 200 IBD patients found poor sleep quality to be significantly associated with poor HRQoL. Patients with self-reported poor sleep quality are also 3 times as likely to have active IBD as compared with patients who reported good sleep quality.[63,64]
Psychotherapy	Several studies have found CBT to positively affect QOL. This effect is most likely secondary to improvements in coping mechanisms, as well as treatment of coexisting anxiety/depression.[65,66]
Hypnotherapy	Hypnotherapy seems to be effective in diseases with a psychosomatic component. In one study, patients with severe IBD refractory to corticosteroids reported an 80% improvement in QOL after 12 sessions of hypnotherapy. Such benefits likely stem from its ability to control emotional symptoms, and possibly improve pain.[67,68]
Social support	Family and social support has been reported by patients as being helpful with managing IBD, particularly with respect to coping and stress management.[69]
Pharmacotherapy	Several RCTs have found the biologics infliximab, adalimumab, certolizumab, and natalizumab to be associated with significant and sustained improvements of HRQoL in IBD patients compared with placebo. This is likely owing to their ability to induce and sustain remission, a factor that has been associated with improved QOL.[70–74] In a recent survey, almost 75% of patients receiving biologics reported QOL improvements.[15] Medication nonadherence can increase the risk of surgery and result in more severe disease with detrimental effects on QOL.[75] Physicians should thus focus their efforts on educating patients, simplifying regimens, and identifying barriers to adherence.

Abbreviations: CBT, cognitive–behavioral therapy; IBD, inflammatory bowel disease; HRQoL, health-related quality of life; QOL, quality of life.

Adapted from Karwowski CA, Keljo D, Szigethy E. Strategies to improve quality of life in adolescents with inflammatory bowel disease. Inflamm Bowel Dis 2009;15(11):1755–64; with permission; and *Data from* Refs.[59–74]

These are all constant and real concerns that can result in loss of feelings of self-worth. How one responds to and copes with IBD seems to be an important determinant of QOL as well as psychiatric comorbidity and disability.

Coping may be broadly defined as the "cognitive and behavioral efforts to manage specific external or internal demands that are appraised as taxing or exceeding the resources of a person."[56] Although coping strategies do not necessarily affect the disease process itself, the use of coping strategies can decrease the extent of disease-related emotional, social, and physiologic distress. Coping has been shown to be an important determinant of outcomes in a number of chronic diseases, including rheumatoid arthritis and sickle cell disease. The relationship between coping and outcome in patients with IBD, however, is variable. A systemic review of all published literature regarding coping strategies of IBD patients found no consistent relationship between coping and psychological outcomes. There was, however, a trend toward better outcomes with problem-focused coping (ie, to alter or eliminate the source of stress) compared with emotion-focused coping (aims to reduce the emotional distress caused by the situation).[57] Not surprisingly, maladaptive behavior such as self-pitying, musing, social withdrawal, and feelings of helplessness contribute to a reduced QOL.[58]

IMPROVING QUALITY OF LIFE IN PATIENTS WITH INFLAMMATORY BOWEL DISEASE

The main psychosocial factors shown to improve QOL are summarized in **Table 3**.[51]

SUMMARY

IBD is a chronic, debilitating disease whose effects spread far beyond the gut. An illness that does not generally result in excess mortality, patients spend many years coping with their condition and its associated morbidity. Screening for the early signs of depression or anxiety and the initiation of pharmacologic or psychological treatment when appropriate can lead to improved functioning and positively impact the course of disease. HRQoL is a major outcome in patients with IBD and can be influenced by a myriad of factors. Factors that seem to have the greatest impact are social and emotional, not physical.[76] A multidisciplinary, evidence-based approach involving psychosocial and medical interventions is of paramount importance to provide optimal care in managing these patients.[77]

REFERENCES

1. Ananthakrishnan AN. Epidemiology and risk factors for IBD. Nat Rev Gastroenterol Hepatol 2015;12(4):205–17.
2. Schoultz M, Atherton I, Hubbard G, et al. Assessment of causal link between psychological factors and symptom exacerbation in inflammatory bowel disease: a protocol for systematic review of prospective cohort studies. Syst Rev 2013;2(1):8.
3. Ghosh S, Mitchell R. Impact of inflammatory bowel disease on quality of life: Results of the European Federation of Crohn's and Ulcerative Colitis Associations (EFCCA) patient survey. J Crohns Colitis 2007;1(1):10–20.
4. Filipovic BR, Filipovic BF. Psychiatric comorbidity in the treatment of patients with inflammatory bowel disease. World J Gastroenterol 2014;20(13):3552.
5. Sajadinejad M, Asgari K, Molavi H, et al. Psychological issues in inflammatory bowel disease: an overview. Gastroenterol Res Pract 2012;2012:106502.
6. Mackner LM, Greenley RN, Szigethy E, et al. Psychosocial issues in pediatric inflammatory bowel disease: a clinical report of the North American Society for

Pediatric Gastroenterology, Hepatology and Nutrition. J Pediatr Gastroenterol Nutr 2013;56(4):449.

7. Kurina L, Goldacre M, Yeates D, et al. Depression and anxiety in people with inflammatory bowel disease. J Epidemiol Community Health 2001;55(10):716–20.

8. Lerebours E, Gower-Rousseau C, Merle V, et al. Stressful life events as a risk factor for inflammatory bowel disease onset: a population-based case–control study. Am J Gastroenterol 2007;102(1):122–31.

9. Fuller-Thomson E, Sulman J. Depression and inflammatory bowel disease: findings from two nationally representative Canadian surveys. Inflamm Bowel Dis 2006;12(8):697–707.

10. Graff LA, Walker JR, Bernstein CN. Depression and anxiety in inflammatory bowel disease: a review of comorbidity and management. Inflamm Bowel Dis 2009; 15(7):1105–18.

11. Association AP. Diagnostic and statistical manual of mental disorders, (DSM-5®). American Psychiatric Pub; 2013.

12. Rosenkranz MA. Substance P at the nexus of mind and body in chronic inflammation and affective disorders. Psychol Bull 2007;133(6):1007.

13. Häuser W, Moser G, Klose P, et al. Psychosocial issues in evidence-based guidelines on inflammatory bowel diseases: a review. World J Gastroenterol 2014;20(13):3663.

14. Angelopoulos N, Mantas C, Dalekos G, et al. Psychiatric factors in patients with ulcerative colitis according to disease activity. Eur J Psychiatry 1996;10(2):87–99.

15. Mikocka-Walus AA, Turnbull DA, Moulding NT, et al. Does psychological status influence clinical outcomes in patients with inflammatory bowel disease (IBD) and other chronic gastroenterological diseases: an observational cohort prospective study. Biopsychosoc Med 2008;2:11.

16. Mardini HE, Kip KE, Wilson JW. Crohn's disease: a two-year prospective study of the association between psychological distress and disease activity. Dig Dis Sci 2004;49(3):492–7.

17. Mittermaier C, Dejaco C, Waldhoer T, et al. Impact of depressive mood on relapse in patients with inflammatory bowel disease: a prospective 18-month follow-up study. Psychosom Med 2004;66(1):79–84.

18. Panara A, Yarur A, Rieders B, et al. The incidence and risk factors for developing depression after being diagnosed with inflammatory bowel disease: a cohort study. Aliment Pharmacol Ther 2014;39(8):802–10.

19. Slavich GM, Irwin MR. From stress to inflammation and major depressive disorder: A social signal transduction theory of depression. Psychol Bull 2014;140(3):774.

20. Raison CL, Rutherford RE, Woolwine BJ, et al. A randomized controlled trial of the tumor necrosis factor antagonist infliximab for treatment-resistant depression: the role of baseline inflammatory biomarkers. JAMA Psychiatry 2013;70(1):31–41.

21. Horst S, Chao A, Rosen M, et al. Treatment with immunosuppressive therapy may improve depressive symptoms in patients with inflammatory bowel disease. Dig Dis Sci 2014;60(2):465–70.

22. Dowlati Y, Herrmann N, Swardfager W, et al. A meta-analysis of cytokines in major depression. Biol Psychiatry 2010;67(5):446–57.

23. Liu Y, Ho RC-M, Mak A. Interleukin (IL)-6, tumour necrosis factor alpha (TNF-α) and soluble interleukin-2 receptors (sIL-2R) are elevated in patients with major depressive disorder: a meta-analysis and meta-regression. J Affect Disord 2012;139(3):230–9.

24. Hannestad J, DellaGioia N, Bloch M. The effect of antidepressant medication treatment on serum levels of inflammatory cytokines: a meta-analysis. Neuropsychopharmacology 2011;36(12):2452–9.

25. Bonaccorso S, Puzella A, Marino V, et al. Immunotherapy with interferon-alpha in patients affected by chronic hepatitis C induces an intercorrelated stimulation of the cytokine network and an increase in depressive and anxiety symptoms. Psychiatry Res 2001;105(1):45–55.
26. Krishnadas R, Cavanagh J. Depression: an inflammatory illness? Journal of Neurology. Neurosurg Psychiatry 2012;83(5):495–502.
27. Aghazadeh R, Zali MR, Bahari A, et al. Inflammatory bowel disease in Iran: a review of 457 cases. J Gastroenterol Hepatol 2005;20(11):1691–5.
28. Wagtmans M, Verspaget H, Lamers C, et al. Crohn's disease in the elderly: a comparison with young adults. J Clin Gastroenterol 1998;27(2):129–33.
29. Srinath AI, Goyal A, Zimmerman LA, et al. Predictors of abdominal pain in depressed pediatric inflammatory bowel disease patients. Inflamm Bowel Dis 2014;20(8):1329–40.
30. Mayer EA, Tillisch K. The brain-gut axis in abdominal pain syndromes. Annu Rev Med 2011;62:381–96.
31. Zimmerman LA, Srinath AI, Goyal A, et al. The overlap of functional abdominal pain in pediatric Crohn's disease. Inflamm Bowel Dis 2013;19(4):826–31.
32. Lewis DA, Smith RE. Steroid-induced psychiatric syndromes: a report of 14 cases and a review of the literature. J Affect Disord 1983;5(4):319–32.
33. Fardet L, Kassar A, Cabane J, et al. Corticosteroid-induced adverse events in adults. Drug Saf 2007;30(10):861–81.
34. Means-Christensen AJ, Sherbourne CD, Roy-Byrne PP, et al. Using five questions to screen for five common mental disorders in primary care: diagnostic accuracy of the Anxiety and Depression Detector. Gen Hosp Psychiatry 2006;28(2):108–18.
35. Mikocka-Walus AA, Turnbull DA, Moulding NT, et al. "It doesn't do any harm, but patients feel better": a qualitative exploratory study on gastroenterologists' perspectives on the role of antidepressants in inflammatory bowel disease. BMC Gastroenterol 2007;7:38.
36. Mikocka-Walus AA, Gordon AL, Stewart BJ, et al. A magic pill? A qualitative analysis of patients' views on the role of antidepressant therapy in inflammatory bowel disease (IBD). BMC Gastroenterol 2012;12:93.
37. Goodhand JR, Greig FI, Koodun Y, et al. Do antidepressants influence the disease course in inflammatory bowel disease? A retrospective case-matched observational study. Inflamm Bowel Dis 2012;18(7):1232–9.
38. Szigethy E, Whitton SW, Levy-Warren A, et al. Cognitive-behavioral therapy for depression in adolescents with inflammatory bowel disease: a pilot study. J Am Acad Child Adolesc Psychiatry 2004;43(12):1469–77.
39. Szigethy E, Youk AO, Gonzalez-Heydrich J, et al. Effect of 2 Psychotherapies on Depression and Disease Activity in Pediatric Crohn's Disease. Inflamm Bowel Dis 2015;21(6):1321–8.
40. Díaz Sibaja MA, Comeche Moreno MI, Mas Hesse B. [Protocolized cognitive-behavioural group therapy for inflammatory bowel disease]. Rev Esp Enferm Dig 2007;99(10):593–8.
41. Timmer A, Preiss JC, Motschall E, et al. Psychological interventions for treatment of inflammatory bowel disease. Cochrane Database Syst Rev 2011;(2):CD006913.
42. Tabibian A, Tabibian JH, Beckman LJ, et al. Predictors of health-related quality of life and adherence in Crohn's disease and ulcerative colitis: implications for clinical management. Dig Dis Sci 2015;60(5):1366–74.
43. Robinson A. Review article: improving adherence to medication in patients with inflammatory bowel disease. Aliment Pharmacol Ther 2008;27(s1):9–14.

44. Gradus JL, Qin P, Lincoln AK, et al. Inflammatory bowel disease and completed suicide in Danish adults. Inflamm Bowel Dis 2010;16(12):2158–61.

45. Gibson PR, Weston AR, Shann A, et al. Relationship between disease severity, quality of life and health-care resource use in a cross-section of Australian patients with Crohn's disease. J Gastroenterol Hepatol 2007;22(8):1306–12.

46. Alrubaiy L, Rikaby I, Dodds P, et al. Systematic review of the health related quality of life (HRQoL) measures for inflammatory bowel disease. J Crohns Colitis 2015; 9(3):284–92.

47. Lonnfors S, Vermeire S, Greco M, et al. IBD and health-related quality of life – discovering the true impact. J Crohns Colitis 2014;8(10):1281–6.

48. Larsson K, Lööf L, Rönnblom A, et al. Quality of life for patients with exacerbation in inflammatory bowel disease and how they cope with disease activity. J Psychosom Res 2008;64(2):139–48.

49. Nordin K, Påhlman L, Larsson K, et al. Health-related quality of life and psychological distress in a population-based sample of Swedish patients with inflammatory bowel disease. Scand J Gastroenterol 2002;37(4):450–7.

50. Bernklev T, Jahnsen J, Schulz T, et al. Course of disease, drug treatment and health-related quality of life in patients with inflammatory bowel disease 5 years after initial diagnosis. Eur J Gastroenterol Hepatol 2005;17(10):1037–45.

51. Karwowski CA, Keljo D, Szigethy E. Strategies to improve quality of life in adolescents with inflammatory bowel disease. Inflamm Bowel Dis 2009;15(11):1755–64.

52. Wright EK, Kamm MA. Impact of drug therapy and surgery on quality of life in Crohn's disease: a systematic review. Anxiety 2014;63:66.

53. Moradkhani A, Beckman LJ, Tabibian JH. Health-related quality of life in inflammatory bowel disease: psychosocial, clinical, socioeconomic, and demographic predictors. J Crohns Colitis 2013;7(6):467–73.

54. van der Have M, van der Aalst KS, Kaptein AA, et al. Determinants of health-related quality of life in Crohn's disease: A systematic review and meta-analysis. J Crohns Colitis 2014;8(2):93–106.

55. Israeli E, Graff LA, Clara I, et al. Low prevalence of disability among patients with inflammatory bowel diseases a decade after diagnosis. Clin Gastroenterol Hepatol 2014;12(8):1330–7.e2.

56. Folkman S. Stress, appraisal, and coping. New York: Springer Publishing Company LLC; 1984.

57. McCombie AM, Mulder RT, Gearry RB. How IBD patients cope with IBD: a systematic review. J Crohns Colitis 2013;7(2):89–106.

58. Mussell M, Böcker U, Nagel N, et al. Predictors of disease-related concerns and other aspects of health-related quality of life in outpatients with inflammatory bowel disease. Eur J Gastroenterol Hepatol 2004;16(12):1273–80.

59. Moser G, Tillinger W, Sachs G, et al. Disease-related worries and concerns: a study on out-patients with inflammatory bowel disease. Eur J Gastroenterol Hepatol 1995;7(9):853–8.

60. Waters BM, Jensen L, Fedorak RN. Effects of formal education for patients with inflammatory bowel disease: a randomized controlled trial. Can J Gastroenterol 2005;19(4):235–44.

61. Kennedy A, Nelson E, Reeves D, et al. A randomised controlled trial to assess the effectiveness and cost of a patient orientated self management approach to chronic inflammatory bowel disease. Gut 2004;53(11):1639–45.

62. Ng V, Millard W, Lebrun C, et al. Low-intensity exercise improves quality of life in patients with Crohn's disease. Clin J Sport Med 2007;17(5):384–8.

63. Ranjbaran Z, Keefer L, Farhadi A, et al. Impact of sleep disturbances in inflammatory bowel disease. J Gastroenterol Hepatol 2007;22(11):1748–53.

64. Ananthakrishnan AN, Long MD, Martin CF, et al. Sleep disturbance and risk of active disease in patients with Crohn's disease and ulcerative colitis. Clin Gastroenterol Hepatol 2013;11(8):965–71.

65. von Wietersheim J, Kessler H. Psychotherapy with chronic inflammatory bowel disease patients: a review. Inflamm Bowel Dis 2006;12(12):1175–84.

66. Jantschek G, Zeitz M, Pritsch M, et al. Effect of psychotherapy on the course of Crohn's disease: results of the German prospective multicenter psychotherapy treatment study on Crohn's disease. Scand J Gastroenterol 1998;33(12): 1289–96.

67. Miller V, Whorwell PJ. Treatment of inflammatory bowel disease: a role for hypnotherapy? Int J Clin Exp Hypn 2008;56(3):306–17.

68. Mawdsley JE, Jenkins DG, Macey MG, et al. The effect of hypnosis on systemic and rectal mucosal measures of inflammation in ulcerative colitis. Am J Gastroenterol 2008;103(6):1460–9.

69. Drossman DA, Patrick DL, Mitchell CM, et al. Health-related quality of life in inflammatory bowel disease. Dig Dis Sci 1989;34(9):1379–86.

70. Vogelaar L, Spijker AV, van der Woude CJ. The impact of biologics on health-related quality of life in patients with inflammatory bowel disease. Clin Exp Gastroenterol 2009;2:101.

71. Feagan BG, Reinisch W, Rutgeerts P, et al. The effects of infliximab therapy on health-related quality of life in ulcerative colitis patients. Am J Gastroenterol 2007;102(4):794–802.

72. Loftus EV, Feagan BG, Colombel J-F, et al. Effects of adalimumab maintenance therapy on health-related quality of life of patients with Crohn's disease: patient-reported outcomes of the CHARM trial. Am J Gastroenterol 2008; 103(12):3132–41.

73. Rutgeerts P, Schreiber S, Feagan B, et al. Certolizumab pegol, a monthly subcutaneously administered Fc-free anti-TNFα, improves health-related quality of life in patients with moderate to severe Crohn's disease. Int J Colorectal Dis 2008; 23(3):289–96.

74. Feagan BG, Sandborn WJ, Hass S, et al. Health-related quality of life during natalizumab maintenance therapy for Crohn's disease. Am J Gastroenterol 2007;102(12):2737–46.

75. Kane S. Systematic review: adherence issues in the treatment of ulcerative colitis. Aliment Pharmacol Ther 2006;23(5):577–85.

76. Han S-W, Gregory W, Nylander D, et al. The SIBDQ: further validation in ulcerative colitis patients. Am J Gastroenterol 2000;95(1):145–51.

77. Panés J, O'Connor M, Peyrin-Biroulet L, et al. Improving quality of care in inflammatory bowel disease: what changes can be made today? J Crohns Colitis 2014;8(9):919–26.

Index

Note: Page numbers of article titles are in **boldface** type.

Surg Clin N Am 95 (2015) 1295–1309
http://dx.doi.org/10.1016/S0039-6109(15)00178-4
0039-6109/15/$ – see front matter © 2015 Elsevier Inc. All rights reserved.

surgical.theclinics.com

Moving?

Make sure your subscription moves with you!

To notify us of your new address, find your **Clinics Account Number** (located on your mailing label above your name), and contact customer service at:

Email: journalscustomerservice-usa@elsevier.com

800-654-2452 (subscribers in the U.S. & Canada)
314-447-8871 (subscribers outside of the U.S. & Canada)

Fax number: 314-447-8029

Elsevier Health Sciences Division
Subscription Customer Service
3251 Riverport Lane
Maryland Heights, MO 63043

*To ensure uninterrupted delivery of your subscription, please notify us at least 4 weeks in advance of move.

Printed and bound by CPI Group (UK) Ltd, Croydon, CR0 4YY

18/10/2024

01775891-0001